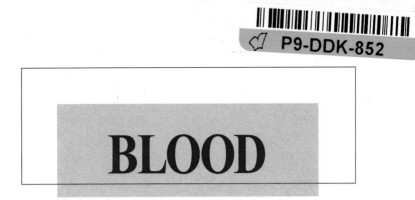

BLOOD

John F. Dailey

Published by
Medical Consulting Group
Arlington, MA 02474
U.S.A.

Editor: Jane E. Manley
Cover Design: Sue Lee
Book Design: George H. McLean
Illustrations: Sue Lee

Note: Although the author and publisher have exhaustively researched all sources to ensure the accuracy and completeness of the information contained in this book, we assume no responsibility for errors, inaccuracies, omissions, or any inconsistency herein. Any slights of people or organizations is unintentional. None of the ideas, procedures, or suggestions are intended as substitutes for customary consultation with your physician. All matters regarding your health require medical supervision.

ISBN: 0-9631819-5-5

Printed in the United States of America
01 00 99 98   10 9 8 7 6 5 4 3 2 1

CONTENTS

FIGURES

PREFACE

The key to understanding human physiology *is* blood, and the reasons for studying blood and its functions are more compelling than ever before.

For example:

- Blood is the most tested tissue in the human body, and is routinely used to diagnose hundreds of illnesses.
- Transfusions, while saving lives, pose the risk of disease transmission and complications.
- Blood-borne pathogens such as hepatitis and AIDS are ongoing threats to public health.
- Medicine uses blood components to treat a variety of pathologic conditions.
- Recombinant technology now provides new treatment modalities, such as growth factors, used to increase blood cell production in bone marrow.
- Treatment protocols make use of the patient's own immune system to combat disease.
- Drug therapies rely on the blood for transport to disease sites.

The study of blood can and should be rewarding. But most hematology texts elicit confusion and dread in the average reader—after all, hematology texts are written for hematologists or for students of this complex topic.

By the late 1980s, John F. Dailey had achieved two decades of practical experience in surgery and industry, including multiple-trauma treatment, operation of the heart bypass pump and other surgical equipment. He worked for medical equipment manufacturers training physicians and allied health personnel on the use of autologous blood recovery systems and conducted clinical trials on blood-related new products. Fascinated with the topic of blood, Dailey became convinced that providing practical, understandable, and easily accessible information on blood would be welcome to a wide audience.

In 1990, he approached Jane E. Manley, an experienced editor and program manager for major publishers in the educational textbook field. Together they established Medical Consulting Group with the express purpose of providing clinicians, allied health personnel, and industry with practical, easy-to-understand information about hematology. The popularity of their first title, *Dailey's Notes on Blood*, confirmed Dailey's basic premise. Medical Consulting Group also provides clinical training seminars in hematology and immunology.

Dailey's background includes a B.A. in Biology, St. Francis College; graduate studies in Biochemistry and Physiology at the University of Rhode Island and Brandeis University; and specialized training in Cardiovascular Perfusion at Northeastern University.

Medical Consulting Group has endeavored to make *Blood* as accurate and easy to understand as *Dailey's Notes on Blood*, our basic hematology text. *Blood* addresses the needs of more advanced readers who require greater detail and additional topics. Therefore, *Blood* devotes entire chapters to topics such as apheresis, bone marrow transplantation, oxygen and carbon dioxide transport, and the major histocompatibility complex molecules, among others. It also includes 78 convenient text-related blood tests. Specialists at the Massachusetts General Hospital and around the country reviewed this book for accuracy, and the author used the most recent texts in hematology, immunology, transfusion therapy, and bone marrow transplantation as references in his research. Editors and designers contributed greatly to what we hope is a very readable text.

ACKNOWLEDGEMENTS

We wish to thank those people whose reviews and thoughtful comments and suggestions helped us develop *Blood*:

Staff members of the Massachusetts General Hospital, Boston, Massachusetts:

David M. Andrews, M.D.

Keith Joung, M.D., Ph.D.

John D. Romo, M.D.

Susan Saidman, Ph.D.

Thomas Spitzer, M.D.

Christopher P. Stowell, M.D., Ph.D.

Zbigniew Szczepiorkowski, M.D., Ph.D.

E.C. Vamvakas, M.D., Ph.D.

Fred Darr, M.D., Director, Medical Affairs, Plasma Operations, American Red Cross

Jerry Ortolano, Ph.D., Senior Scientist, Vice President, CardioVascular Group, Pall Medical

Mortimer Greenberg, M.D., Hematologist, Consulting Staff, Mount Auburn Hospital, Cambridge, Massachusetts

Gary Reeder, CP, Visiting Research Assistant Professor of Surgery, McGowen Center for Artificial Organ Development, Artificial Heart and Lung Program, University of Pittsburgh School of Medicine; Chairman: Transfusion Practices, AmSECT

The Clinical Laboratory at Emerson Hospital, Concord, Massachusetts, for reviewing the Blood Tests

We also thank Sue Lee for conceptualizing and rendering the illustrations as well as laying out the book, Kathleen Dailey and George McLean for the clarity of the book design, and Kathy Massimini for her valuable editorial suggestions.

Very special thanks are due friends and family whose encouragement and support made this project possible.

CHAPTER **1**

The Concept of Blood

Introduction

A thorough understanding of human physiology can only be achieved with a knowledge of hematology, which is the science and study of blood. The tissue that composes blood provides an amazingly wide array of life-supporting functions in the human body: (1) it delivers oxygen, hormones, nutrients, and minerals to body cells and picks up waste products; (2) it prevents blood loss and heals wounds through hemostasis; and (3) it acts as the primary carrier of immunity.

Vital organs such as the brain, heart, liver, and kidneys depend on a steady supply of blood for health. For example, the heart pumps enormous amounts of blood throughout the body and because of this the heart muscle itself requires a steady supply of blood, the kidneys filter out impurities, the liver breaks down nutrients and produces the majority of plasma proteins, and the lungs function in the exchange of oxygen and carbon dioxide between blood and the external environment. The brain is very dependent on blood flow; without blood flow to the brain death occurs within minutes. The spleen removes dead and damaged blood cells.

Blood is a transportation system, with the vessels of the circulatory system (arteries, veins, and capillaries) functioning as roadways. As blood travels throughout the body, it transports oxygen from the lungs to all body cells. From the intestine, blood absorbs and then distributes digestive products used for cellular metabolism. Blood also removes waste products, such as carbon dioxide and other by-products of cellular metabolism, and transports them to the lungs, kidneys, and skin for excretion.

1

total blood volume

plasma

The average adult has 4 to 6 liters (1L = 1000 mL or 1.06 qts) of blood, which accounts for approximately 7% of total body weight. The amount of blood in the circulatory system is referred to as the total blood volume. Formed elements compose 45% of this total volume, whereas plasma constitutes 55%. Plasma is a clear, straw-colored, viscous (sticky) fluid made up of 90% water (H_2O) and about 10% solid matter. The solid matter consists of proteins (clotting proteins, immunoglobulins, complement proteins, albumin), carbohydrates, such as glucose, electrolytes (salts), such as sodium, potassium, and others, vitamins, of which there are many, and other substances. Cellular components *and* plasma constitute what is referred to as whole blood.

whole blood

hematology

formed elements:
red cells
white cells
platelets

Hematology includes the study of blood-forming tissues, blood's functions, blood diseases, and blood use in therapy. It is concerned with the formed elements that make up blood—red blood cells (erythrocytes), white blood cells (leukocytes), and platelets (thrombocytes)—all of which are suspended in the liquid medium of blood called plasma.

Blood Cell Development

A Cell

A cell is a microscopic structure that forms the tissues of an organism, including blood. It is surrounded by an outer membrane called the cell membrane or plasma membrane that contains the cell's cytoplasm, a jellylike substance holding cellular bodies called organelles. Organelles include such structures as mitochondria, Golgi apparatus, and ribosomes, among others. The cell nucleus is the organelle that controls cellular functions. Within the nucleus lie the genes. Genes are hereditary molecules made up of deoxyribonucleic acid (DNA) and are responsible for all of an individual's characteristics, such as eye color and hair color.

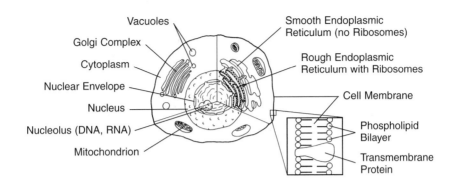

FIGURE 1.1 Typical Body Cell

This typical cell structure simulates most found throughout the body. Via interstitial fluid, substances from the capillaries move into the cell for use in many biochemical reactions. Capillaries and lymphatic vessels take up cellular waste products via interstitial fluid and transport them to the lungs, kidneys, and skin for excretion. Although the formed elements of blood are called "cells," the only true cellular components of blood are the white cells, because they have a nucleus, the cellular organelle where DNA is located.

The Blood Cells

Like other cells, the formed elements of blood have a plasma membrane, cytoplasm, and organelles. Only white cells have a nucleus, which allows them to react quickly to carry out immune functions continuously and relentlessly. Neither red cells nor platelets have a nucleus. Once they are released from the bone marrow into the circulation, red cells and platelets do not require a nucleus to carry out their specialized functions.

plasma membrane, cytoplasm, organelles, nucleus

Production of Blood Cells

The term hematopoiesis refers to the production of mature blood cells from primitive cells in the bone marrow called stem cells. There are many stages of blood cell development, more than can be addressed in this book. The development of blood cells is under the control of protein hormones called hematopoietic growth factors, which belong to a broad class of glycoprotein

hematopoiesis

stem cells

hematopoietic growth factors

cytokines molecules called cytokines. Blood cell production is an ongoing process in which blood cells are constantly regenerated. Each day 1 trillion blood cells are produced to replace those past their life span. The number of blood cells in a healthy individual is constant because the production and destruction of cells are relatively balanced.

Certain conditions stimulate an increase in the production of blood cells. For example, hypoxia, a low level of oxygen in the tissues, increases red cell production. Infection leads to an increase in white cell production, and blood loss to an increase in platelets.

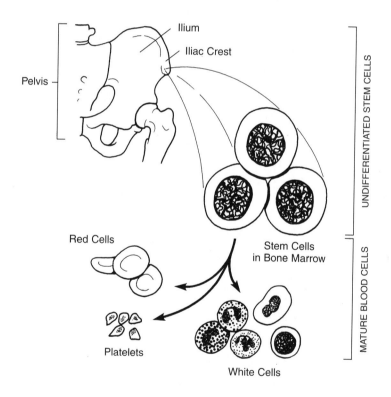

FIGURE 1.2 Stem Cell Production in Bone Marrow
The development of stem cells in hematopoietic bone marrow is called intramedullary hematopoiesis. Stem cells ultimately give rise to mature blood cells.

Stem Cells

Within the hematopoietic marrow is a finite number of specialized precursor cells called stem cells. Through a process called differentiation stem cells develop into mature blood cells. During differentiation blood cells undergo a number of cell divisions in order to become capable of carrying out their intended functions. Stem cells are undifferentiated cells that have two functions: (1) to produce more stem cells (to self-renew their numbers) and (2) to generate mature blood cells.

differentiation

functions of undifferentiated cells: self-renewal and generation

Another term sometimes used synonymously with stem cells is progenitor cells, although most medical professionals consider progenitor cells to be somewhat more mature precursor cells than stem cells. Progenitor cells have retained the ability to self-renew and pro-duce mature blood cells. They are found outside the bone marrow.

progenitor cells

Pluripotential Stem Cells

Pluripotential stem cells, which exist predominantly in hematopoietic marrow, are few in number. They are the precursors to all blood cells, giving rise to both the myeloid and lymphoid cell lines. Blood cells that become committed to the myeloid line differentiate into red cells, platelets, and certain white cells, namely, granulocytes, and monocytes/macrophages. Lymphoid stem cells differentiate into mature white cells called lymphocytes. There are two types of lymphocytes: T lymphocytes and B lymphocytes, also called T cells and B cells. Pluripotential stem cells have been difficult to characterize and identify; much of our knowledge about them is theoretical, that is, implied by their behavior.

blood cell precursors myeloid and lymphoid cell lines

lymphocytes: T cells B cells

Multipotential Stem Cells

"Multipotential" refers to the ability of stem cells to differentiate into any of the mature blood cell types. Hematopoiesis involves the differentiation of multipotential stem cells into unipotential stem cells that, in turn, develop into mature blood cells. Once a multipotential stem cell becomes committed to the development of a particular blood cell type, it is referred to as a unipotential stem cell.

Unipotential Stem Cells

A unipotential cell is not a fully differentiated, mature blood cell but it is committed to developing into a specific blood cell type, such as a red cell. Unipotential stem cells have lost the ability to self-renew.

Molecules Necessary for Blood Cell Development

Cytokines

Cytokine molecules are a broad class of glycoprotein hormones released by many cell types, such as endothelial cells, monocytes, macrophages, fibroblasts, and lymphocytes. They have many important and overlapping physiological functions in the body and do the following:

endothelial cells, monocytes, macrophages, fibroblasts, lymphocytes, other cells
↓
cytokine release

- control the growth and differentiation of stem and progenitor cells
- regulate the immune response
- play a role in inflammation
- aid in the functions of mature blood cells

Examples of cytokines and their functions include:

hematopoietic growth factors

- Hematopoietic growth factors are crucial to the growth and differentiation of stem and progenitor cells. An example is the colony-stimulating factors.

inflammatory response cytokines

- Inflammatory response cytokines are necessary in the inflammation response to tissue injury and foreign matter. They are mainly interleukins, interferons, and tumor necrosis factors.

interleukins

- Interleukins (ILs) affect and enhance the functions of mature blood cells.

interferons

- Interferons (INFs) are essential in the immune response to viral antigens and also for white cell function.

tumor necrosis factors

- Tumor necrosis factors (TNFs) help protect the body against malignant cells.

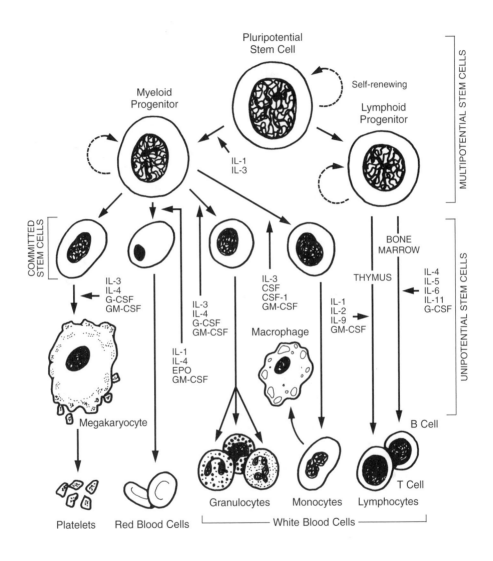

FIGURE 1.3 **Stem Cell Differentiation**

Stem cells in hematopoietic marrow develop and mature into functional blood cells. Growth factors IL, EPO, G-CSF, and GM-CSF work in combination to bring about the development of mature blood cells from primitive stem cells. Fully differentiated blood cells are released into circulation, with each blood cell having a specific function or functions. As they mature into blood cells, stem cells undergo many more steps than shown in this schematic representation.

Hematopoietic Growth Factors

Growth and development of blood cells depend on the action of growth factors, which work in combination either with or against one another. Hematopoietic growth factors include: the interleukins (ILs), colony-stimulating-factors (CSFs), and erythropoietin (EPO), a hormone released by kidney cells.

ILs
CSFs, EPO

Hematopoietic growth factors act on stem and progenitor cells causing them to either undergo self-renewal or to further differentiate into mature functioning blood cells. They bring about these changes by binding to receptors on stem and progenitor cells. Hematopoietic growth factors are produced by a number of cell types, such as endothelial cells, B cells, T cells, monocytes, fibroblasts. Kidney cells produce only erythropoietin.

Interleukins   There are thirteen interleukin molecules, numbered IL-1 to IL-13. Interleukins, such as IL-1 and IL-6, cause stem cells to produce precursors to red cells, granulocytes, lymphocytes, monocytes, and platelets.

Colony-stimulating-factors   There are several colony-stimulating factors. The ones most often referred to are granulocyte-colony-stimulating factor (G-CSF) and granulocyte-macrophage colony-stimulating factor (GM-CSF). Both factors cause stem and progenitor cells to produce many blood cell types.

G-CSF

GM-CSF

Thrombopoietins   The thrombopoietins are used to describe all molecules responsible for the development of platelets from megakaryocytes. Examples of thrombopoietins include: IL-3, IL-6, and GM-CSF, among others.

Erythropoietin

renal hormone

The production of red cells is dependent on the renal hormone erythropoietin. This molecule is released by the peritubular cells of the kidneys. During fetal life erythropoietin is produced in the liver, which continues to produce about 10% of this hormone after birth. Stimulated by the release of erythropoietin, stem cells committed to red cell production increase in numbers.

Other Molecules Necessary for Blood Cell Development

In addition to hematopoietic growth factors, other molecules are necessary for blood cell development. These include: (1) many vitamins, such as B_{12} and folic acid, among others; (2) metals, such as iron, cobalt, and manganese; (3) amino acids; (4) hormones, such as thyroxin. If any of these is not present, abnormal or decreased blood cell production occurs.

Bone Marrow

Hematopoiesis takes place in bone marrow, a highly complex tissue in the center of bones. There are two types of bone marrow: red, preferentially called hematopoietic, and yellow. Both are composed of a spongy, fibrous matrix composed of endothelial cells, macrophages, fibroblasts (precursors of connective tissue cells), and fat cells and an extensive capillary network. Yellow marrow is 96% fat and not involved with hematopoiesis. Hematopoietic marrow is where the development of red cells, white cells, and platelets takes place. Unlike yellow marrow, hematopoietic marrow contains stem cells in its stroma, a spongy, fibrous material. This marrow appears as a gelatinous mass and is 25% solid matter and 75% water.

marrow: hematopoietic and yellow

stroma

Intramedullary and Extramedullary Hematopoiesis

Blood cell formation that occurs in bone marrow is called intramedullary hematopoiesis. When it takes place in tissue other than bone marrow, for example, in the yolk sac, liver, spleen, and thymus, it is called extramedullary hematopoiesis. This kind of hematopoiesis is normal in the embryo. In the adult it is abnormal and bone marrow dysfunction is indicated:

the hematopoietic marrow cannot produce enough blood cells to sustain normal blood cell counts. Causes of adult extramedullary hematopoiesis include: tumors, diseases, chemotherapies, ionizing radiation, and certain congenital disorders.

Diseased or defective marrow can be replaced with healthy marrow from another individual (donor) in a bone marrow transplant procedure (see Ch. 20, Bone Marrow Transplantation).

Sites of Blood Cell Development

Blood cell growth and development occurs in different sites at various stages of human development. In the early embryo, it occurs in blood islands found in a membranous structure called the yolk sac. These blood islands are the precursors of blood cells and also the beginnings of the vascular system (blood vessels). By the third month of fetal growth, blood cell production moves from the blood islands to the liver. The liver is the main organ of fetal blood cell development until the seventh month. Subsequently during the third

blood islands
yolk sac

liver

FIGURE 1.4 Sites of Blood Cell Development in the Fetus, Child, and Adult

The sites shown for the fetus indicate the order of blood cell development during fetal growth. In the child, almost all bones of the body produce blood cells. As one ages, the sites become fewer.

THIRD WEEK:
   Yolk Sac
THIRD MONTH:
   Liver
   Spleen
   Thymus
FOURTH MONTH:
   Bone Marrow

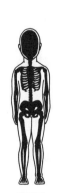

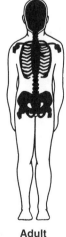

Fetus   **Child**   **Adult**

month, it also occurs in the thymus and spleen.   thymus, spleen
The thymus is responsible only for T lymphocyte
development. By the fourth month, bone marrow joins
the other organ systems that produce blood cells and
continues to do so throughout life. The embryonic
sites of blood cell development overlap with one
another until birth when bone marrow becomes the
site of hematopoiesis and the others stop producing
blood cells.

At birth, almost all bones of the body produce blood
cells. During childhood the long bones of the arms and   long bones
legs stop producing blood cells and the stroma becomes
replaced with fat. By adolescence and continuing into
adulthood, only the flat bones of the central skeleton   flat bones of the
—the skull, sternum, vertebrae, ribs, and pelvis—are   central skeleton
involved in blood cell development. In the elderly the
hematopoietic marrow of the cranium becomes
jellylike forming what is called gelatinous marrow and   gelatinous marrow
no longer plays a role in hematopoiesis.

Types of Blood Cells

Each type of blood cell has special functions and differs
morphologically (in size and shape) from the others.   white cells:
White cells are components of the immune system,   immune system
which protects the body against foreign matter.   red cells:
Red cells transport oxygen and carbon dioxide.   oxygen and carbon
Platelets are essential in preventing blood loss because   dioxide transport
they form a platelet plug, which is one of the initial   platelets:
steps in hemostasis (clotting).   hemostasis

Just as human beings go through the different stages of
the life cycle, from birth to death, so do blood cells. Each
type of blood cell has a characteristic life span. Some cells
function for a few hours, days, or months, whereas others
stay in the body for years or possibly for a lifetime. Blood
cells must be fully mature before they can carry out their
intended functions. Mature blood cells predominate in
the circulation of healthy individuals. In persons with
disease states, immature and abnormal blood cells may be
present in greater numbers.

Leukocytes, the white cells, protect the body against foreign matter. There are many different types of leukocytes.

Granulocytes   These cells are characterized by granules within their cytoplasm.

Neutrophil   Eosinophil   Basophil

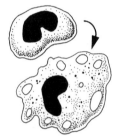

Monocytes and Macrophages
A monocyte gives rise to a macrophage.

Lymphocytes
T and B cells and their subsets make up the lymphocytes.

Erythrocytes, or red cells, transport oxygen and carbon dioxide to and from all body cells.

Thrombocytes, the platelets, prevent blood loss by forming a platelet plug at the site of injury until a stable clot forms.

FIGURE 1.5 **Individual Blood Cells, or Formed Elements**

▪ QUESTIONS ▪

1. What are the three major functions of blood tissue?

2. How is cellular metabolism dependent on blood?

3. How much blood does an average adult have?

4. What is the amount of blood in the circulatory system called?

5. Blood is composed of plasma and what three formed elements? Plasma is composed of water and what four major substances?

6. What is a cell? Describe its structure.

7. Blood cells share characteristics with other body cells. In what major cellular characteristics are blood cells different from other body cells?

8. Explain the term hematopoiesis.

9. How many blood cells are produced each day in an individual?

10. List three conditions that can cause an increase in blood cell production.

11. Identify another term often used for stem cells. What are the differences between the two cells?

12. Describe the three major phases of stem cell differentiation.

13. Multipotential stem cells and unipotential stem cells are both involved in hematopoiesis. Which comes first?

14. Identify molecules necessary for blood cell development.

15. How many kinds of interleukin molecules are there? What role do they play in hematopoiesis?

16. Explain the role of thrombopoietins in blood cell development.

17. The production of red cells is dependent on a hormone. What is this hormone? and where is it produced?

18. What is the function of the hematopoietic growth factors? and where are they produced?

19. In addition to hematopoietic growth factors, other molecules are necessary for blood cell development. List four of these.

20. Two types of bone marrow are found in bones: hematopoietic (red) and yellow. How do they compare with one another?

21. What clinical conditions may cause hematopoiesis to occur outside the marrow in an adult?

22. In the early embryo, where do blood cell growth and development occur?

23. In later embryonic development, blood cell growth and development move on to other sites. When does this happen and what are the sites?

24. What occurs with blood cell development at birth?

25. When does the cranium cease producing blood cells? and what replaces the hematopoietic marrow?

26. What are the three main types of blood cells and their major functions?

27. Mature blood cells predominate in the circulation of persons with disease states. True or False? Explain your answer.

28. List six kinds of white cells (leukocytes).

CHAPTER 2

The Circulatory System

Introduction

The circulatory system, also called the vascular system or vascular space, provides a roadway of tubes through which blood travels as it delivers oxygen and nutrients to organs and tissues and removes waste products of cellular metabolism. This system is made up of two closed loops: (1) a major systemic one that delivers blood to body cells and (2) a minor one, the pulmonary, that delivers blood to the lungs. In the circulatory system, blood leaves the heart and returns to it, which is why the entire circulatory system can be referred to as a closed-loop system. Blood requires constant circulation to carry out its functions; it clots if it remains stagnant. The heart is the pump that propels blood throughout the vascular system. Normally, blood does not leave the vessels of the vascular system and is said to be intravascular. Extravascular blood refers to blood outside the vascular space, and results from trauma.

vascular space

closed-loop system

intravascular blood
extravascular blood

The tubes of the vascular system consist of blood vessels—arteries, arterioles, capillaries, venules, veins—and, indirectly, the lymphatic system (see p. 23). All blood and lymphatic vessels are lined with a layer of flat, endothelial cells called the endothelium.

endothelium

Arteries

Function and Location

Arteries are conducting and distributing vessels that carry blood away from the heart. The major artery of the circulatory system is the aorta, which arises from

aorta

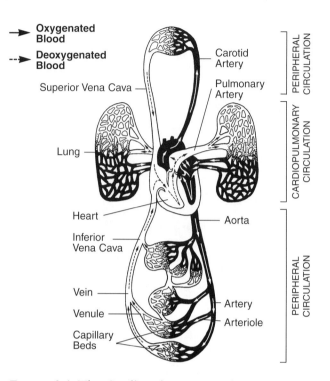

→ **Oxygenated Blood**

--→ **Deoxygenated Blood**

Carotid Artery

Superior Vena Cava

Pulmonary Artery

Lung

Heart

Aorta

Inferior Vena Cava

Vein

Venule

Artery

Arteriole

Capillary Beds

PERIPHERAL CIRCULATION

CARDIOPULMONARY CIRCULATION

PERIPHERAL CIRCULATION

FIGURE 2.1 **The Cardiopulmonary and Peripheral Circulation**

This schematic representation shows the closed-loop arrangement of the vascular system. The arteries carry blood away from the heart, and the veins return blood to the heart. The heart is the connecting point in the closed loop.

the left ventricle of the heart. Major arteries branch from the aorta to supply blood to body organs. The pulmonary artery, however, bifurcates going directly from the right ventricle to the lungs. As arteries branch from the aorta they increase in number and decrease in internal diameter. Arteries lie deep within the body's interior where they are protected from damage caused by trauma. As they approach organs and tissues, arteries decrease in size and become arterioles. Arterioles are known as resistance vessels because of their small size and the increased muscle tissue surrounding them. Once inside organs and tissues, arterioles further

arteries

arterioles
resistance vessels

branch into capillaries, the smallest vessels of the vascular system.

capillaries

The aorta assists the movement of blood through the vasculature. Blood that leaves the heart is under pressure. When the left ventricle ejects blood into the aorta, the elastic fibers within the aorta allow the aorta to expand. As the aorta retracts to its normal size, the blood is propelled forward. The expansion and contraction of the aorta is called the Windkessel effect.

Windkessel effect

Structure

All arteries have muscle and elastic tissue surrounding their thick walls in order to accommodate the blood that enters them. Arteries have three tissue layers: the adventitia (outer), the media (middle), and the intima (inner). The media of large arteries has elastic tissue and very few muscle fibers. In small arteries and arterioles the media has very little elastic tissue but many muscle

tissue layers:
adventitia
media
intima

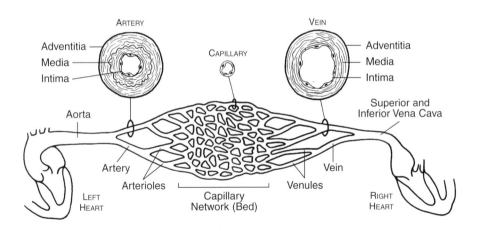

FIGURE 2.2 **The Vascular System**

Blood leaves the left side of the heart and travels through the aorta, arteries, and arterioles to capillary networks throughout the body. Venules and veins return blood to the right heart. Blood flows from the left heart and returns to the right heart in a continuous closed-loop cycle.

fibers innervated (connected) with nerve fibers that cause the blood vessels either to constrict or dilate. The action of nerve impulses on muscle fibers regulates the flow of blood within the body. When muscle fibers in arterial vessels constrict, less blood flows through to reach the tissues. When they dilate, more blood flows through to reach the tissues.

Capillaries

Function

exchange vessels

Capillaries are the smallest blood vessels in the body. They are referred to as exchange vessels because they are the only circulatory vessels in which the movement of substances takes place between the blood and tissues. Blood enters a capillary through an arteriole to deliver oxygen, nutrients, hormones, vitamins, and other substances to cells. Blood that carries cellular waste products, such as carbon dioxide (CO_2), exits the capillary bed through a venule.

Structure and Location

An individual capillary measures 1 mm long and 7 to 9μ in diameter. It is only one cell layer thick, which allows for the easy exchange of substances across its membrane. Capillaries penetrate and abound in every

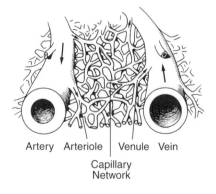

FIGURE 2.3 The Capillary Network

Capillaries make up dense networks of blood vessels located throughout the body. Capillary networks are in close proximity to all body cells, a relationship that facilitates the movement of substances into and out of the cell. Substances that leave the capillaries have less than a millimeter to move into the cells.

Artery   Arteriole | Venule   Vein

Capillary
Network

organ and tissue and, therefore, capillaries lie in close proximity to body cells. Capillaries embedded within organs and tissues are referred to as a capillary bed, a capillary network, or the microvasculature.

capillary bed
capillary network
microvasculature

Interstitial Fluid

Function

Nutrients and other substances dissolved in blood are transported from capillaries to body cells by interstitial fluid. This fluid is composed of water, electrolytes, vitamins, and other substances that filter out of the plasma. Proteins usually are not found in interstitial fluid. Due to their size, proteins cannot leave the vascular space. Interstitial fluid is filtered from plasma through the capillary pores into the interstitial space, which is the microscopic area surrounding cells. Being constantly bathed by interstitial fluid, body cells take up vital substances needed for cellular activity. In turn, waste products from these cells are picked up by the interstitial fluid and returned to the blood.

plasma minus proteins

interstitial space

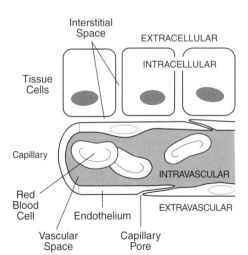

FIGURE 2.4 Blood-tissue Interface

As fluid circulates throughout the vascular system, it continually moves back and forth between the vascular space and cells. Depicted here are basic terms used to describe the locations and movement of substances and fluid between the vascular space and the cells. Substances and fluid within the blood are intravascular. They become extravascular when they leave the vascular space and move into the interstitial space. Once inside the cell they become intracellular. On leaving the cell for return to the vascular space they become extravascular.

Hydrostatic and Osmotic Pressure

The movement of fluid between capillaries (the vascular space) and body cells (tissues) is the result of pressure differences between the blood and tissue spaces. The pressures are hydrostatic and osmotic. Blood entering a capillary is under hydrostatic (blood) pressure. Because this pressure is greater than the osmotic pressure within tissues, fluid (water) is forced from the capillary into the interstitial space. As water moves out of the plasma into the interstitial space, the protein concentration of plasma increases. Because proteins do not leave the vascular space, the concentration of plasma proteins increases and exerts osmotic pressure in capillary blood. Some fluid is thus pulled back into the vascular space. The rate of tissue fluid formation generally exceeds the capillary re-uptake.

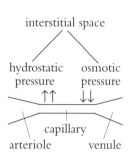

lymphatic system

The lymphatic system drains excess fluid (see p. 23). The network of vessels that make up the lymphatic system aids the vascular system in maintaining fluid volume. Continuous movement of fluid between the blood and interstitial space is essential for normal physiological processes and therefore for health.

fluid volume

Veins

Functions

Veins are vessels that return blood to the heart. The smallest veins are called venules. They form at the distal (farthest) end of capillaries. As they return to the heart and extend farther from capillary networks, venules become progressively larger to form veins. As veins approach the heart they decrease in number and increase in internal diameter. The two major veins of the body are the superior vena cava and the inferior vena cava. Both veins enter the right atrium of the heart. The superior vena cava receives venous blood

venules

superior vena cava
inferior vena cava

from the head and upper extremities of the body. The inferior vena cava receives venous blood from the organs and lower extremities of the body.

Structure

Veins have thinner walls than arteries because they must expand to receive large volumes of blood from organs. For this reason, veins are known as capacitance vessels. Although they have the same tissue layers as arteries: intima, media, and adventitia, the muscle fibers of the media are not as well developed. Elastic tissue within their walls expands to accommodate large volumes of blood.

capacitance vessels

Location

Veins are found throughout the body in many locations. Superficial veins lie beneath the skin close to the surface. Deep veins lie within interior body tissues. Examples of superficial veins of the lower extremities are the greater and lesser saphenous veins. Two deep veins of the leg are the popliteal vein and femoral vein. Deep veins derive their names from the arteries that they accompany.

superficial veins
deep veins

Venous Blood Flow to the Heart

Venous blood is assisted in its return to the heart. As blood leaves the capillary, its movement is slow because the arterial pressure that propelled blood into the capillary has drastically diminished by the time it reaches a venule. Two mechanisms assist venous return: (1) the skeletal muscles of the lower extremities contract during body movement and force the blood forward and (2) the one-way valves within the veins prevent the backflow of blood, which would occur in the lower extremities due to the pull of gravity. The system of valves is essential for returning blood from the lower body. When valves break down or become nonfunctional, a condition known as varicose veins develop.

skeletal muscles

one-way valves

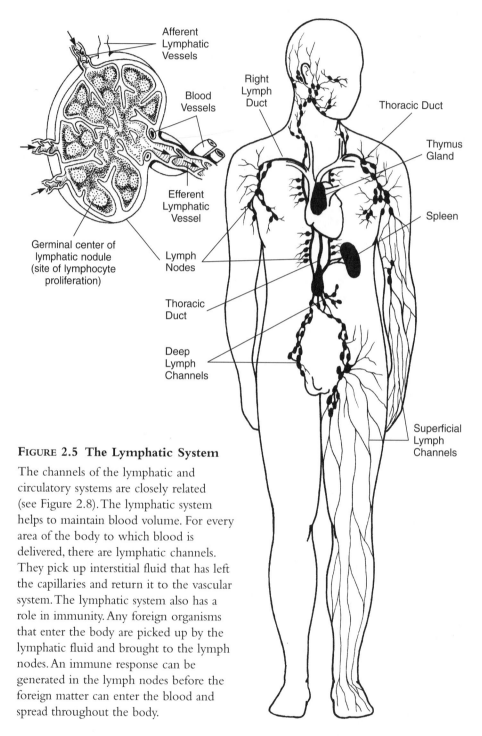

FIGURE 2.5 **The Lymphatic System**

The channels of the lymphatic and
circulatory systems are closely related
(see Figure 2.8). The lymphatic system
helps to maintain blood volume. For every
area of the body to which blood is
delivered, there are lymphatic channels.
They pick up interstitial fluid that has left
the capillaries and return it to the vascular
system. The lymphatic system also has a
role in immunity. Any foreign organisms
that enter the body are picked up by the
lymphatic fluid and brought to the lymph
nodes. An immune response can be
generated in the lymph nodes before the
foreign matter can enter the blood and
spread throughout the body.

The Lymphatic System

Functions

The lymphatic system has important functions related to the blood's vascular system. It maintains blood volume and assists with immunity.

blood volume
immunity

Any fluid that leaves the vascular system and enters the interstitial space must ultimately be returned to the bloodstream by either the lymphatic or vascular capillaries. The lymphatic system picks up fluid that is not transported to the heart via the veins and returns it to the vascular system. If fluid were to remain in the interstitial space, blood volume would be depleted. When abnormal amounts of fluid remain in body tissues, the individual develops a swollen appearance, a condition called edema. There are many causes of edema.

edema

The lymphatic system also has a vital role in the body's immune system. Lymphatic fluid carries foreign matter to the lymph nodes, which are small filtering stations that remove foreign matter, such as cell debris and antigens, from lymphatic fluid. Lymph nodes contain T and B cells and other white cells that help destroy foreign matter (see Ch. 9, The Immune System).

lymph nodes

Structure and Location

Like the vascular system, the lymphatic system is made up of a roadway of tubes. However, it is not a closed-loop system. It originates within body tissues, drains into chest veins, and has no direct connecting point like the heart. Fluid in the lymphatic system is called lymph. Lymphatic vessels begin as tiny, unconnected capillarylike structures within body tissues. These vessels merge to form progressively larger tubes that are interrupted by lymph nodes at various sites throughout the body. All lymphatic vessels drain into two large lymphatic vessels, the thoracic duct on the left side of the body and the right lymphatic duct on the right side. These two ducts empty into veins of the upper chest that return lymphatic fluid to the bloodstream.

lymph

thoracic duct
right lymphatic duct

The Cardiopulmonary System

Function

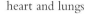 heart and lungs

respiratory gases:
O_2 and CO_2

The cardiopulmonary system refers to the heart and lungs as they function together. As the heart pumps blood through the lungs, the blood releases carbon dioxide (CO_2) and takes up oxygen (O_2). O_2 and CO_2 are called respiratory gases. The lungs are large, pink, spongy organs in which O_2 from the outside environment is taken up by the blood and CO_2 is

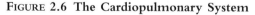

FROM HEAD
AND UPPER
EXTREMITIES

TO HEAD
AND UPPER
EXTREMITIES

→ **Oxygenated Blood**

- → **Deoxygenated Blood**

Right Lung

Left Lung

Capillaries

Alveolus

CO_2 — Alveolus

O_2

Capillary

Red
Blood
Cell

FROM TRUNK
AND LOWER
EXTREMITIES

TO TRUNK
AND LOWER
EXTREMITIES

FIGURE 2.6 The Cardiopulmonary System

The heart and lungs function together to exhange O_2 and CO_2 between the blood and the atmosphere. The capillary network of the lungs is extremely dense and totally encompasses the alveoli. This relationship makes possible a rapid exchange of O_2 and CO_2 between the alveoli and capillary blood. This exchange takes place in three quarters of a second.

released from the blood to the outside through the act of breathing.

Respiratory Gas Exchange

The exchange of respiratory gases in the lungs occurs in structures called alveoli, which are tiny air sacs that form grapelike clusters at the end of the small airways of the lungs. There are approximately 300 million alveoli. Each alveolus is surrounded by a dense network of capillaries. The entire alveolar-capillary network is very large. In fact, if this microvasculature were removed and spread out, it would be the size of a tennis court. The area comprised by the alveolar-capillary network allows for the maximum exchange of respiratory gases.

alveoli

alveolar-capillary network

Deoxygenated Blood

Blood returning from body organs and tissues is deoxygenated, that is, low in O_2 and high in CO_2. As a result, it has a deep purple color. Carbon dioxide, a waste product of cellular metabolism produced in body cells and tissues, is removed from the body via the lungs. On its way to the lungs, deoxygenated blood enters the heart via the inferior and superior venae cavae. The blood fills the right atrium (RA) of the heart and from there flows through the tricuspid valve to the right ventricle (RV). It is then pumped out through the pulmonary valve (PV) into the pulmonary artery (PA) and into the lungs. Once blood is in the alveolar-capillary network, CO_2 leaves and O_2 enters. As blood is oxygenated, it becomes bright red due to the increased saturation of hemoglobin by O_2.

carbon dioxide

blood flow:
heart
↓
RA
↓
tricuspid valve
↓
RV
↓
PV
↓
PA
↓
lungs

Oxygenated Blood

Once the exchange of CO_2 and O_2 has taken place in the lungs, the pulmonary veins return oxygen–rich blood from the lungs to the left atrium (LA) of the heart. From there, it flows through the mitral valve (MV; also called bicuspid valve) into the left ventricle (LV). The left ventricle ejects blood through the aortic valve (AV) into the aorta (Ao). Oxygenated blood is

blood flow:
lungs
↓
pulmonary veins
↓
LA
↓
MV
↓
LV
↓
AV
↓
aorta

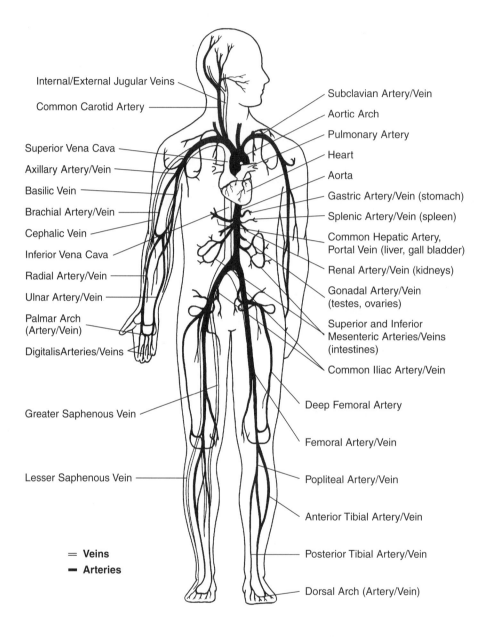

FIGURE 2.7 The Circulatory System

The circulatory system is an enormous network of blood vessels. Blood leaves the heart through the arteries and returns by the veins.

then distributed throughout the body to all organs and tissues via arteries, arterioles, and capillaries.

The Peripheral Circulation

The vascular system includes blood vessels of both the cardiopulmonary and peripheral circulatory (systemic) systems. The cardiopulmonary system includes the heart and the great vessels: venae cavae, pulmonary arteries, pulmonary veins, and aorta. The peripheral circulatory (systemic) system includes all vessels outside the chest cavity, which is also known as the thorax. These include all vessels that are not a part of the cardiopulmonary system.

heart, great vessels

▪ QUESTIONS ▪

1. Describe the two closed loops of the circulatory system.

2. What can cause blood to be found outside the vascular space?

3. List five types of blood vessels.

4. Where is endothelium found?

5. What is the major artery of the circulatory system?

6. Where are arteries and arterioles in the circulatory system?

7. Arterioles are known as resistance vessels. Explain the reasons why.

8. What is the Windkessel effect? Explain when it occurs.

9. Describe the anatomic characteristics of arteries. How do they differ from the arterioles?

10. How is blood flow regulated?

11. How do capillaries function as exchange vessels?

12. Nutrients and other substances dissolved in the bloodstream are transported from the capillaries to body cells by interstitial fluid. What is the composition of this fluid?

13. Where is interstitial fluid? What does it do?

14. What happens to proteins in the vascular system?

15. What are the dynamics of the movement of fluid between the capillaries and the body cells?

16. Identify the two major veins of the body.

17. Compare the function, structure, and location of veins and venules with arteries and arterioles.

18. Explain the difference between resistance and capacitance vessels.

19. How do varicose veins develop?

20. What are the two main functions of the lymphatic system, and why is it not a closed–loop system like the vascular system?

21. What is edema?

22. What is the cardiopulmonary system? and how are the respiratory gases involved?

23. Describe the appearance of the lungs.

24. The alveolar-capillary network for the exchange of respirator gases is very large. How many alveoli exist in an individual's lungs?

25. How and when does the color of blood in the body change?

26. Describe the pathway of oxygenated blood.

27. Describe how the peripheral circulation is different from the cardiopulmonary circulation.

CHAPTER **3**

Special Circulations:
CARDIAC, RENAL, HEPATIC, AND FETAL

Introduction

Blood is a tissue that every organ in the body relies on to function. In turn, organs process, regulate, and assist blood in some way. This chapter focuses on the circulatory patterns of the heart, kidneys, liver, and fetus, as well as their importance and uniqueness in physiology.

The heart is the pump for the entire circulatory system, making adequate cardiac (coronary) circulation fundamental to life. If the heart cannot pump blood adequately, an individual becomes ill or dies. Coronary artery disease affects the vasculature of the heart and is among the leading causes of death in adults. Renal circulation cleanses the blood of impurities and produces urine, functions that are critical to normal physiology. As the chemical processing plant of the body, the liver performs an extraordinary range of important functions, one of which is to detoxify all harmful substances in blood. The liver also produces the majority of the plasma proteins, including the clotting proteins. In fetal circulation, oxygenation of blood does not take place in the lungs. The developing fetus obtains its oxygen supply through the mother's placenta.

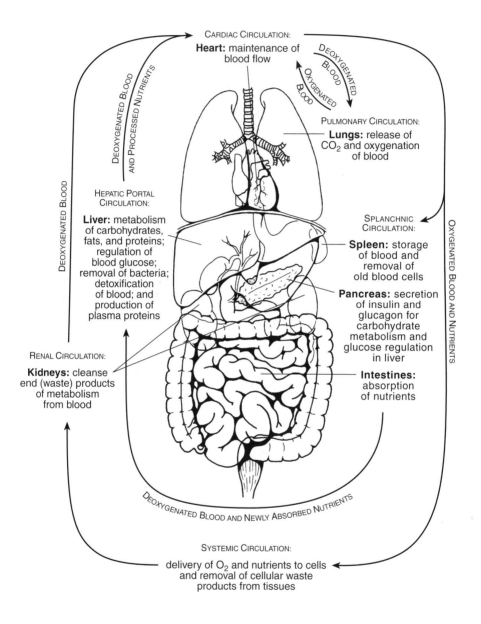

CARDIAC CIRCULATION:
Heart: maintenance of blood flow

DEOXYGENATED BLOOD AND PROCESSED NUTRIENTS

DEOXYGENATED BLOOD

OXYGENATED BLOOD

DEOXYGENATED BLOOD

OXYGENATED BLOOD AND NUTRIENTS

PULMONARY CIRCULATION:
Lungs: release of CO_2 and oxygenation of blood

HEPATIC PORTAL CIRCULATION:
Liver: metabolism of carbohydrates, fats, and proteins; regulation of blood glucose; removal of bacteria; detoxification of blood; and production of plasma proteins

SPLANCHNIC CIRCULATION:
Spleen: storage of blood and removal of old blood cells

Pancreas: secretion of insulin and glucagon for carbohydrate metabolism and glucose regulation in liver

RENAL CIRCULATION:
Kidneys: cleanse end (waste) products of metabolism from blood

Intestines: absorption of nutrients

DEOXYGENATED BLOOD AND NEWLY ABSORBED NUTRIENTS

SYSTEMIC CIRCULATION:
delivery of O_2 and nutrients to cells and removal of cellular waste products from tissues

FIGURE 3.1 Schematic Relationship of Vital Organs and Blood Flow

THE HEART AND CORONARY CIRCULATION

Introduction

The main function of the heart is to pump blood through the circulatory system to all organs of the body. Blood pumped from the heart delivers oxygen, nutrients, hormones, and other important life-sustaining substances. For the heart to carry out this demanding task, a disease-free coronary circulation is essential. Coronary circulation refers to the circulatory system of the heart. As a hardworking muscular pump responsible for the circulation of blood throughout the body, the heart itself needs a large amount of oxygen to meet the enormous demand placed on it.

Throughout one's life, the heart beats continuously and contracts rhythmically due to electrical impulses. Each day it pumps about 1800 gallons (7200 L) of blood through the body and beats approximately 100,000 times.

Heart Structure

The heart is a four-chambered organ that lies within the thorax (chest cavity). It is about the size of a clenched fist and weighs around 300 grams (g; 454 g = 1 lb). There are three layers of the heart: the outer layer, or epicardium; the middle muscle layer, or myocardium; and the inner layer, or endocardium. Like blood vessels, the endocardium is lined with endothelium.

outer layer: epicardium
middle layer: myocardium
inner layer: endocardium

Although the heart appears to be a single organ, it is actually two organs in one. A muscle wall called the septum divides it structurally into two sides, commonly referred to as the left and right hearts. Each side has an upper chamber, the atrium, and a lower chamber, the ventricle. The two hearts have interdependent yet different functions. Although they both receive and pump blood, the right heart pumps blood to the pulmonary system and the left heart pumps blood systemically, that is, throughout the rest of the body.

septum

right heart
left heart

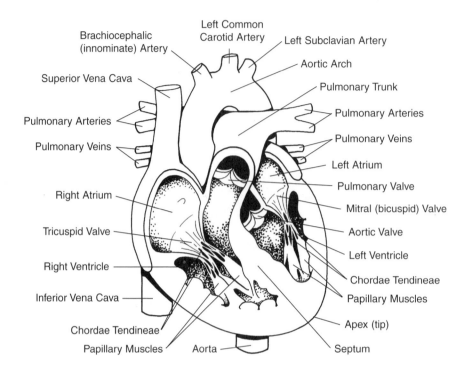

FIGURE 3.2 Anatomy of the Heart and Great Vessels

The sole function of the heart is to pump blood throughout the body. Although the heart appears to be a single organ, it actually consists of two: the left and right hearts. Each heart consists of two chambers, an atrium and a ventricle. Great vessels refer to all the major arteries and veins entering and exiting the heart.

Right Heart

receives deoxygenated blood from inferior and superior venae cavae

pumps blood to pulmonary system

The right heart receives deoxygenated blood from the body via the inferior and superior venae cavae for delivery to the lungs. The inferior vena cava returns blood from the organs and lower extremities, and the superior vena cava returns blood from the head and upper extremities. This side of the heart consists of the right atrium, tricuspid valve, right ventricle, pulmonary valve, and pulmonary artery. Blood from the venae cavae enters the right atrium and flows through the tricuspid valve into the right ventricle.

The pulmonary artery transports deoxygenated blood from the right ventricle to the lungs. Deoxygenated blood gives off carbon dioxide in the lungs and picks up oxygen.

pulmonary artery

Left Heart

The left heart receives oxygenated blood from the lungs. This side of the heart consists of the left atrium, mitral valve, left ventricle, aortic valve, and aorta. Pulmonary veins, two from the right lung and two from the left lung, carry blood to the left atrium. Blood flows from this chamber through the mitral valve into the left ventricle where it is pumped through the aorta and delivered to all body tissues. Because the left heart pumps blood systemically, the muscle wall of the left ventricle is three times (x3) thicker than the muscle wall of the right ventricle. The left ventricle exerts high pressure on the blood thus ensuring that blood reaches cells distant from the heart. At the same time, this pressure assists the return of blood to the heart through the veins.

receives oxygenated blood from lungs

pulmonary veins

pumps blood systemically

Coronary Circulation

The coronary arteries form an extensive and well-branched network of vessels supplying the myocardium. Vessels of the heart include the left and right coronary arteries (LCA and RCA) along with a system of arterioles, veins, venules, and a microvascular network. Arterial vessels deliver oxygen to the myocardium, and venous vessels return deoxygenated blood to the right and left atria of the heart. The volume of blood flow through the coronary arteries is regulated by the blood pressure and the internal diameter of the coronary arteries. If an artery's diameter is decreased due to blockage, less blood reaches the myocardium.

coronary arteries supply myocardium

Coronary Blood Flow and Disease

Disease states, such as atherosclerosis and thrombotic (blood clot) disorders, affect coronary blood flow. When coronary flow is diminished, the heart cannot contract normally. Heart disease affects blood pressure and blood flow resulting in a decrease in oxygen delivery to body tissues. Vascular diseases, such as atheroma, alters the diameter of the coronary vessels, thereby restricting blood flow. When the supply of blood to the heart is reduced, an individual is likely to show signs of ischemia and experience chest

ischemia   pain. Ischemia refers to a decrease in blood flow to tissue caused by blockage in a blood vessel. Ischemia and associated chest pain form the complex called

angina pectoris   angina pectoris.

Right and Left Coronary Arteries

RCA and LCA
deliver oxygenated
blood to myocardium

ostia

The right and left coronary arteries and their respective branches deliver oxygenated blood to the myocardium. The right coronary artery and the left coronary artery are the first vessels to arise (branch) from the aorta. Ostia are the openings of the coronary arteries in the wall of the aorta.

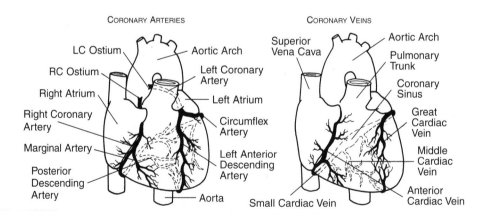

FIGURE 3.3 Arteries and Veins of Coronary Circulation

The heart must perform unfailingly; therefore, it needs a large blood supply to deliver oxygen and nutrients to its cells and remove cellular waste products. The vasculature of the heart is extensive and well branched.

Right Coronary Artery

The right coronary artery (RCA) carries oxygenated blood to the right side of the heart. The ostium of this artery arises in the anterior wall of the aorta. As the RCA travels down the anterior (front) surface of the heart, it gives off many branches to ensure that all areas of the right heart are well supplied with blood. As the RCA approaches the apex (tip) of the heart, it curves around to the posterior (back) surface of the heart where it becomes the posterior descending artery (PDA).

carries oxygenated blood to right heart

posterior descending artery

Left Coronary Artery

The left coronary artery (LCA) delivers oxygenated blood to the left side of the heart. The ostium of this artery arises in the posterior wall of the aorta. Somewhat longer in length than the RCA, the LCA divides almost immediately to form the left anterior descending artery (LAD) and the circumflex artery (Cx). The LAD travels down the anterior surface of the heart through the interventricular sulcus, the area between the ventricles. The circumflex branch travels to the lateral (side) and posterior surfaces of the heart.

delivers oxygenated blood to left heart

left anterior descending artery, circumflex artery

Conus Artery

There is considerable variation among individuals with respect to the distribution of coronary arteries and to the areas of the heart that they perfuse. Some individuals have a third coronary artery called the conus. This artery may have its own ostium in the aorta or may share an ostium with the RCA. If the conus artery is present, it usually supplies blood to the anterior wall of the right ventricle.

Coronary Venous System

The cardiac veins return deoxygenated blood from the myocardium to both the left and right atria of the heart. The coronary venous system consists of the

returns deoxygenated blood from myocardium

coronary sinus
anterior cardiac
venous system

coronary sinus on the posterior surface of the heart and the anterior cardiac venous system. The coronary sinus receives blood from the surface (superficial) veins of the heart and delivers it the right atrium near the tricuspid valve. Veins that drain into the coronary sinus include the great cardiac vein, the left marginal vein, and the left posterior vein.

The anterior cardiac venous system is made up of veins that originate in the front and side (anterolateral) surface of the right ventricle and empty into the left atrium. The anterior cardiac venous system includes the right marginal vein, the small cardiac vein, and other smaller branches.

Microvasculature of the Heart

Many different types of small capillarylike vessels supply the myocardium. These vessels deliver nutrients and oxygen to the myocardium and return carbon dioxide and waste products to the coronary veins. A rich supply of these vessels provides the walls of the myocardium with an adequate blood supply to meet the metabolic demands of the heart.

Heart Disease

There are many causes of heart disease. They include: coronary artery disease (CAD), congenital conditions, acquired abnormalities, and bacterial or viral infections.

Coronary Artery Disease

atheroma
atherosclerosis

coronary artery disease

As individuals age, the diameter of their coronary arteries often become narrowed due to the buildup of plaque, called atheroma, in the arteries. This condition is known as atherosclerosis, the heart disease state caused by atheroma. Atherosclerosis in the coronary arteries is called coronary artery disease (CAD). All arteries in the body can be affected by atherosclerosis.

Many factors are responsible for atheroma: genetics, hypertension, gender (males are more prone to CAD), diabetes mellitus, cholesterol level, diet, and smoking.

Ischemia and Angina Pectoris

Atheroma is formed in coronary arteries when plaque is deposited on the endothelial surface of these arteries. As the amount of plaque increases, blood flow through an artery decreases because the vessel diameter has been narrowed. The section of heart muscle supplied by that artery and its tributaries receives less oxygen and fewer nutrients. When blood flow is restricted enough, an individual develops ischemia because oxygen delivery to the heart tissue is not sufficient enough to meet metabolic demands.

Angina pectoris is one of the most frequent and obvious signs of ischemia. Although angina is not the same as a myocardial infarction (MI; heart attack), it indicates that the heart muscle is not receiving adequate blood flow to meet its metabolic demands. A myocardial infarction can develop from persistent or prolonged ischemia.

Myocardial Infarction

An individual can experience a myocardial infarction (MI) when plaque ruptures within a coronary artery and a thrombus (blood clot) forms. Plaque rupture causes platelets to adhere to the damaged endothelium of the artery (see Ch. 9, Hemostasis). As platelets become activated, they release chemicals that initiate the clotting process (see Ch. 10, Coagulation). Clotting proteins in plasma interact with platelets to form a thrombus. Once a thrombus forms in the artery, blood flow distal to (farthest from) the thrombus is virtually nonexistent. When blood flow to the myocardium is nonexistent, an infarct occurs. Irreversible injury to the heart muscle occurs if the thrombotic occlusion (blockage) lasts for more than 15 to 20 minutes.

plaque rupture
↓
platelet adherence
↓
clotting process
↓
thrombus/blood clot

Most MIs develop in the endocardium and spread outward through the myocardium to the epicardium. An infarct causes scar tissue, or tissue necrosis (tissue

tissue necrosis

death), to form several days afterwards. Because scar tissue cannot transmit electrical impulses that stimulate muscle contraction, wall motion of the infarcted area is hampered and the heart muscle does not contract normally. Cardiac output, referring to the amount of blood pumped from the left ventricle per minute, is decreased as is cardiac function.

cardiac output

cardiac function

Most MIs occur between the hours of 6 A.M. and 12 P.M. Physicians feel that increased levels of epinephrine (adrenaline), increased levels of fibrinogen (clotting protein), and increased platelet adhesiveness to arterial endothelium occur during these hours.

Symptoms   The symptoms of an infarct include chest pain, diaphoresis (sweating), dyspnea (shortness of breath), nausea, and vomiting. Patients can experience pain in the chest, and upper back, down the left arm, and/or into the neck and jaw.

Treatment   Muscle damage to the heart can be minimized if the infarct is treated within 4 to 6 hours after it occurs. Most damage following an infarct occurs within the first 2 to 3 hours. When the infarct is treated within this time frame, myocardial salvage is possible. The longer treatment is delayed, the more irreversible the myocardial damage. If an individual reaches the hospital soon enough after an infarct has occurred,

myocardial salvage

FIGURE 3.4 Saphenous Vein Bypass

When plaque builds up in an artery, blood flow is restricted. Heart tissue does not receive adequate amounts of oxygen and tissue necrosis results. The saphenous vein bypass is used to deliver blood from the aorta past the area of blockage.

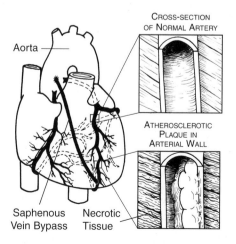

thrombolytic (clot-lysing or clot-dissolving) drugs, such as streptokinase, urokinase, or tPA (tissue plasminogen activator) can be administered to dissolve the thrombus. If blood flow can be restored to the infarcted area, there is a good chance that damage can be minimized.

thrombolytic drugs

In some instances, however, infarcts can be fatal. Death occurs when greater than 40% of the heart muscle is destroyed. The major factor in MI morbidity is the infarct size, or the amount of muscle that has been damaged. Any increase in myocardial oxygen demand or stress put on the heart during the infarct increases the infarct size.

CAD Treatment Modalities   There are a number of therapeutic modalities (options) for individuals with CAD. These patients are treated with medication, angioplasty, or bypass, depending on the type and severity of the disease.

When angina is first discovered, physicians initially try treating it with medication. If medication does not relieve the symptoms, an individual may be a candidate for coronary angioplasty or bypass. Angioplasty is a fairly common treatment. The procedure does not remove plaque but does increase the arterial lumen by the use of a balloon catheter. If successful, more blood reaches the ischemic area, whereupon angina eases. Angioplasty is usually a temporary measure often followed by a coronary bypass. A bypass is a surgical procedure used to treat individuals with advanced CAD by reestablishing blood flow to the myocardium. Veins are taken from the individual's body and grafted below the arterial obstruction and extended to the aorta.

angioplasty

coronary bypass

THE KIDNEYS AND RENAL BLOOD FLOW

Renal Function

The kidneys are vital organs. Their main function is to cleanse the blood of impurities and produce urine in the process. Only a small amount of urine, between

1 to 2 mL, is produced from the liter (or somewhat more) of blood that flows through the kidneys every minute. The rate of blood flow through the kidneys is high. The kidneys are exceptionally efficient at filtering and reabsorbing fluid and solutes (plasma substances) from the blood. Some renal functions include the following:

- filtering of blood
- regulation of fluid balance
- responding to the release of antidiuretic hormone and aldosterone
- release of erythropoietin
- production of renin, a hormone that regulates blood pressure
- pH balance
- regulation of electrolytes

Structure of the Kidneys

The kidneys are two separate reddish-brown, bean-shaped organs. They lie on either side of the vertebral column (spine) in the retroperitoneum (posterior abdomen). This region is referred to as the flank. Normally there are two kidneys, but only one is needed to maintain health. Each kidney is about the size of a clenched fist (12 cm x 6 cm x 3 cm).

capsule
outer cortex
inner medulla

nephrons

The outer covering of each kidney consists of a smooth, tough, fibrous capsule. Lying beneath the capsule are two separate and distinct regions: the outer cortex and the inner medulla. Within the cortex and medulla are the functional filtering units of the kidneys called nephrons. At birth, each kidney contains about 1 million nephrons, but this number decreases as an individual ages.

Nephrons

Each nephron is a tubular structure composed of several parts. These parts simultaneously filter blood, remove impurities, and maintain fluid volume. The parts of the nephron are:

- The glomerulus, a mass of capillaries that forms the first "in series" capillary bed

  glomerulus

- The cup-shaped Bowman's capsule, a structure that forms a reservoir around the glomerulus

  Bowman's capsule

- The renal corpuscle, a structure made up of the glomerulus and Bowman's capsule

  renal corpuscle

- The renal tubule, a structure with several discreet sections, each of which is specifically designed to filter and reabsorb substances within the blood: the proximal convoluted tubule, the loop of Henle, the distal convoluted tubule, and the collecting duct

  renal tubule

- The peritubular capillaries, which weave around the renal tubule reabsorbing solutes and water from it to form the second "in series" capillary bed

  peritubular capillaries

Route of Renal Blood Flow

Blood flow through the kidneys is somewhat different from blood flow through other organs of the body. Most organs have an "in parallel" capillary arrangement. As blood enters an organ through an artery, it flows into arterioles and then into capillary networks within the organ. Deoxygenated blood leaves the capillaries through venules that empty into veins, which transport blood to the venae cavae. In contrast, the capillary arrangement of the kidneys is structured "in series," which means that one capillary network is followed by another capillary network. Specifically, within each nephron are two capillary beds (the glomerulus and the peritubular), and blood flows through one and then the other.

in parallel
capillary arrangement

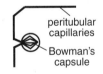

in series
capillary arrangement

Blood enters the kidneys through the renal artery and eventually flows into the nephrons via the afferent arteriole. Blood from the afferent arteriole enters a highly porous tuft of capillaries within the nephron called the glomerulus. This structure forms the first of the "in series" capillary beds.

afferent arteriole

glomerulus

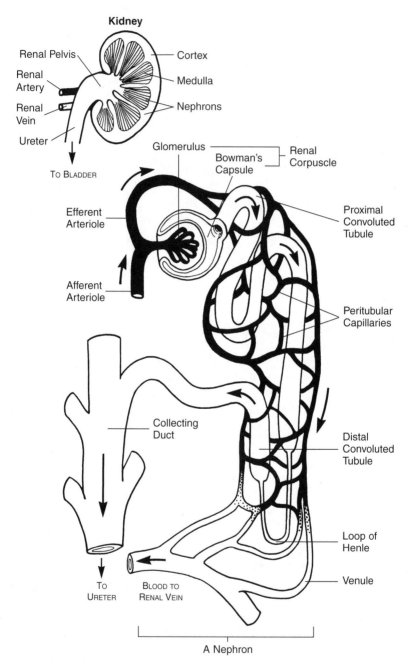

FIGURE 3.5 **Anatomy of a Nephron**

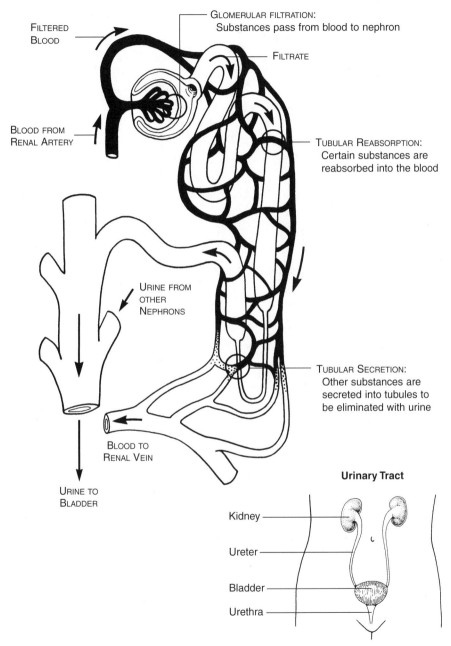

FILTERED BLOOD

GLOMERULAR FILTRATION:
Substances pass from blood to nephron

FILTRATE

BLOOD FROM RENAL ARTERY

TUBULAR REABSORPTION:
Certain substances are reabsorbed into the blood

URINE FROM OTHER NEPHRONS

TUBULAR SECRETION:
Other substances are secreted into tubules to be eliminated with urine

BLOOD TO RENAL VEIN

URINE TO BLADDER

Urinary Tract

Kidney

Ureter

Bladder

Urethra

FIGURE 3.6 **Circulation Through a Nephron**

As blood flows through the kidneys, it undergoes filtration and reabsorption. Through these regulatory processes, the kidneys remove waste products and excess water and electrolytes from the blood.

Blood entering the glomerulus is under high pressure. This pressure forces water and solutes dissolved in plasma (such as salts, amino acids, minerals, vitamins, hormones, glucose, and electrolytes) to be filtered out of the blood into Bowman's capsule.

The wall of the renal corpuscle promotes the movement and filtration of fluid and solutes between the glomerulus and Bowman's capsule. This wall is one cell layer thick and acts as a semipermeable membrane that allows some solutes through and not others, usually according to molecular size. Formed elements and plasma proteins remain in the bloodstream. Fluid that is filtered into

filtrate

Bowman's capsule is called filtrate. It is similar to plasma but has no blood cells and few if any proteins.

After filtration takes place in Bowman's capsule, blood and filtrate follow different but parallel routes. The filtrate enters the proximal convoluted tubule and passes through the loop of Henle, the distal convoluted tubule, and finally into the collecting duct. Blood that has been filtered in Bowman's capsule leaves the

efferent arteriole

glomerulus via the efferent arteriole. It passes into the peritubular capillaries that compose the second "in series" capillary bed within the kidneys. The peritubular capillaries are attached to the efferent arteriole and surround the renal tubule.

Reabsorption takes place in the peritubular capillaries and is the process by which the blood takes up solutes and water that the body needs from the filtrate within the renal tubule. For example, when the body needs water, the blood reabsorbs more water from the filtrate. Water and solutes are constantly shuffled back and forth between blood in the peritubular capillaries and fluid in the renal tubule. Fluid remaining in the renal tubule that is not reabsorbed by the blood becomes urine. Low pressure and plasma proteins in the peritubular capillaries favor reabsorption.

Movement of fluid and substances between the peritubular capillaries and renal tubule occurs as the

filtration

result of filtration, osmosis, and reabsorption. Filtration refers to the movement of fluid due to pressure.

Osmosis refers to the movement of water from a region of lower solute concentration to one of higher solute concentration. Reabsorption is the process of fluid return into the capillary by filtration and osmosis.

osmosis

reabsorption

Blood and filtrate leave the kidneys via separate routes. Blood flows from the peritubular capillaries into venules that eventually join the renal vein. Blood leaves the kidneys through the renal vein and flows to the heart via the inferior vena cava. The filtrate in a nephron empties into a collecting duct. Many nephrons are attached to a single collecting duct. All collecting ducts empty their contents into the renal pelvis. Fluid in the renal pelvis drains through the ureter into the bladder to be stored until it is excreted as urine.

Blood Volume

In the process of filtering and reabsorbing water and solutes, the kidneys help regulate the amount of water and solutes in the body. Blood volume in the vascular system is determined by the amount of water and solutes in the blood. If the body is dehydrated (low in water or fluid volume), the kidneys reabsorb water from the renal tubule into the blood with the aid of two hormones, antidiuretic hormone (ADH) and aldosterone. Blood volume increases and dehydration abates. If the body has too much water, the kidneys filter excess water from the blood into the renal tubule to be excreted in urine.

Renal Failure

There are many types of kidney diseases. Some interfere with kidney function by preventing the production of urine and the removal of waste products from the blood. With renal failure the kidneys are unable to cleanse the blood of its impurities. Waste products, excess water, acids, and electrolytes accumulate in the bloodstream and cause uremia, a form of blood poisoning. Untreated uremia leads to death.

uremia

Renal failure can be acute or chronic. Individuals with end-stage renal failure must receive hemodialysis, the

end-stage renal failure
hemodialysis

dialyzer

process by which an artificial kidney cleanses the blood. The artificial kidney is referred to as a dialyzer. Individuals with renal failure cannot survive unless they receive hemodialysis or a kidney transplant.

THE LIVER AND HEPATIC CIRCULATION

Introduction

As well as being a fascinating organ the liver is essential to life. The liver is unique in that it is the only organ in the body that has a dual blood supply. It is the largest organ in the abdominal cavity and has more functions than any other organ in the body, but describing all of them is beyond the scope of this book.

Liver Functions

As the body's main chemical processing plant, the liver is responsible for synthesizing (manufacturing) and metabolizing (breaking down) chemical substances that are utilized by all body cells for life, growth, and reproduction. The liver also removes and detoxifies harmful substances from the body, such as bacteria and toxins.

Liver functions include the following:

- Metabolism and synthesis, involving the
  - breakdown of nutrients into simpler molecules
  - production of bile
  - production of most plasma proteins
  - breakdown of hormones
  - regulation of blood glucose and glycogen levels
- The storage of
  - blood in the sinusoids (spaces in the liver)
  - glycogen
  - vitamins A, D, E, K, and B_{12}
  - ferritin (iron compound)
  - bile is stored in the gallbladder (a sac on the underside of the liver)

- The detoxification of
  - toxic substances
  - drugs
  - waste products (ammonia)
  - alcohol
- Others, including the
  - maintenance of hormone balance
  - removal of excess calcium (Ca^{++})
  - phagocytosis of microorganisms
  - production of fetal blood cells
  - regeneration of its own tissue

Anatomy and Circulation of the Liver

The liver is a mahogany-colored, smooth-surfaced, triangular-shaped organ. It weighs between 1200 and 2000 g (1.2 and 2.0 kg or 2.5 and 3.0 lbs) and makes up 2.5% of total body weight. The liver lies in the upper right quadrant of the abdomen just under the ribs and below the diaphragm, the large flat muscle that separates the chest and abdominal cavities. The upper border of the liver extends to the level of the nipples. The rib cage helps protect the liver from damage due to trauma.

The liver is divided into right and left lobes, with the right lobe being six times (x6) larger than the left lobe. The right lobe is dome shaped, whereas the left lobe tapers to a point. The two lobes are separated by a fold of peritoneum called the falciform ligament. The ligamentum venosum, which is the remnant of the atrophied, fetal ductus venosus, anchors the liver to the abdominal wall.

right and left lobes

Lobules and Hepatocytes

The functional unit of the liver is called a lobule. The liver contains from 50,000 to 100,000 lobules within it. Hepatocytes are liver cells that make up a lobule. The lobules are grouped together and surround a central vein. All chemical reactions within the liver take place within the hepatocytes. These metabolically active cells process numerous substances, such as carbohydrates, lipids, and proteins, that are taken up by the blood and

lobule

hepatocytes
central vein

transported to other body organs. These substances are then used by body cells to produce energy and other life-sustaining chemical reactions. Some molecules broken down by hepatocytes are released into the bloodstream, whereas bile produced in hepatocytes is released into the canaliculi. Blood exits a lobule through the central vein, which empties blood into the hepatic vein. Blood within the hepatic vein flows into the inferior vena cava and then onto the heart.

hepatic vein

Canaliculi

bile
bile duct
gallbladder

The canaliculi are tiny tubes that transport bile. Canaliculi merge with others and form the bile duct, which transports bile to the gallbladder for storage until it is needed for digestion.

Hepatic Blood Flow

hepatic artery
portal vein

Blood flow to the liver is unique in that it receives blood via two distinct and separate sources, the hepatic artery and the portal vein. The hepatic artery branches from the celiac artery that branches from the aorta carrying oxygenated blood to the liver. The portal vein delivers deoxygenated, nutrient-rich blood from the stomach, intestines, spleen, and pancreas to the liver for

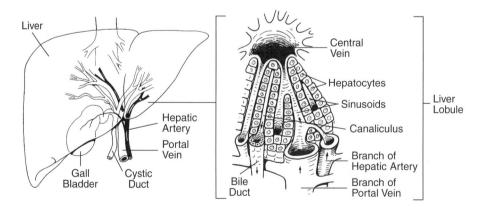

FIGURE 3.7 Anatomy of the Liver

The liver is made up of approximately 100,000 lobules, which are the liver's functional units.

processing nutrients before being distributed to other body organs and tissues. Nutrients are of no value to body cells until they have been processed by the liver.

The hepatic artery and portal vein enter the liver inferiorly (from below) in the area called the porta hepatis, or hilus. Each vessel branches many times to supply blood to both lobes of the liver. Approximately 30% (350 mL) of the blood flow to the liver is supplied by the hepatic artery, whereas 60% (1150 mL) is supplied by the portal vein. Total blood supply to the liver is 1500 mL/minute.

porta hepatis, or hilus

Sinusoids

Blood from the hepatic artery and portal vein mix in the liver sinusoids (cavities). The sinusoids are lined with epithelial cells and Kupffer's cells. Kupffer's cells (tissue macrophages, or histiocytes) of the liver remove foreign matter, such as bacteria and other microorganisms, picked up in the intestinal tract and brought to the liver by the portal blood. The Kupffer's cells prevent bacteria from entering the bloodstream and spreading throughout the body. Due to its numerous sinusoids, the liver also has the capacity to store a large volume of blood (450 mL).

Kupffer's cells

Vascular and Lymphatic Capillaries

The pores in most capillaries of the body are too small to allow proteins to escape from the bloodstream; therefore, proteins remain in the circulatory system and exert osmotic pressure. Proteins in hepatic capillaries, however, enter the hepatocytes of the liver. The size of hepatic capillary pores, which are larger (1 mm or more) than pores in other capillaries, accommodates protein absorption by the hepatocytes. Proteins that enter the hepatocytes are metabolized into simpler compounds called amino acids. These amino acids are then transported via the vascular system to other body cells for use.

amino acids

The liver is inundated with lymphatic capillaries that drain the interstitial spaces in the liver. Because hepatic capillaries are more porous they allow proteins to pass through them. Therefore, lymphatic drainage from the liver has a very high protein content. The liver is responsible for half the total amount of lymph produced in the body.

Plasma Protein Production

plasma proteins
coagulation factors

The liver produces most of the plasma proteins, such as albumin, and the coagulation factors: fibrinogen, II, V, VII, VIII, IX, X, antithrombin III, proteins C and S, and plasminogen, among others.

albumin

Albumin's main functions include: (1) the transport of substances within the blood and (2) the generation of osmotic pressure that helps maintain normal blood volume. The coagulation factors are necessary for fibrin clot formation. Antithrombin III and proteins C and S inactivate activated coagulation factors to prevent inappropriate clot formation. Fibrinogen is the coagulation factor activated by thrombin to produce fibrin.

plasminogen
plasmin
FSPs

The liver also produces plasminogen, which is the inactive form of plasmin. Plasmin breaks down fibrin clots that release fibrin split products (FSPs) into the bloodstream. Fibrin split products are removed from the circulation by Kupffer's cells.

When the liver becomes diseased for whatever reason, plasma protein production is decreased or deficient. Decreased or deficient plasma proteins, especially coagulation proteins, causes blood clotting problems in patients. A decreased level of albumin interferes with osmotic pressure production and transport of substances in the blood.

Bile Production

Bile is produced in the hepatocytes and released into the canaliculi that transport it to the gallbladder, an organ that stores bile. Bile is released into the intestine where it breaks down fat molecules. Many substances are excreted in the bile and then eliminated from the body with feces. A breakdown product of hemoglobin called bilirubin is excreted in bile.

bilirubin

Disorders of the Liver

Like all organs of the body, the liver is susceptible to many diseases and disorders. A major disease of the liver is cirrhosis, which is caused by excessive alcohol consumption, infection, poisons, and other diseases. Other conditions affecting the liver include: congenital defects, autoimmune disorders, metabolic disorders, and tumors. The most frequent and obvious signs of liver disease are jaundice and hepatomegaly (enlargement of the liver). Jaundice is characterized by a yellow color to the whites of the eyes and skin.

cirrhosis

jaundice, hepatomegaly

FETAL CIRCULATION

Introduction

Fetal circulation is quite different from the adult's because oxygenation of blood does not take place in the lungs. The lungs of the fetus are deflated, and, therefore, they resist blood flow and are unable to exchange respiratory gases. Being enclosed in the fluid-filled amniotic sac, the fetus receives its supply of oxygen from maternal circulation via the placenta, which is sometimes referred to as the fetal lung. The placenta is an organ attached to the lining of the uterus and connected to the fetus by the umbilical cord. Richly endowed with maternal blood vessels, the placenta enables the fetus to exchange oxygen and nutrients and remove carbon dioxide and other waste products through its mother's circulation. Fetal extraction of oxygen from maternal blood is also made possible by fetal hemoglobin (Hgb F). This molecule has a greater affinity for oxygen than adult hemoglobin (Hgb A) and can extract oxygen from Hgb A.

placenta/fetal lung

fetal hemoglobin (Hgb F), adult hemoglobin (Hgb A)

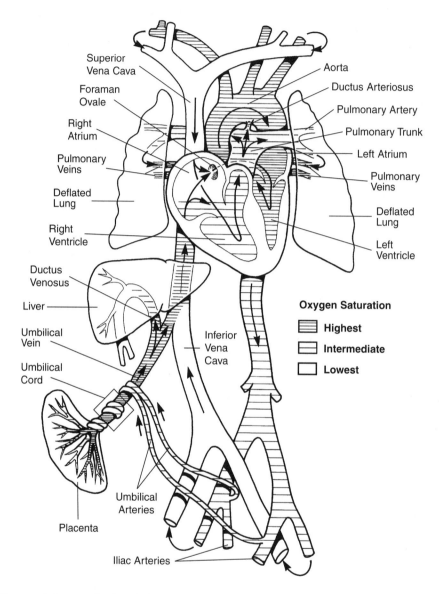

FIGURE 3.8 Fetal Circulation

Fetal lungs are nonfunctional. The fetus receives richly oxygenated blood via the placenta. Blood from the placenta is about 80% saturated with oxygen. This oxygen-rich blood travels to the head and upper body. Blood returning to the heart has a lower oxygen saturation of about 65%. This blood is pumped to the lower body. The foramen ovale and the ductus arteriosus are the two major structures that distinguish fetal circulation from the adult's. During gestation, they permit blood to bypass the deflated lungs of the fetus.

Route of Fetal Blood Flow

The route of blood flow through the fetus is unique. Oxygen-rich blood from the placenta circulates through the fetus. The foramen ovale and ductus arteriosus are two openings in fetal circulation that permit blood flow to bypass the fetal lungs. The foramen ovale is an opening in the atrium of the heart, and the ductus arteriosus is an opening between the aorta and the pulmonary artery.

foramen ovale
ductus arteriosus

The flow of blood from the placenta to the fetus begins in the umbilical cord. Within the umbilical cord lie the umbilical arteries and vein. A fetal vein called the ductus venosus connects the umbilical vein to the inferior vena cava of the fetus. Blood empties into the right atrium of the fetal heart, but rather than moving from this chamber into the right ventricle for passage to the lungs, blood is shunted through the foramen ovale into the left atrium. Because of blood flow dynamics and position of the inferior vena cava, the foramen ovale diverts blood from entering the right ventricle and hence the nonbreathing lungs. Blood in the left atrium flows through the mitral valve into the left ventricle and out the aorta to be circulated to the head and upper body. This blood has the highest concentration of oxygen in fetal circulation. A developing brain is very dependent on a rich oxygen supply.

umbilical cord

ductus venosus

Blood returns from the head and upper body of the fetus through the superior vena cava into the right atrium. This blood has a lower oxygen concentration because the brain has extracted some oxygen from it. Due to blood flow dynamics and position of the superior vena cava, blood returning from the head and upper body travels through the tricuspid valve into the right ventricle and is not diverted through the foramen ovale. The right ventricle ejects this blood through the pulmonary valve into the pulmonary artery. Rather than entering the lungs, this blood with its lower oxygen concentration is shunted out the ductus arteriosus into the aorta to be circulated to the organs and lower extremities, a region less dependent on oxygen than the brain. Blood bypasses the aortic arch, at which the head and upper body vessels are joined.

Deoxygenated blood leaves the fetus's lower body via the umbilical arteries for transport to the placenta. The placenta removes carbon dioxide and other waste products of fetal metabolism. The umbilical arteries branch from the iliac arteries which branch from the aorta.

Fetal Circulation at Birth

At the time of birth, the newborn's cardiopulmonary system undergoes important structural changes. As breathing inflates the infant's lungs, resistance to blood flow in the lungs decreases and blood begins circulating through them. Neonatal circulation is like the adult's because blood goes to the lungs and is no longer diverted from them.

Other structural changes take place in the fetal circulation at birth. The foramen ovale closes and becomes the fossa ovalis. The ductus arteriosus atrophies into the nonfunctional ligamentum arteriosum. Because the placenta no longer supplies blood to the fetus, the ductus venosus closes and becomes the ligamentum venosum. It fibroses forming the ligament that anchors the liver to the abdominal wall.

fossa ovalis
ligamentum arteriosum

ligamentum venosum

Congenital Defects

If either the foramen ovale or ductus arteriosus does not close, the newborn receives less oxygenated blood and may develop cyanosis, a condition in which the newborn turns blue from decreased oxygen in the blood. Surgery may be required to correct these defects. When the foramen ovale remains open, blood is shunted between the atria rather than following the normal path of blood flow. The amount of blood flow and oxygen delivered to body tissues is therefore decreased. This condition is known as a patent foramen

cyanosis

ovale, also referred to as an atrial septal defect. The foramen ovale is usually closed surgically with a patch of tissue taken from the pericardium, the sac in which the heart lies.

patent foramen ovale

When the ductus arteriosus remains open, some blood in the pulmonary artery is shunted into the aorta or from the aorta into the pulmonary artery. Therefore, the systemic blood supply has a lower oxygen content than normal, which causes the infant to become cyanotic. This condition, known as patent ductus arteriosus (PDA), is the most common congenital vascular defect occurring in newborns and is more common in females than in males.

patent ductus
arteriosus (PDA)

Signs and Symptoms of PDA

Signs and symptoms of PDA are pounding pulse and increased pulse pressure. PDA may be treated with drugs or tied off surgically. The drug used to close a PDA is indomethacin, which can be given either by mouth or by injection. The prognosis for patent foramen ovale and patent ductus arteriosus is usually favorable. Once the patent foramen ovale is patched, an infant usually has an unremarkable recovery. Infants with PDA can experience complications later in life, usually in their third or fourth decade. These individuals can develop pulmonary hypertension or congestive heart failure (CHF).

▪ QUESTIONS ▪

1. What are the main functions of the heart? the kidneys? the liver?

2. How does oxygenation of the blood in fetal circulation differ from that in adult circulation?

3. How much blood does the average heart pump per day?

4. Describe the anatomical structure of the heart.

5. How does the function of the right side of the heart differ from the left side?

6. How does the anatomy of the right side of the heart differ from the left side?

7. Identify two diseases associated with the coronary circulation. Explain their related physiology.

8. Identify the two major arteries of the heart and explain their functions.

9. Name four other, lesser arteries involved in the coronary circulation.

10. Define the ostia in the coronary circulation.

11. Briefly describe the coronary venous system and how it operates.

12. List seven factors associated with coronary artery disease.

13. How is atherosclerosis associated with CAD?

14. How may atheroma, or the buildup of plaque in arteries, lead to coronary ischemia and angina pectoris?

15. Define cardiac output.

16. What is an MI (myocardial infarction) and how does it affect cardiac output and function?

17. How is an MI treated? What are the defining factors in the prognosis for an individual?

18. Explain the treatment modalities for CAD and how they relate to one another.

19. List six functions of the kidneys.

20. Describe the anatomic structure and position of the kidneys.

21. What are the functional filtering units of the kidneys? Identify five anatomical entities that make up these units.

22. How does renal blood flow differ from that of other organs?

23. Define the terms filtration, osmosis, and reabsorption as they relate to renal circulation.

24. What is urine?

25. What happens when an individual becomes dehydrated?

26. What is renal failure? and how may it cause uremia?

27. What is the process by which an artificial kidney cleanses the blood called?

28. How is the liver unique among the organs of the body?

29. The liver is responsible for the synthesis of many substances. Identify two.

30. What vitamins are stored in the liver?

31. Name two substances detoxified by the liver.

32. Where are fetal blood cells produced?

33. Where is the liver located? Describe its basic anatomy.

34. What is a lobule? What is it made up of?

35. Explain the role of canaliculi in the liver.

36. How does the liver receive its blood supply?

37. What are the sinusoids? What are their functions?

38. How are amino acids produced in the body?

39. List five plasma proteins produced by the liver.

40. What breakdown product of hemoglobin is excreted in the bile?

41. How is fetal hemoglobin (Hgb F) different from adult hemoglobin (Hgb A)?

42. How does fetal circulation differ from adult circulation?

43. What are the two openings in the fetal circulation that permit blood flow to bypass the fetal lungs called?

44. Where in the fetal circulation is the highest concentration of oxygen?

45. What occurs to the fetal circulation at birth?

46. What two possible defects in the circulation can compromise the life of a newborn?

CHAPTER 4

Red Blood Cells

Introduction

Red blood cells are called erythrocytes or red corpuscles. They are released from hematopoietic bone marrow into the circulation as fully mature blood cells. At this time, they are ready to perform their major function of transporting the respiratory gases, oxygen (O_2) and carbon dioxide (CO_2). Red cells transport O_2 from the lungs to body tissues and CO_2 from body tissues to the lungs. As fully differentiated cells, red cells do not require a nucleus and therefore do not undergo cell division. Oxygen and carbon dioxide, hemoglobin molecules, and cellular organelles occupy the entire space of a red cell. If nucleated red cells are found in the circulation, extramedullary hematopoiesis is taking place.

erythrocytes

respiratory gases: O_2 and CO_2

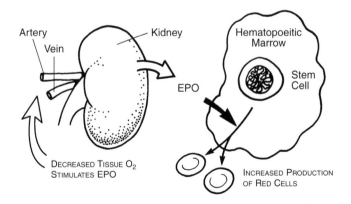

FIGURE **4.1 Release of Erythropoietin (EPO)**

Blood low in O_2 flows through the kidneys, which stimulates the release of EPO. In turn, EPO stimulates stem cells in the bone marrow to produce red cells. An increase in the numbers of red cells increases the ability to transport O_2.

Erythropoiesis

erythropoietin

Production of red cells by bone marrow is called erythropoiesis. Blood low in O_2 passing through the kidneys stimulates red cell production. Renal (kidney) peritubular cells sense the decreased O_2 and release the hormone erythropoietin (EPO). This hormone circulates in the plasma to hematopoietic marrow and activates stem cells to produce red cells. Additional erythrocytes increase the O_2-carrying capacity of the blood by elevating the hemoglobin concentration (see p. 65).

Shape

rouleaux formation

A red cell is a flexible, biconcave disk with a diameter of 7μ and a thickness of 2μ. This shape imparts a maximum surface area for the transfer of respiratory gases into and out of red cells. The flexibility of erythrocytes enables them to change shape as they flow through capillaries, which have a slightly larger diameter than a red cell. As red cells flow through the capillaries they do so in single file like a stack of coins in what is called rouleaux formation.

Life Span

120 days

reticulocytes

Once a red cell is released into the circulation, it has a life span of approximately 120 days. Immature red cells sometimes found in the circulation are called reticulocytes. They are released into the bloodstream

FIGURE 4.2 Erythrocyte

An erythrocyte is a flexible, biconcave disk without a nucleus. Its disk shape allows a maximum surface area to transport respiratory gases into and out of the cell. The red cell's flexibility allows it to alter its shape as it flows through capillaries.

**Side View
of Erythrocyte**

following blood loss or therapy for anemia, among other reasons. When red cells are hemolyzed (ruptured) or near the end of their life cycle, they are removed from circulation by macrophages (white cells) in the liver and spleen, which are organs located in the abdominal cavity. Remnants of ruptured red cells are called ghosts or red cell stroma.

ghosts/red cell stroma

Number of Red Cells

The number range of red cells in the average adult is 4.2 to 6.2 x 10^6/uL (4.2 to 6.2 x 10^{12}/L). The average is 5.5 x 10^6/uL (5.5 x 10^{12}/L) for males and 4.5 x 10^6/uL (4.5 x 10^{12}/L) for females. These numbers are considered standard, and any major deviation suggests a problem.

4 million to 6 million per microliter

Erythrocytosis, or Polycythemia

Erythrocytosis and polycythemia are synonymous terms that refer to an elevated red cell count signifying an excess of red cells in the circulation. The term polycythemia is usually used in reference to an elevated red cell count due to pathologic reasons (see below). Erythrocytosis is the compensatory increase of red cells due to diseases and conditions, such as vascular or pulmonary disease, that affects O_2 delivery to the tissues.

elevated red cell count

Polycythemia Vera

Polycythemia vera (PV), also called erythema, is an extremely high red cell count. In this case, hemoglobin is greater than 18 g/dl, the red cell count is greater than 6.2 X 10^{12}/L, and the hematocrit (see p. 70) is greater than 0.55. Polycythemia vera is a myeloproliferative blood disease resulting from a stem cell disorder in which the red cells are produced in very high numbers. The condition is usually found in older patients. Polycythemia vera can present circulatory problems for a patient because the blood may be so thick that it blocks the microvasculature of the lungs and kidneys.

erythema

high red cell count

myeloproliferative blood disease

It may also cause increased numbers of platelets and granulocytes within the circulation. Thrombosis and hemorrhage occur frequently and vascular accidents are a major cause of death in persons with PV. Thrombosis is caused by hypeviscous plasma, decreased blood flow, and increased platelet numbers. Hemorrhage is caused by poor platelet function, vascular abnormalities, and infarcts (necrosis) of the microvasculature.

Symptoms   Symptoms of PV include: night sweats, itching after a hot bath, splenomegaly, plethora (facial redness), hemorrhage or thrombosis, blurred vision, and hypertension.

phlebotomy
cytotoxic drugs

Treatments   Treatment aims at maintaining normal red cell numbers through phlebotomy or the use of cytotoxic drugs. The prognosis for patients affected by polycythemia vera is between 10 to 16 years.

Anemia

low red cell count

A low red cell count indicates anemia. This condition is defined as a hemoglobin content of less than 13 g/dL in males and 11 g/dL in females. Anemia is not a disease of the blood but rather an indication of a disease process elsewhere in the body.

There are many causes of anemia, such as iron deficiency and vitamin deficiencies, hemolysis (rupture of red cell membrane), and autoimmune diseases. With all anemias, there are not enough red cells (hemoglobin) in circulation to supply adequate O_2 to body tissues. Therefore, other body systems have to compensate. For example, the heart beats faster to circulate more blood and breathing becomes more rapid, causing the lungs to take in more O_2.

Anemia is a condition often seen in patients with end-stage renal (kidney) disease or in those receiving chemotherapy or radiation to treat malignancies. Anemia may also occur following major blood loss, pregnancy, and with increased plasma volume.

Symptoms

Symptoms of anemia include: dyspnea, weakness, pale color of the mucous membranes, headaches, heart palpitations, and sluggishness. Older individuals can experience cardiac failure, angina pectoris, confusion, and claudication (impaired blood flow) in the legs.

Treatments

The treatment for anemia is aimed at increasing the number of red cells in circulation. This can be through the transfusion of red cells or administration of recombinant erythropoietin.

Hemoglobin

All cells of the body require O_2 to carry out their metabolic processes. The hemoglobin (Hgb) molecule in red cells makes it possible for blood to transport sufficient amounts of O_2 to body cells. Along with O_2 transport, Hgb has other important and essential functions, such as transport of some CO_2 and the buffering (prevention of pH changes) of hydrogen ions within the red cell.

Hgb

O_2 and CO_2 transport

buffering

The Hemoglobin Molecule

Hemoglobin is a chemically complex protein molecule produced within mitochondria (cellular organelles) of immature red cells. The presence of approximately 300 million Hgb molecules in each red cell virtually makes the cell a membrane-bound sac filled with Hgb. After a mature red cell is released into circulation, it no longer synthesizes Hgb.

The Hgb molecule is made up of four individual polypeptide chains of amino acids linked together in a specific linear arrangement. The polypeptide chains in adult Hgb, called Hgb A, are designated as alpha (α) and beta (β). There are two of both kinds in every Hgb molecule. A single molecule of heme is attached to each polypeptide chain. The heme molecule is the site at which O_2 binds to Hgb. Because it contains an

polypeptide chains of amino acids

Hgb A

heme molecule

FIGURE 4.3 Structure of Hemoglobin Molecule

This schematic representation of a hemoglobin molecule shows the location of the individual polypeptide chains, two alpha and two beta, and the O_2 binding sites attached to each chain. An atom of iron is present within each binding site. There are approximately 300 million molecules of hemoglobin in a single red cell.

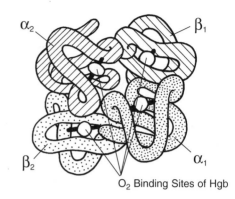

O_2 Binding Sites of Hgb

iron (Fe) atom

iron (Fe) atom, the heme molecule is responsible for the red color of blood. When the red color is brightest, red cells are saturated with O_2.

Oxygenated Blood   Blood returns to the lungs low in O_2 and transporting CO_2. Within the lungs, red cells release CO_2 and pick up O_2 via Hgb in the pulmonary capillaries surrounding the alveoli. Oxygen diffuses into the red cells and binds with Hgb molecules. Oxygenated blood is ready for delivery to body tissues. As red cells perfuse systemic capillary beds, O_2 is released from Hgb molecules into body tissues. The exchange of O_2 and CO_2 occurs approximately 200,000 times in the average life span of a red cell.

Deoxygenated Blood   The loss of O_2 to body tissues causes blood to take on a purplish color. Deoxygenated blood (blood low in oxygen) picks up CO_2 from body tissues and transports it to the lungs. Carbon dioxide is not transported in the same way as O_2 (see Ch. 5, Oxygen and Carbon Dioxide Transport).

Hemoglobin Saturation

Each Hgb molecule has four heme sites and therefore is able to bind four O_2 molecules. When a Hgb molecule contains four O_2 molecules it is considered fully saturated. Hemoglobin saturated with O_2 is called oxyhemoglobin. Hemoglobin that has released O_2 is called deoxyhemoglobin, sometimes referred to as reduced hemoglobin. The latter term is actually

oxyhemoglobin
deoxyhemoglobin

incorrect, but is still used. The percentage of Hgb that is bound to O_2 in arterial blood is called the oxygen saturation (SaO_2) of arterial blood. The saturation is a measure of the amount of O_2 combined with Hgb and not the amount of Hgb in the blood.

SaO_2 of arterial blood

Hemoglobin's Oxygen Affinity

Hemoglobin's ability to pick up and release O_2 to body tissues depends on its affinity for O_2. Affinity is the ability either to bind (hold on to, pick up) or to release (give up) O_2. Certain conditions in the lungs and other body tissues influence the affinity of Hgb for O_2. When tissues have a decreased pH (increased H^+ ion concentration) and an increased CO_2 concentration, as occurs in metabolically active tissues, Hgb has less affinity for O_2 and thus releases it into body tissues. In the lungs, where there is an increased pH (decreased hydrogen ion concentration) and a decreased CO_2 concentration, Hgb binds (picks up) O_2 more easily. The influence of pH and CO_2 on Hgb's affinity to bind and release O_2 is known as the Bohr effect.

affinity:
binding or release
of O_2

Bohr effect:
decreased pH and
increased CO_2
↓
O_2 release

increased pH and
decreased CO_2
↓
O_2 binding

Hypoxia

A decreased concentration of O_2 in body tissues is called hypoxia. It can develop for a number of reasons. A low concentration of Hgb, for example, causes the blood to carry less O_2. Therefore, body tissues may not receive adequate O_2, which presents problems over time. Inadequate O_2 delivery to tissues leads to poor wound healing and may also increase the workload on the heart. Hypoxia stimulates the kidneys to release erythropoietin, which increases the red cell numbers.

decreased
concentration of O_2

hypoxia
↓
erythropoietin
↓
increase of red cells

Blood Test for Hgb Concentration

The oxygen-carrying capacity of blood is indicated by the test that measures the concentration of Hgb in blood (see Appendix, Blood Tests). The Hgb concentration in adult males is 13.5 to 18 g/dL and in females 12 to 16 g/dL. The Hgb concentration in newborns is greater than in adults, between 15 to 24 g/dL.

Fetal Hemoglobin

Types

Gower I and Gower II
Portland

Hgb F

During the phases of embryonic development, different types of Hgb molecules are produced. The earliest is called Gower I, followed by Gower II, which in turn is replaced by hemoglobin Portland. By the time red cell production moves from the yolk sac to the liver (fourth month), hemoglobin F (fetal Hgb) is produced by the immature red cells in bone marrow.

Adult and fetal Hgb molecules differ in their polypetide chains. Hemoglobin F molecules are designed to extract O_2 from maternal red cells at the placenta. They have a greater affinity for O_2 than hemoglobin A (adult Hgb). Between the third and sixth months following birth, most Hgb F has been replaced by Hgb A.

Abnormal Hemoglobin Molecules

HgbA:
α and β chains

Abnormal Hgb molecules transport O_2 poorly. In the red cells of normal adults, the globin (protein part of hemoglobin) of Hgb A consists of two alpha (α) chains and two beta (β) chains. Each alpha chain contains 141 amino acids and each beta chain 146 amino acids arranged in a specific sequence. Any variation in the amino acid sequence of either chain produces an abnormal Hgb molecule. Whether or not abnormal Hgb presents oxygenation problems depends on the location of the amino acid defect in the polypeptide chain. If the defect is at a crucial point, such as the O_2 binding site, O_2 transport is hampered.

There are about 400 different or abnormal Hgb molecules. Not all of them present clinical oxygenation problems, but some do (see below).

Hemoglobin S

Sickle-cell Anemia   Hemoglobin S is a congenital disorder resulting in sickle-cell anemia, a disease found predominately among African Americans. Sickle-cell anemia is a hemolytic anemia, which means that red cells rupture. This type of anemia presents many health problems for affected individuals. Sickle-cell disease is found in individuals homozygous for Hgb S, that is, they have have two defective genes that code for the hemoglobin molecule. Individuals with one defective gene for Hgb S are heterozygous. In this case, the normal Hgb gene produces enough normal Hgb. Heterozygous individuals do not usually have symptoms of the disease but are carriers of the defective gene and can transmit the defective gene to their offspring. Hemoglobin S results from a substitution of the amino acid valine by glutamic acid in position 6 in the beta chains.

hemolytic anemia

Oxygen Transport Hemoglobin S transports O_2 normally. However, when it releases O_2 into body tissues, Hgb crystallizes and causes red cells to take on the classic sickle shape. Distorted red cells become trapped or are easily hemolyzed in the microvasculature of many organs (heart, lungs, kidneys, joints, eyes, and others) and cause multiple problems. For example, if the capillaries in joints become blocked, an individual experiences discomfort and joint pain. Other complications caused by Hgb S include: retinal degeneration, ulcerations of the lower legs, infarctions of organs, such as the liver and spleen, and priapisms (constant erection caused by occluded blood vessels in the penis).

Thalassemias

Other abnormal forms of hemoglobins are classified under the name of thalassemia. Thalassemias are caused by a genetic defect in which an individual's Hgb molecules show production of only one type of polypeptide chain. If the individual produces only alpha chains, he or she is said to have beta thalassemia (minor). If only beta chains are produced, the individual has alpha thalassemia (major). Thalassemias are most prevalent in persons of Mediterranean or Asian ancestry. Depending on the severity of the

beta thalassemia (minor)
alpha thalassemia (major)

condition, individuals with thalassemias experience low Hgb concentration and fatigue. Thalassemia major requires the use of blood transfusions, whereas thalassemia minor is usually symptomless and presents few if any problems.

2,3-Diphosphoglycerate

Hgb release of O$_2$

The 2,3-diphosphoglycerate (2,3-DPG) molecule is produced within the red cell by the metabolic breakdown of glucose. This molecule has the same concentration in red cells as Hgb and is bound to it. The function of 2,3-DPG is to allow Hgb to release O$_2$ to the tissues more easily.

In Stored Blood

The discovery of 2,3-DPG function in O$_2$ release provided clinical medicine with insights about stored blood. Stored blood has very low levels of 2,3-DPG. Some patients transfused with stored blood are compromised because O$_2$ release to body tissues is minimal. Transfused cells depleted of 2,3-DPG can recover only half their normal level within a 24-hour period, possibly not rapidly enough for a compromised or severely ill individual.

reversible storage lesion
storage lesion

After stored blood is infused into a patient, the recovery of 2,3-DPG is one of the reversible storage lesions of blood. A storage lesion is damage incurred by blood in storage. Nothing is gained, however, by adding 2,3-DPG to stored blood because the red cell membrane is impermeable to this molecule.

The Hematocrit

Hct
index of red cell concentration

The hematocrit (Hct) is the percentage of whole blood occupied by red cells. It is an important index of red cell concentration, and thus an indirect measure of the oxygen carrying capacity of blood. In adults, the Hct is between 0.38 to 0.54. This indicates that 38 to 54% of

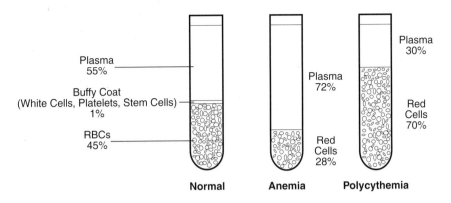

FIGURE 4.4 Hematocrits

The hematocrit (Hct) represents the percentage of whole blood occupied by red cells. If a tube of anticoagulated blood is allowed to stand, the blood components separate into plasma (55%) and formed elements (45%). These hematocrit tubes show the relationship between the level of red cells and plasma, depending on the health status of the individual. The Hct provides information about the volume of red cells and is an approximate indication of the O_2-carrying capacity of blood.

whole blood is made up of red cells. The Hct in females ranges from 0.38 to 0.46, and in males from 0.42 to 0.54. The Hct of infants is higher than adults at birth the range is from 0.55 to 0.68. The Hct in children changes to adult levels at about 10 years of age.

The Hct is sometimes referred to as the crit or packed cell volume. A transfusion of red cells into the average-sized adult elevates the Hct by 0.03 to 0.04 (3 to 4%). For example, a unit of Packed Red Cells raises a Hct from 0.35 to 0.38.

the crit/
packed cell volume

Red Cell Hemolysis

The term hemolysis refers to the lysis of the red cell membrane. Hemolyzed cells, no matter what the cause, present serious problems in patients. When a red cell ruptures, Hgb is released as plasma-free hemoglobin. In

hemolysis

plasma-free hemoglobin

this state, Hgb can no longer transport O_2, and the ability of blood to oxygenate body tissues is decreased. In addition, remnants of ruptured red cells (red cell stroma, or ghosts) can activate the clotting cascade. Blood clots and stroma can lodge in the microvasculature of the lung and kidneys, possibly causing these organs to fail.

The following conditions cause hemolysis:

- Immune responses caused by transfusions
- Sepsis, a serious bacterial or viral infection
- Red cell membrane stress from mechanical causes, such as a cardiopulmonary bypass pump, hemodialysis machine, or high-suction pressure during autologous blood recovery
- Medications and toxins, such as alcohol
- Aging red cells, which makes membranes fragile and more susceptible to hemolysis
- Activation of the complement system by antigen-antibody complexes, which stimulates complement proteins in plasma to bind to the red cell membrane thus causing hemolysis
- Enzyme deficiencies, such as glucose-6-phosphate dehydrogenase

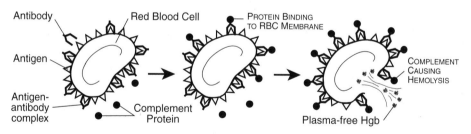

FIGURE 4.5 Red Cell Hemolysis

Hemolysis is the destruction of the red cell membrane and the release of hemoglobin into plasma. There are many causes of hemolysis. This schematic representation shows hemolysis caused by antibody and complement proteins (components of the immune response). Because plasma-free hemoglobin cannot transport O_2, it is quickly broken down into bilirubin and metabolized by the liver. If hemolysis is severe, the liver may not be able to metabolize all the bilirubin, which may accumulate in body tissues and cause jaundice.

Bilirubin

Hemoglobin that is released from red cells is broken down into bilirubin by the liver. If hemolysis is significant, the liver is unable to excrete bilirubin. Bilirubin then accumulates in the bloodstream and leaks into the tissues giving the skin and eyes a yellow color referred to as jaundice.   jaundice

▪ QUESTIONS ▪

1. What is the term used for red blood cells?

2. Where are red cells formed? and what is their approximate life span?

3. What are the main functions of red cells?

4. Red cells do not have a nucleus. True or False?

5. Explain the term erythropoiesis.

6. Describe the shape of a red cell. Why is it important?

7. What is the life span of a red cell? and then what happens to it after its life span is over?

8. What are the terms used for an elevated red cell count?

9. What are the signs and symptoms of polycythemia? and how is it treated?

10. What are the signs and symptoms of anemia? and how is it treated?

11. What are the three functions of hemoglobin (Hgb)?

12. Where does O_2 bind with Hgb in the circulatory system?

13. Why is blood colored red? Why is it sometimes purple in color?

14. What is the oxygen saturation (SaO_2) of arterial blood?

15. Explain the Bohr effect.

16. What is the condition called when body tissues receive an inadequate oxygen supply? What physiological event does this condition stimulate?

17. What are the normal Hgb values in males? in females?

18. How does fetal Hgb differ from adult Hgb?

19. What is the disease caused by the abnormal Hgb molecule Hgb S? How does it present? and what are the implications for the patient?

20. Identify and describe the major symptom of another disease caused by an abnormal Hgb molecule.

21. How is 2,3-DPG produced? and what is its function?

22. What is a storage lesion?

23. What is the hematocrit? and why is it important?

24. What are the normal laboratory values for the hematocrit?

25. What is hemolysis? and what are its two major effects?

26. What can cause hemolysis?

27. What are the symptoms of a patient with a high bilirubin level?

CHAPTER 5

Oxygen and Carbon Dioxide Transport

Introduction

The transport and release of oxygen (O_2) to body tissues and the return of carbon dioxide (CO_2), the end product of cellular metabolism, to the lungs requires complex processes involving red cells. Transport of the respiratory gases, O_2 and CO_2, is essential to human life. Exchange of the respiratory gases is called respiration.

respiratory gases: O_2 and CO_2
respiration

The term respiration is often used to mean "breathing." Technically, however, it refers to the exchange of respiratory gases between the lungs and body tissues. Breathing refers to the movement of air into and out of the lungs and is the process of ventilation. Ventilation has two phases: (1) inspiration, the movement of air into the lungs, and (2) expiration, the movement of air out of the lungs.

ventilation: inspiration
expiration

Movement of O_2 and CO_2 into and out of the lungs depends on other systems and organs as well. The respiratory muscles, consisting of the intercostal muscles and the diaphragm, must work properly. Because the heart pumps blood around the body, it is an essential organ in O_2 and CO_2 transport also. When the heart is damaged, exchange of O_2 and CO_2 is impaired and the quality of life jeopardized. Some diseases are associated with impaired O_2 and CO_2 exchange. These include: emphysema, chronic obstructive pulmonary disease (COPD), congestive heart failure (CHF), and pneumonias.

77

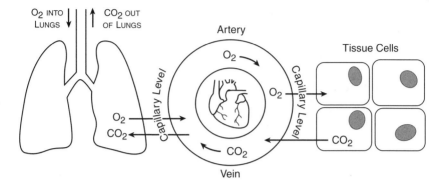

FIGURE 5.1 Oxygen (O_2) and Carbon Dioxide (CO_2) Transfer

In respiration, O_2 picked up in the lungs is distributed to body tissues. Carbon dioxide produced in body tissues is delivered to the lungs. Exchange of respiratory gases takes place between the lungs and body tissues.

Role of Hemoglobin in Respiration

Transport of O_2 to body tissues and CO_2 to the lungs requires that specific events take place involving ventilation, red cells, and hemoglobin molecules. When O_2 is inhaled from the atmosphere, it enters the alveoli of the lungs and combines with Hgb in pulmonary capillary blood. Hemoglobin molecules are responsible for delivering an adequate amount (supply) of O_2 to body cells in order to meet cellular requirements (demand) for O_2. If it were not for Hgb, body tissues would receive an insufficient supply of O_2.

carboxyhemoglobin

Carbon dioxide produced by body tissues enters systemic capillary blood. Within these capillaries, some CO_2 becomes attached to Hgb molecules, called carboxyhemoglobin, while the remainder is transported by plasma to the lungs. Through ventilation, it is exhaled from the lungs into the atmosphere. Hemoglobin is essential for the transport of both O_2 and CO_2 as well as the buffering of hydrogen ions.

Diffusion and Partial Pressure

Diffusion and partial pressure are fundamental processes involved in the transport and exchange of the respiratory gases. Gases are colorless and sometimes odorless atoms or molecules with little mass (weight) and no specific shape. They have the ability to expand and contract with changes in pressure and temperature. The atmosphere is made up of many gases, the two predominant ones being nitrogen (N_2; 78%) and oxygen (O_2; 21%).

Diffusion is the process whereby atoms or molecules move from a region of higher partial pressure (concentration) to a region of lower partial pressure.

The individual pressure exerted by each gas in the atmosphere is called partial pressure, which is represented by "P" followed by the symbol for the gas. For example, the partial pressure of O_2 is represented as PO_2.

partial pressure

The difference in partial pressures between two areas is referred to as the diffusion gradient. The greater the gradient the greater the movement of gas, and vice versa.

diffusion gradient

The combined partial pressures of the gases of the atmosphere create the total pressure called barometric, or atmospheric, pressure. Barometric pressure is greatest at sea level and becomes progressively less going up into the atmosphere.

barometric or atmospheric pressure

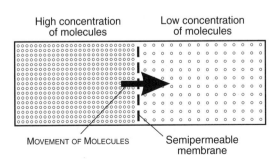

High concentration of molecules   Low concentration of molecules

MOVEMENT OF MOLECULES   Semipermeable membrane

FIGURE 5.2 Principle of Diffusion

Atoms and molecules move from an area of higher concentration to an area of lower concentration through a semipermeable membrane. In the case of respiration, diffusion is dependent on the partial pressures of O_2 and CO_2.

Pressure is measured in mm Hg (millimeters of mercury). At sea level, atmospheric pressure equals 760 mm Hg, also referred to as 760 torr. Atmospheric pressure is determined by the following equation:

Atmospheric pressure = PN_2 + PO_2 + P (other trace gases, such as carbon dioxide).

partial pressure of O_2 (PO_2)

The partial pressure of O_2 (PO_2) is an important concept in respiration. It is the driving force that moves O_2 from the lungs into red cells during external respiration and O_2 from red cells into tissues cells during internal respiration. The partial pressure of CO_2 (PCO_2) is responsible for the movement of CO_2 between tissue cells and blood and between blood and alveoli. During respiration, O_2 and CO_2 diffuse between alveoli and blood and between blood and body tissues.

The Oxyhemoglobin Dissociation Curve

The loading and unloading of O_2 on to and off the Hgb molecule is described by the oxyhemoglobin dissociation curve. The curve is a conceptual model that relates the PO_2 of blood to the O_2 saturation (SaO_2), or amount of O_2 bound to Hgb. In the lungs, where the PO_2 (100 mm Hg) is greater, O_2 is loaded on to Hgb (upper portion of the curve; called the association portion).

Conversely, in the tissues, where the PO_2 is lower (40 mm Hg), O_2 is unloaded to the tissues (lower portion of the curve; called the dissociation portion). The relationship between PO_2 and SaO_2 forms an S-shaped, or sigmoid-shaped, curve.

Association Portion and Oxygen Loading

The upper portion of the curve is referred to as the association portion. It pertains to the lungs where deoxygenated blood in the pulmonary capillaries goes from a PO_2 of 40 mm Hg to a PO_2 of 100 mm Hg (oxygen loading). Oxygen is loaded onto the Hgb molecule thereby saturating it.

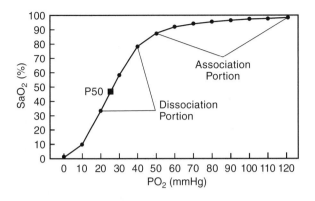

FIGURE 5.3 **Oxyhemoglobin Dissociation Curve**

Dissociation Portion and Oxygen Unloading

The lower portion of the curve is called the dissociation portion. This portion pertains to the systemic capillaries where the PO_2 goes from 100 mm Hg to a PO_2 of 40 mm Hg (oxygen unloading). Oxygen is released from Hgb and diffuses into the tissues. At a PO_2 of 40 mm Hg the curve shows that Hgb is 75% saturated with O_2.

A Physiologic Advantage

Hgb does not release all of its O_2 to the tissues. Hgb has the ability to save some O_2, which is called a physiologic advantage, should the tissues increase their metabolic demand. In other words, if the tissues need more O_2, Hgb can release additional O_2. When the metabolic rate of the tissues increases, such as during heavy exertion by the muscles, more O_2 can be released from Hgb.

The Affinity of O_2 for Hgb

The oxyhemoglobin dissociation curve shows how PO_2 affects the binding of O_2 to Hgb. It describes the affinity of O_2 for Hgb. The actual affinity of O_2 for Hgb can be determined by measuring the PO_2 at which 50% of the Hgb is saturated. This is called the P50. The normal P50 is approximately 26 mm Hg.

P50

The affinity of O_2 for Hgb, or how Hgb binds or releases O_2, is affected by the following: (1) the hydrogen ion concentration (pH), (2) PCO_2, (3) temperature, and (4) the amount of 2,3-diphosphoglycerate (2,3-DPG) in the red cells.

Left Shift of the Curve   Oxygen has an increased affinity for Hgb, shown by a shift of the curve to the left and occurs when there is a decrease in one or more of the following: (1) hydrogen ion concentration (increased pH), (2) PCO_2, (3) amount of 2,3-DPG, and (4) temperature. The increased affinity is shown by a shift in the curve to the left. With a left shift, O_2 has greater affinity for Hgb and less O_2 is released to the tissues.

O_2:
greater affinity for Hgb
less O_2 release

Clinical conditions that shift the curve to the left include hypothermia (decreased body temperature), some abnormal types of Hgb, alkalosis (increased pH), and transfusions of bank blood, among others.

Right Shift of the Curve   A decreased affinity of O_2 for Hgb is indicated by a shift of the curve to the right and occurs when there is an increase in (1) hydrogen ion concentration (decreased pH), (2) PCO_2, (3) 2,3-DPG, and (4) temperature. A right shift indicates that O_2 has less affinity for Hgb and O_2 release to the tissues is enhanced. A right shift occurs because either the metabolic demand is increased or blood flow to the tissues is decreased.

O_2:
less affinity for Hgb
more O_2 release

Clinical conditions associated with a right shift of the curve include: hyperthermia, acidemia, some types of heart disease, increased amounts of CO_2, and pulmonary disease, among others.

External and Internal Respiration

The process of O_2 binding to Hgb in the lungs and the release of O_2 from Hgb in the tissues is called respiration. Respiration is separated into external and internal phases: (1) external respiration is the diffusion of CO_2 from the pulmonary capillary blood into the

respiration

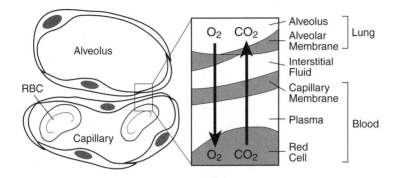

FIGURE 5.4 Alveolar Gas Exchange

To carry out respiration, O_2 and CO_2 must diffuse across various layers of tissue. The distance the respiratory gases have to travel between an alveolus and a pulmonary capillary is approximately 1 mm. With chronic lung disease,.the space between the alveolus and pulmonary capillary increases and interferes with the transfer of gases across their membranes; therefore, an individual experiences difficulty breathing.

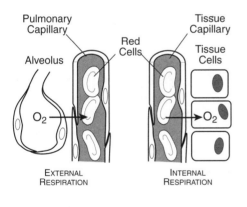

FIGURE 5.5 Transport of Respiratory Gases

In external respiration, O_2 moves from the alveolus in the lungs into red cells within the pulmonary capillaries. In internal respiration, O_2 moves from red cells in tissue capillaries into body tissue cells.

alveoli and the diffusion of O_2 in the alveoli into red cells within pulmonary capillaries; (2) internal respiration is the diffusion of CO_2 from the tissues into the blood and the diffusion of O_2 from the systemic capillaries into body tissues. The diffusion of O_2 and CO_2 happen almost simultaneously, taking place in a fraction of a second.

In this discussion of external and internal respiration only the diffusion of O_2 will be addressed. For diffusion of CO_2, see CO_2 Transport, this chapter.

External Respiration and O_2 Transport

External respiration is the diffusion of O_2 from the alveoli of the lungs into pulmonary capillary blood. Diffusion of O_2 depends on the difference in PO_2 between the alveoli and the blood. Blood returning from body tissues is low in O_2 and high in CO_2. The PO_2 in the alveoli (100 mm Hg) is greater than the PO_2 in pulmonary capillary blood (40 mm Hg). The partial pressure diffusion gradient (60 mm Hg) forces O_2 to diffuse from the alveoli into the blood as the blood circulates through the pulmonary capillaries. At this time, O_2 diffuses into the red cell and binds to Hgb. Hemoglobin becomes saturated with O_2 and the blood is ready to deliver O_2 to body tissues.

Once O_2 dissolves in the plasma it is transported in two ways:

1. About 1% of O_2 remains in a dissolved state in plasma.

2. About 99% combines reversibly with Hgb in red cells. "Combines reversibly" means that O_2 can be released from Hgb when blood reaches body cells. Hemoglobin only carries O_2; it does not react with it.

FIGURE 5.6 External Respiration and O_2 Transport

In external respiration, O_2 moves from the alveoli in the lungs into red cells within the pulmonary capillaries. When O_2 diffuses into the pulmonary capillary blood the PO_2 increases to 100 mm Hg.

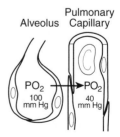

Alveolus   Pulmonary Capillary

PO_2 100 mm Hg PO_2 40 mm Hg

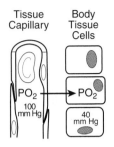

Tissue Capillary | Body Tissue Cells

FIGURE **5.7 Internal Respiration and O₂ Transport**

In internal respiration, the difference in PO_2 between tissue capillaries and body tissues is the driving force that moves O_2 from the blood to tissue cells. When O_2 diffuses into the tissue cells the PO_2 increases to 100 mm Hg.

Internal Respiration

Internal respiration is the movement of O_2 from blood within systemic capillaries into body tissues. It is the process by which O_2 leaves Hgb and diffuses into tissue cells. Diffusion occurs because the PO_2 in red cells (100 mm Hg) is greater than the PO_2 in body tissues (about 40 mm Hg). The diffusion gradient (60 mm Hg) forces O_2 to diffuse from red cells to the interstitial space and into body cells where it is used in cellular reactions within mitochondria (cellular organelles). Oxygen is eventually reduced through a series of chemical reactions and, with the metabolism of glucose, it forms high-energy compounds, such as ATP. High-energy compounds are used by cells to provide energy for cellular reactions.

The amount of O_2 that tissues receive depends on three factors:

1. The amount of blood flow to tissues

2. The Hgb concentration in blood

3. The affinity of Hgb for O_2

If any one of these factors is abnormal, the body may not receive enough O_2. However, the body automatically compensates for this by adjusting one, two, or all three factors to maintain optimal tissue perfusion. For example, if the Hgb concentration is low, heart rate increases, which in turn increases blood flow to body tissues.

CO_2 Transport to the Lungs

As O_2 is released to tissue cells, the blood picks up CO_2 and transports it to the lungs. Carbon dioxide forms in tissue cells as the result of cellular metabolism (breakdown of proteins, carbohydrates, and lipids). Metabolism increases the levels of CO_2 in tissue cells to a PCO_2 of about 46 mm Hg. Because the PCO_2 of blood in tissue capillaries is lower (40 mm Hg) than in tissue cells, CO_2 diffuses from tissue cells into capillary blood. Venous blood transports CO_2 to the lungs where it is released and exhaled into the atmosphere.

Transport of CO_2 by blood is somewhat more complicated than transport of O_2. Whereas O_2 is transported in two ways, CO_2 is transported in three ways once it diffuses from tissue cells into plasma.

1. Five percent of CO_2 is dissolved in plasma.

2. Thirty percent of CO_2 enters red cells where it binds to certain amino acids in the Hgb molecule.

3. Sixty-five percent of CO_2 is transported as bicarbonate ions (HCO_3^-) via plasma to the lungs.

FIGURE 5.8 CO_2 Diffusion Into Tissue Capillary Blood

Because of the difference in PCO_2 between body tissues and blood, CO_2 moves from interstitial fluid into capillary blood. When CO_2 diffuses into the tissue capillary blood the PCO_2 increases to 46 mm Hg.

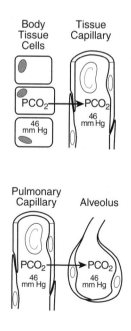

FIGURE 5.9 CO_2 Diffusion in the Alveoli

The greater PCO_2 of blood returning from the tissues drives CO_2 from the pulmonary capillaries into the alveoli. CO_2 is released from red cells into the alveoli and exhaled from the lungs.

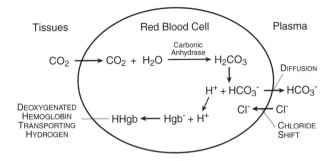

FIGURE 5.10 Conversion of CO$_2$ to HCO$_3^-$

CO$_2$ produced in cellular metabolism diffuses into red cells and combines with H$_2$O in the presence of carbonic anhydrase (CA) to form carbonic acid (H$_2$CO$_3$). Carbonic acid dissociates into H$^+$ and HCO$_3^-$. Hydrogen ions are buffered (bound; picked up) by Hgb. Bicarbonate diffuses from the red blood cells into the plasma. Chloride ions (Cl$^-$) diffuse into the red cells from plasma to maintain electrical neutrality.

Bicarbonate Ion Production in CO$_2$ Transport

Conversion of CO$_2$ into HCO$_3^-$ (bicarbonate ions) is complex and involves several chemical reactions. After CO$_2$ enters red cells, it combines with water (H$_2$O). In the presence of the enzyme carbonic anhydrase (CA), which is found in the cytoplasm of red cells and renal tubular cells, CO$_2$ and H$_2$O form carbonic acid (H$_2$CO$_3$). In a liquid solution such as plasma, acids dissociate (separate) into free ions not bound to one another chemically. Dissociation of H$_2$CO$_3$ produces two ions: H$^+$ (hydrogen ion) and HCO$_3^-$ (bicarbonate ion). Both H$^+$ and HCO$_3^-$ are transported to the lungs, allowing for the removal of CO$_2$.

In the transport process, however, any free H$^+$ must be removed (buffered) to prevent drastic changes in pH, a measure of the acidity of a solution. Hydrogen ions in solution make the solution more acidic (lower pH); thus pH refers to the concentration of H$^+$ in a solution. A change in blood pH has serious consequences because it affects the enzyme-dependent reactions of the body and alters normal physiology. For normal body functions, the pH of blood must remain in the range of 7.35 to 7.45, slightly basic.

Chemicals in blood that prevent changes in pH are called buffers. They remove excess H^+ by "soaking them up," thereby preventing changes in blood pH. The main buffers in blood are Hgb and HCO_3^-. Hemoglobin binds H^+ as these ions are produced in red cells (see Appendix, Blood Gases).

Conversion of CO_2 to HCO_3^- allows for the transport of CO_2 to the lungs without altering the pH of blood to a significant degree. As CO_2 is converted to HCO_3^- in red cells, HCO_3^- diffuses into the plasma. In a reaction that takes place in a fraction of a second within red cells, CA allows CO_2 and H_2O to form H_2CO_3. H_2CO_3 then dissociates into $H+$ and HCO_3^-. Hemoglobin binds $H+$ while HCO_3^- diffuses into the plasma. As HCO_3^- leaves

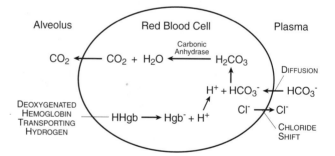

FIGURE 5.11 CO_2 Removal from the Lungs

For CO_2 to be exhaled from the lungs, HCO_3^- must be converted back into CO_2. This occurs when HCO_3^- diffuses back into the red cells and Hgb within these cells releases H^+. Bicarbonate ions and H^+ ions form H_2CO_3, which is broken down into CO_2 and H_2O in the presence of CA. Carbon dioxide then diffuses into the alveoli and is exhaled from the lungs. Water molecules remain in the red cells, and Cl^- diffuses out to maintain electrical neutrality.

the red cells, Cl^- (chloride ion) in the plasma moves into the red cells. This reaction is called the chloride shift, which maintains electrical neutrality between red cells and plasma because one negative ion (HCO_3^-) leaves the red cell and enters the plasma while another negative ion (Cl^-) leaves the plasma and enters the red cell. In other words, one negative ion is exchanged for another negative ion.

Once CO_2 is transported to the pulmonary capillaries it diffuses into the alveoli of the lungs. The gas is released by red cells in the following steps:

1. Bicarbonate ions (HCO_3^-) diffuse from plasma back into red cells. To maintain electrical neutrality chloride ions (Cl^-) move from the red cells into plasma (called the chloride shift).

2. Hemoglobin molecules release H^+.

3. Hydrogen ions and HCO_3^- rejoin to form H_2CO_3, which forms CO_2 and H_2O in the presence of CA. Carbon dioxide enters the alveoli and is exhaled in the next breath. Water stays within the red cells.

▪ QUESTIONS ▪

1. Describe the important differences between respiration and ventilation.

2. What three muscles (or muscle groups) are essential in the respiratory process?

3. The quality of life diminishes in diseases of impaired O_2 and CO_2 exchange. List four of these diseases.

4. Hemoglobin (Hgb) is important in the respiration process. What are its three major roles?

5. Explain the principle of diffusion.

6. Explain partial pressure.

7. What is the difference in partial pressures between two areas called?

8. What is barometric pressure?

9. How is atmospheric (or barometric) pressure determined?

10. What role does the partial pressure of O_2 (PO_2) play during respiration? The partial pressure of CO_2 (PCO_2)?

11. Explain the oxyhemoglobin dissociation curve.

12. Explain the physiologic advantage of hemoglobin.

13. What does P50 measure, and what is its normal value?

14. What four factors determine the affinity of O_2 for Hgb or how Hgb binds or releases O_2?

15. How does the oxyhemoglobin dissociation curve shift in alkalosis? In acidemia?

16. Explain the difference between external and internal respiration.

17. What is the significance of the fact that O_2 "combines reversibly" with Hgb in the red cells?

18. During internal respiration what three factors determine the amount of O_2 that body tissues receive?

19. What causes CO_2 to form in the cells of various body tissues?

20. In what three steps is CO_2 transported once it diffuses from the tissue cells into the plasma?

21. What is the enzyme found in the cytoplasm of red cells and in renal tubular cells that is important in the production of HCO_3^-?

22. What is the pH, and why is it important?

23. What is the normal range of the body's pH? Is it acidic or basic?

24. There are two main buffers in the blood. What are they? and what do they do?

25. How does the chloride shift affect bicarbonate ion transport?

26. How is CO_2 released by the red cells?

CHAPTER **6**

White Blood Cells

Introduction

White cells, called leukocytes, are the cellular components of the immune system, which provides protection against foreign matter. For the purpose of this text, all nonself material (foreign matter) is referred to as antigen (Ag). Antigen includes: bacteria, viruses, fungi, parasites, transfused or transplanted allogeneic cells (cells from a genetically dissimilar individual), infected cells, and tumor cells. On entering the body, antigen evokes an immune response by activating white cells, antibody, and complement proteins. Antibody and complement proteins are molecules that aid in antigen destruction (see Ch. 7, Antigen, Antibody, and Complement).

leukocytes

antigen
↓
white cells
antibody
complement proteins
↓
immune response

There are several types of white cells, each having special functions related to seeking out and destroying antigen. White cells communicate among themselves via a highly complex network of glycoprotein molecules called cytokines. These molecules play an important role in inflammation and the immune response (see Ch. 9, The Immune System).

cytokines

Locations and Life Spans

All white cells originate from stem cells in hematopoietic bone marrow, but some complete maturation in other sites. Most white cells circulate within the vascular and lymphatic channels; however, some reside in body tissues. White cells have varying life spans that range from a few hours to years, possibly for one's lifetime.

93

Number of White Cells

4,500 to 11,000
per microliter

The number range of white cells in an adult is 4.5 to 11 x 10^3/μL (4.5 to 11 x 10^9/L). These numbers are higher at birth—15 to 25 x 10^3/μL (15 to 25 x 10^9/L)—but gradually decrease and attain adult levels during early adolescence.

Leukocytosis

increase in white cells

An increase in white cells is called leukocytosis, a classic sign of infection. Depending on the length of time an infection is present, the white cell count may rise to 21 x 10^3/μL (21 x 10^9/L) or higher. There are numerous reasons for an increased white cell count, infection is one of many, leukemia is another.

Leukopenia

decrease in white cells

A decrease in white cells is called leukopenia. When the white cell count drops below 4.5 x 10^3/μL (4.5 x 10^9/L), individuals are more susceptible to infections. Leukopenia results from conditions that cause decreased production or increased destruction of white cells. Decreased production within bone marrow occurs with stem cell disorders, chemotherapies, and radiation therapy. Increased destruction of white cells occurs with hypersplenism (increased removal of blood cells from circulation), autoimmune disorders, and some drugs.

Types of White Cells

The three major groups of white cells are:

granulocytes:
neutrophils,
eosinophils, basophils

monocyte→macrophage

lymphocytes:
T and B cells

(1) Granulocytes. This group includes: neutrophils, eosinophils, and basophils.

(2) Monocytes. A monocyte leaves the blood to enter tissues where it matures and becomes a macrophage.

(3) Lymphocytes. This group includes T and B cells, which direct the immune response.

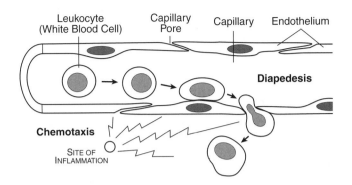

FIGURE 6.1 Diapedesis and Chemotaxis

Diapedesis refers to the movement of white cells to the site where antigen has invaded the body. Chemotaxis is the release of cytokines, complement proteins, and bacterial toxins that stimulate white cells to move into the area of antigen invasion.

Properties of White Cells

White cells have special properties that aid them in destroying antigen: diapedesis, chemotaxis, and phagocytosis. All three perform important and continuous roles in antigen destruction.

diapedesis, chemotaxis, phagocytosis

Diapedesis and Chemotaxis

Diapedesis refers to the movement, or migration, of neutrophils and monocytes through capillary pores into body tissues in response to antigen. Chemotaxis is the release of cytokines, complement proteins, and bacterial toxins that stimulate white cells to move into (diapedesis) the area of antigen invasion. In response to chemotaxis, capillary pores expand, allowing white cells to leave the vasculature and enter the tissue space in order to destroy antigen.

Defects Associated with Chemotaxis

Congenital and acquired abnormalities associated with chemotaxis include: lazy leukocyte syndrome (Chediak-Higashi syndrome), which is rare; absent or decreased complement protein production, which results in hereditary angioedema (hives and swelling within tissues); systemic lupus erythematosus, which is an autoimmune disorder that affects the skin, kidneys, and other organs; leukemia; defective bone marrow; and others.

Phagocytosis

The term phagocytosis is derived from the Greek language and means "to eat cells." Phagocytosis is enhanced by opsonization, which is the coating of antigen by antibody and/or complement proteins that make the antigen more palatable to phagocytic white cells. Receptors on white cell membranes are binding sites for antibody and complement. Receptors allow white cells to attach to antigen opsonized with antibody and/or complement. The Fc receptor is the attachment point for antibody, and the C3 receptor is the attachment point for complement (see Ch. 7, Antigen, Antibody, and Complement).

opsonization

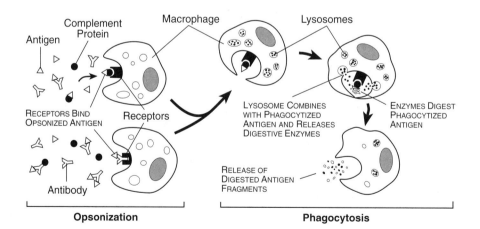

FIGURE 6.2 Opsonization and Phagocytosis

Opsonization of antigen by antibody and/or complement enhances phagocytosis. Once antigen is phagocytized, it is degraded by chemicals in the lysosomes within the phagocytic cell.

Neutrophils, monocytes, and macrophages are the body's main phagocytic white cells. Phagocytosis is the ongoing process by which phagocytic cells engulf antigens through the following steps: (1) attachment of opsonized antigen to receptors on the white cell membrane, (2) ingestion of antigen by the phagocyte, and (3) the killing and digestion of antigen via degradative (digestive) enzymes released from cytoplasmic granules. These enzymes are powerfully destructive oxygen-derived molecules, such as superoxides, myeloperoxidases, and oxygen-free radicals.

Defects Associated with Phagocytosis

There are several congenital and acquired defects of phagocytic white cells that interfere with their ability to destroy antigen. Defects involve a decrease in degradative enzyme production and/or opsonization.

Defective phagocytosis usually is congenital and is associated with decreased or absent production of degradative enzymes, such as superoxides and myeloperoxidases. In these instances, the antigen can be phagocytized, but it is not digested and destroyed. Chronic granulomatous disease is an example of a congenital defect resulting in the lack of digestive enzymes.

Phagocytosis also is impaired if opsonization cannot take place. Defective opsonization is due to (1) decreased or absent production of antibody (hypogammaglobulinemia or agammaglobulinemia) and (2) decreased or absent production of complement proteins.

The chemotactic and phagocytic disorders described above make individuals susceptible to a wide range of chronic bacterial and fungal infections, from mild skin irritations to severe systemic infections.

Myeloid and Lymphoid Cell Lines

All blood cells develop from one of two separate but related lines of stem cells called the myeloid and lymphoid lineages (see Ch. 1, The Concept of Blood,

Fig. 1.3). The myeloid lineage gives rise to monocytes, macrophages, and granulocytes. These are the phagocytic cells that provide the first line of cellular defense antigen encounters when it breaches the physical and chemical barriers of the body. These white cells continuously scavenge the body for antigen and damaged and dead cells. They are nonspecific and attack any and all antigen.

myeloid white cells: provide first line defense

nonspecific attack

The lymphoid lineage gives rise to lymphocytes that direct the body's immune response to antigen. These cells develop from a cell line separate from the myeloid white cells. Lymphocytes are immunologically competent cells that assist other white cells in antigen destruction and generate a specific response to antigen. These immunologically active cells are immature in neonatal life and mature as individuals are exposed to different antigens.

lymphoid cells: direct the immune response

specific response

White Cells of the Myeloid Lineage

Granulocytes

Granulocytes are named for the numerous granules present within their cytoplasm. These granules contain digestive enzymes. The number of immature granulocytes in the bone marrow is greater than the number found circulating in the blood. This bone marrow reserve provides additional granulocytes needed to fight infection. Granulocytes are further divided into neutrophils, eosinophils, and basophils.

granules

digestive/degradative enzymes

Neutrophils

Functions Neutrophils are the body's primary phagocytic defense against bacterial antigens. They respond to many types of injuries, such as burns, trauma, and foreign bodies (for example, a splinter), but they are ineffective against protein toxins produced by microorganisms. Neutrophils act quickly and in vast numbers in response to inflammation and infection. These cells are very sensitive to chemotactic molecules and can detect as little as 1nM (nanomolar; billionth

respond to bacterial antigens, injuries, foreign bodies

of a mole) of chemotactic factor in tissues. Neutrophils are strongly phagocytic and their membranes have Fc and C3 receptors that bind antibody and complement. Binding of antibody and complement enhances phagocytosis.

strongly phagocytic
Fc and C3 receptors

Once neutrophils fulfill their function in an area of antigenic invasion, they die and release chemicals that lead to pus formation. Dead neutrophils are removed by macrophages.

Size Neutrophils measure 10 to 15μ in diameter. They are also referred to as polymorphonuclear leukocytes because of their multilobed nucleus, which can have 2 to 5 lobes.

polymorphonuclear
leukocytes

Life Span The life cycle of neutrophils takes place in bone marrow, blood, and body tissues. Neutrophils are short lived, living from a few hours to a few days and spending about 10 to 12 hours in the blood before moving into the tissues. It is believed that they spend approximately 5 to 6 days within the tissues. Although there are millions of neutrophils in circulation, they tire quickly when fighting infection and need assistance from macrophages, which are more effective phagocytes due to their longer life span.

life span in tissue:
5 to 6 days

Bands Immature neutrophils released from bone marrow into circulation are referred to as bands. They are called bands because their nucleus is rectangular and nonsegmented in shape. Some physicians believe that the presence of bands in circulation is one of several classic signs of infection. A white cell count in which bands are detected is called a "shift to the left."

immature neutrophils

shift to the left

Location After neutrophils mature and enter the bloodstream, 50% circulate within the vascular and lymphatic channels and 50% adhere to the endothelial lining of capillaries, which is called margination. This property allows neutrophils to move into tissues in response to chemotactic factors. Neutrophils travel freely between the blood and tissues.

vascular and
lymphatic channels
capillary endothelium
margination

Numbers Neutrophils are the most abundant white cells and compose about 70% (1900 to 8300/μL) of the body's white cells. The number of neutrophils in

70% of white cells

circulation varies. Individuals of Middle Eastern and African American ancestry normally have lower numbers (1.5 x $10^3/\mu L$; 1.5 x $10^9/L$) of neutrophils.

Neutrophils are immature in premature infants and low in number during neonatal life. Premature infants and neonates are therefore more susceptible to bacterial and fungal infections.

increase of neutrophils

Neutrophilia An increase in the number of neutrophils is called neutrophilia. The following diseases and conditions cause neutrophilia: bacterial infections, heavy exercise, inflammation, malignancies, hemorrhage, hemolysis, myeloproliferative disorders, chronic granulocytic leukemia, administration of hematopoietic growth factors, metabolic disorders, corticosteroid and epinephrine (adrenalin) injections, convulsive seizures, pain, nausea, and vomiting.

decrease of neutrophils

Neutropenia A decrease in the number of neutrophils is called neutropenia. Situations that cause decreased numbers of neutrophils include: congenital stem cell disorders, chemotherapies, radiation therapies, certain antibiotics, aplastic anemia, hypersplenism, anti-inflammatory drugs, autoimmune disorders, viral and certain bacterial infections, and bone marrow failure, among others. Neutropenia is associated with infections and ulcerations of the nasopharynx (nose and throat).

Eosinophils

foreign proteins, parasites, allergic reactions

Fc and C3 receptors

weakly phagocytic

MBP

Functions Eosinophils attack foreign proteins and parasites, and function in allergic reactions. Armed with Fc and C3 receptors for antibody and complement proteins, eosinophils can bind and phagocytize opsonized antigens. These white cells are only weakly phagocytic, however. They usually destroy antigen by releasing a chemical called major basic protein (MBP). Major basic protein is found in the eosinophil's cytoplasmic granules. It binds to antigen and lyses the antigen's membrane. It is toxic to all antigen, being especially effective against parasitic worms, called helminths.

Size and Life Span   Eosinophils measure 12 to 17μ in diameter. Their cytoplasmic granules have a coarse appearance under the microscope. The life span of eosinophils is anywhere from 12 to 24 hours.

life span: 12 to 24 hours

Numbers   Eosinophils make up about 2 to 5% (10 to 760/μL) of white cells. The number of eosinophils varies under different conditions. An increase of eosinophils, called eosinophilia, occurs with exercise, allergic reactions (asthma, hay fever), chronic renal disease, collagen vascular disease, radiation therapy, parasitic infections, pneumocystis pneumonia, Hodgkin's disease, certain drugs, skin diseases, and following histamine release by basophils. Emotional stress, administration of steroids, viral infections, acute bacterial infections, burns, and shock, among others, cause a decrease of eosinophils.

2 to 5% of white cells

eosinophilia:
increase in numbers

Location   Eosinophils mature in bone marrow. Rather than circulate, they reside in various tissues of the body, such as the skin and bronchi and bronchioles (airways of the lungs). On release from bone marrow, eosinophils circulate in the blood for a day before entering the tissue spaces.

body tissues

Basophils

Functions   Basophils exhibit chemotaxis and very little if any phagocytic activity. Although their main function is not well known, it is believed that they release molecules of histamine and heparin into the area of antigen invasion. Basophils have high affinity Fc receptors for IgE antibody and C3 receptors for complement components called anaphylatoxins. When basophils bind either IgE or anaphylatoxins, these molecules cause the release of histamine from the basophils' intracellular granules.

very weakly phagocytic

histamine and
heparin release
Fc and C3 receptors
anaphylatoxins

Histamine   Histamine promotes (1) increased vascular permeability, which causes fluid to leak from capillaries into tissue spaces (edema); (2) smooth muscle contraction, or constriction, of the blood vessels, gastrointestinal tract, and airways of the lungs; and

(3) chemotaxis, which attracts white cells to the area of antigen invasion.

In type I hypersensitivity reactions, such as allergic and anaphylactic reactions, basophils bound by IgE release histamine. Histamine is the causative agent of the symptoms of type I hypersensitivity reactions (see Ch. 9, The Immune System).

Heparin   An anticoagulant released by basophils, heparin prevents blood from clotting in the area of antigen invasion. If blood clots, phagocytes cannot reach antigen to destroy it and the infected tissue necroses (dies).

mast cells/
tissue basophils

Size and Location   Basophils measure 5 to 7µ in diameter and are found in blood and body tissues. Those found in body tissues are called mast cells. These cells measure about 10 to 15µ. Mast cells reside in connective tissue, specifically in the intestine, skin, lungs, and mucosa of the nasal cavity.

0.5% of white cells

basophilia:
increase in numbers

Numbers   Basophils are the least common of the white cells, making up less than 0.5% (10 to 250/µL) of the total number. Increased numbers of basophils, called basophilia, are rare but are found in individuals with chronic myeloid leukemia, postsplenectomy, inflammatory states, polycythemia vera, ulcerative colitis, and in newborns. Decreased numbers occur with the use of steroid hormones.

Monocytes

tissue macrophages/
histiocytes

Location   Monocytes are released into circulation from bone marrow at an immature stage. They circulate for a day or two and then move into tissue spaces where they mature into tissue macrophages, also called histiocytes.

Size, Shape, and Life Span   Monocytes measure 12 to 20µ in diameter and are larger than other blood cells. These cells can be identified under the microscope by their nucleus, which is centrally located, large, and indented in shape like a horseshoe. A monocyte has many lysosomes (membrane-bound sacs within the cytoplasm). As monocytes develop into macrophages, the number of intracellular lysosomes increases. Digestive juices

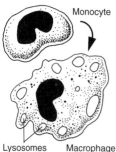

Lysosomes   Macrophage

in lysosomes called lysozymes, or lysosomal enzymes, allow macrophages to digest antigen. Macrophages are also 12 to 20μ in diameter and similar in appearance to monocytes. In the tissues, macrophages may live anywhere from months to years.

Numbers Monocytes make up about 5% (20 to 1000/μL) of all circulating white cells. Conditions and diseases that cause increased numbers, called monocytosis, are rare but include chronic bacterial infections (especially tuberculosis), some protozoan infections, inflammatory reactions, myeloproliferative disorders, Hodgkin's disease, decreased neutrophils, and some leukemias, among others.

Functions of Macrophages

Humans cannot live without macrophages. In their defense against antigen, macrophages are the most important of the phagocytic white cells. Scattered throughout the body, they most commonly line the sinusoids (spaces) of the liver, spleen, and lungs where they can reside for years. They not only engulf antigen but they also release many important chemicals needed for antigen destruction, such as digestive enzymes and cytokines.

The Reticuloendothelial System Tissue macrophages make up the reticuloendothelial system (RES), also referred to as the mononuclear phagocytic system (MPS). These phagocytic cells include: endothelial cells of the spleen, lymph nodes, and thymus, among others. Macrophages of the RES typically have a life span of 2 to 4 months. RES cells have a role in the inflammatory process, and they continuously remove dead, old, damaged, or altered cells from body tissues.

It takes about 7 to 10 days for the number of tissue macrophages to reach sufficient levels to destroy antigen. Although they are slower to respond than neutrophils, they remain much longer at the site of inflammation, until antigen is destroyed.

Sites Tissue macrophages are named according to the organ in which they are found. In the liver, they are

---

lysozymes

life span:
months to years

monocytosis:
increase in numbers

strongly phagocytic

found in sinusoids

life span: years

tissue macrophages:
RES, or MPS

life span:
2 to 4 months

Kupffer's cells

alveolar macrophages
microglial cells
spleen macrophages
dendritic cells
peritoneal macrophages

called Kupffer's cells. In the lungs, where they are a major player in respiratory defense, they are known as alveolar macrophages. They form microglial cells of the brain and spleen macrophages in the spleen. In bone marrow, macrophages are referred to as dendritic cells. In the gastrointestinal tract, they are found in Peyer's patches and called peritoneal macrophages.

Antigen-Presenting Cells Macrophages belong to a specialized group of cells called antigen-presenting

APCs

cells (APCs). As the name suggests, antigen-presenting cells present pieces of antigen to helper T lymphocytes (white cells). APCs phagocytize and break down antigens into small fragments called antigenic

antigenic peptides

peptides (proteins) that can then be recognized by helper T cells, leading to antigen destruction.

Cells other than macrophages can function as antigen-presenting cells. Endothelial cells, dendritic cells, B lymphocytes, and Langerhans' cells of the pancreas are examples of APCs.

Cells of the Lymphoid Lineage

T and B lymphocytes
and subsets

The lymphoid cell line consists of T and B lymphocytes, also known as T and B cells, and their subsets. Lymphocytes are the most complex of the white cells. Along with macrophages and granulocytes, lymphocytes help prevent disease and infection. Lymphocytes add specificity to the attack on antigen; that is, they direct the immune response because they have the ability to recognize, respond to, and retain memory for individual antigens, unlike myeloid white cells. The ability of lymphocytes to distinguish self-tissue from nonself tissue (1) allows for recognition of foreign molecules and (2) is the basis of cell-mediated immunity (the

cell-mediated and
humoral immunity

response to antigen by T cells) and humoral immunity (antibody production by B cells).

Size

Lymphocytes are 5 to 12μ in diameter and have a large round nucleus that takes up almost the entire cell area. Microscopically T and B cells are virtually indistinguishable from one another. Therefore, for certain blood tests, lymphocytes must be separated from one another. This is accomplished using specially prepared antibodies (called monoclonal antibodies) that bind to either T cells or B cells.

Numbers

Lymphocytes compose about 25% (650 to 4500/μL) of the total number of white cells. T cells make up the majority of circulating lymphocytes (75%).

25% of white cells

Lymphocytosis Increased numbers of lymphocytes is referred to as lymphocytosis. It is most often found in infants and young children in response to infectious organisms. Other causes of lymphocytosis include many types of leukemias, Hodgkin's disease, chronic bacterial infections, viral infections, allergic reactions, tuberculosis, and syphilis, among others.

increase of lymphocytes

Lymphopenia Decreased numbers of lymphocytes within the circulation is referred to as lymphopenia. It can be caused by the following: bone marrow failure, chemotherapy and radiation therapy, AIDS/HIV, a variety of immune deficiency disorders, uremia, alcoholism, steroids, and immunosuppressive drug therapy, among others.

decrease of lymphocytes

T Lymphocytes

Functions T cells are the white cells that direct the immune response against protein antigen, which make up the majority of antigen. They are responsible for the type of white cells that respond to protein antigen as well as for how these cells react. The response to antigen by T cells is called cell-mediated immunity. Before protein antigen can be destroyed, T cells must

immune response to protein antigen

cell-mediated immunity

have antigen fragments presented to them for recognition. T cells in turn activate other white cells necessary to destroy antigen.

T cells carry out cell-mediated immunity in the following ways:

- They direct the immune response.
- They assist phagocytosis by releasing cytokines that activate phagocytic white cells.
- They destroy malignant cells, allogeneic cells, and infected cells through lysis.
- They aid B cells/plasma cells in antibody production in response to protein antigens (humoral immunity).
- They are involved in delayed hypersensitivity immune reactions (see Ch. 9, The Immune Response).
- They cause some types of graft rejection in organ and tissue transplantation.
- They are involved in graft-versus-host disease (see Ch. 20, Bone Marrow Transplantation).
- They are responsible for certain types of autoimmune disorders.

maturation in the thymus

Location   T cells originate in bone marrow from pluripotential stem cells but mature in the thymus, a gland that lies on the heart and atrophies with age. The T in T cell stands for thymus-derived. The thymus educates T cells to distinguish and tolerate self-tissue from nonself tissue. During maturation in the thymus, T cells that mistakenly recognize self-tissue as foreign are destroyed to prevent them from attacking and destroying one's own tissue.

secondary lymphatic organs

Once T lymphocytes leave the thymus, the majority of them travel to the secondary lymphatic organs, such as lymph nodes, spleen, and tonsils, where they reside. Lymph nodes are conglomerations of lymphatic tissue found throughout the body. They are most palpable in the armpits, neck, and groin. It is in the lymph nodes that T lymphocytes first encounter antigen and where APCs present antigen to T cells for destruction.

lymph nodes

T Lymphocyte Subsets

T lymphocytes are categorized into subsets according to the protein molecules on the cell membrane that distinguish one type of T cell from another. The distinguishing protein molecule is referred to as CD and stands for "cluster of differentiation." All CD8+ T cells have the CD8 protein as their cell surface marker, and all CD4+ T cells have the CD4 protein as their marker. The major subsets are helper, usually CD4, and cytotoxic and suppressor, usually CD8. The CD marker of a T cell membrane determines the class of major histocompatibility complex (MHC) molecule that a T cell can bind to through its T cell receptor.

CD molecule

T cell subsets:
helper cells—
CD4 marker
cytotoxic and
suppressor cells—
CD8 marker

MHC molecules are found on most body cells. They are divided into class I and II molecules, which have significant roles in the immune response to protein antigen. CD4+ T cells respond only to antigen fragments bound to class II molecules, and CD8+ T cells respond only to antigen fragments bound to class I molecules (see Ch. 8, The Major Histocompatibility Molecules).

MHC molecules

CD4+ T cells and
class II MHC molecules
CD8+ T cells and
class I MHC molecules

Helper T Cells

Functions   There are two subsets of CD4+ helper T cells, referred to as T^{H1} and T^{H2}. Helper T cells are called helper because they assist or activate other white cells in response to antigen. Helper T cells do not destroy antigen directly, but through the release of cytokines, they direct other immune cells— granulocytes, monocytes/macrophages, B cells, and other T cells—to respond to antigen. However, before helper T cells can assist these cells, they have to have protein antigen presented to them in combination with MHC class II molecules. The antigen-MHC complex must attach themselves to the T cell receptor for antigen recognition to occur.

CD4+ helper T subsets:

T^{H1}	T^{H2}
↓	↓
cytokine release	
↓	↓
inactive	B cell
T cells	activation
↓	and
cytotoxic	antibody
T cells	production
↓	↓
target cell	opsonization
destruction	↓
by lysis	phagocytosis

The two subsets of helper T cells have similar yet different functions. The T^{H1} subset, called the inflammatory helper cell, releases cytokines that

inflammatory
helper cell

convert inactive T cells into cytotoxic T cells that lyse target cells (allogeneic cells, tumor cells, and infected cells). TH2 helper cells release cytokines necessary for B cell activation and antibody secretion. If TH2 helper cells did not stimulate B cells, antibody production against protein antigen would be minimal.

Cytotoxic T Cells

MHC class I
and antigen
↓
CD8+ cytotoxic
T cells
↓
target cell destruction

Cytotoxic T cells release lytic molecules that rupture target cells. Before cytotoxic T cells can destroy target cells, however, they are transformed from inactive CD8+ T lymphocytes into cytotoxic T lymphocytes (CTLs). Transformation of cytotoxic T cells from inactive CD8+ T cells occurs when (1) they respond to cytokines released by TH1 cells and (2) the CD8+ T cell receptor recognizes antigen combined with MHC class I molecules.

Suppressor T Cells

Once antigen has been destroyed, suppressor T cells are activated to stop the immune response. Unless suppression occurs, the immune response would continue and destroy normal tissue. Suppressor T cells are thought to carry the CD8 marker.

Memory T Cells

anamnestic response
primary response/
immunization

Most T cells die within a few days after an infection, but those that are left retain memory for the offending antigen. Memory T cells live for many years, possibly for an individual's lifetime, and reside in lymph nodes. Memory T cells respond more rapidly on subsequent exposure to antigens to which they have been immunized. This second exposure is called the anamnestic response and is a more rapid immune response than the primary response, known as immunization or sensitization.

T Cell Receptor

TCR

The T cell receptor (TCR) is a protein complex on the outer membranes of T cells. This protein receptor is

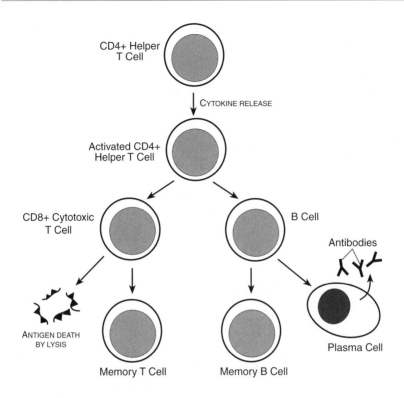

FIGURE 6.3 T Cell Function in Immunity

This is a schematic representation of the CD4+ helper
T cell response to protein antigen.

designed so that the MHC-antigen complex fits into
it like a key fits into a lock. When the T cell receptor
and the MHC complex join, the T cell can recognize
the antigen. Each T cell receptor is specific in that
it will recognize only one antigen's configuration
bound by MHC. Therefore each T cell will only
recognize one specific antigen.

B Lymphocytes

Functions B cells produce antibody in response to
antigen. Production of antibody is called humoral
immunity. Antibody opsonizes microorganisms, tumor
cells, and allogeneic cells, leading to their destruction.
Once microorganisms (viruses) enter a cell, they are safe

humoral immunity:
antibody production
↓
opsonization of
allogeneic cells, tumor
cells, microorganisms

from antibody because antibody cannot penetrate the cell membrane.

antigen recognition:
whole or fragmented

Unlike T cells, B cells have the ability to recognize whole or soluble (dissolved) carbohydrate and lipid antigens through their B cell surface receptors. Carbohydrate and lipid antigens do not have to be recognized by T cells in order for B cells to recognize and respond to them. Lipid and carbohydrate antigens are called T cell-independent antigens. However, B cells cannot recognize protein antigen; they must be activated by helper CD4+ T^{H2} cells to produce antibody against protein antigen. For this reason, protein antigen is referred to as T cell-dependent antigen.

soluble lipid and
carbohydrate antigens:
T cell-independent

protein antigen:
T cell-dependent

B Cell Receptors B cells have membrane/surface receptors that allow them to attach to and recognize soluble or whole antigen. B cell receptors are immunoglobulins M and D that are embedded in the B cell membrane.

immunoglobulins
M and D

Location B lymphocytes mature in bone marrow. When released from marrow, they reside in lymph nodes where they lie in wait for antigen. Although B cells are concentrated in lymph nodes, they are also found throughout the lymphatic and vascular systems. The letter B is derived from the discovery of these immune cells in the bursa of Fabricius, which is a gland associated with the intestine of birds.

lymph nodes

lymphatic and
vascular systems

Plasma Cells

life span:
days to weeks
immunoglobulins/
antibodies

Once B cells are activated by antigen or CD4+ T^{H2} lymphocytes, they undergo rapid proliferation and differentiate into a plasma cells, which have a life span of a few days to weeks. Plasma cells are the only cells in the body capable of producing immunoglobulins, which are called antibodies when secreted from plasma cells. A plasma cell produces antibody specific for the stimulating antigen. It also undergoes cloning in order to produce antibody in large amounts. Antibody production continues until the antigen has been destroyed. Once plasma cells fulfill their function, they die.

Memory B Cells

Memory B cells are generated when plasma cells produce antibodies. Following an infection, memory B cells possibly live for the rest of one's life. Like memory T cells, they recognize antigen faster when responding the second time and can, therefore, initiate antibody production sooner.

Killer and Natural Killer Cells

Killer (K) and natural killer (NK) cells are large lymphocytelike cells with the ability to destroy target cells. Both cells are distinct from T and B cells. Killer cells destroy target cells opsonized with antibody. Macrophages and eosinophils have some K cell activity. Natural killer cells have the ability to destroy infected cells, tumor cells, and parasitic organisms. Natural killer cells do not need prior exposure to antigen to destroy antigen.

Autoimmunity

T and B cells that destroy self-tissue are responsible for autoimmune diseases. With an autoimmune disease, the body does not recognize and protect its own cells. This phenomenon is called loss of self-tolerance. Rheumatoid arthritis, multiple sclerosis (MS), some types of diabetes mellitus, and some hemolytic anemias are examples of autoimmune diseases (see Ch. 9, The Immune System).

loss of self-tolerance

■ **QUESTIONS** ■

1. Define antigen. Give at least five examples used in this book.

2. Identify the three major components of the immune response.

3. Define cytokines and the major role they play in the immune response.

4. There are three sites in the body where white cells reside. Where are they?

5. An increase in white cells is called leukopenia. True or False?

6. Give two reasons for an increased white cell count.

7. Identify two causes of decreased white cells in the body.

8. List the three groups of white cells and give an example of each.

9. White cells are affected by both diapedisis and chemotaxis. How do these two phenomena relate to one another?

10. What autoimmune disorder that affects the skin, kidneys, and other organs is associated with defective chemotaxis?

11. How do phagocytes engulf antigens? Describe the process in three steps.

12. How does opsonization interfere with phagocytosis?

13. Compare and contrast the white cells of the myeloid lineage with those of the lymphoid lineage.

14. Neutrophils, eosinophils, and basophils make up one group of white cells. What is this group? and how did it get its name?

15. Describe pus formation.

16. Explain the "shift to the left" as it relates to neutrophils.

17. Where in the body do the neutrophils that respond so quickly to chemotactic factors reside?

18. List five conditions that cause neutrophilia.

19. MBP is a major chemical released by eosinophils. What is it? and what is its function?

20. Basophils release two chemicals. Name them.

21. Why is it essential that clotting not take place in an infected area?

22. Which of the granulocytes are the most prevalent? the least?

23. Explain what happens to monocytes when they leave the blood.

24. Why can't humans live without macrophages?

25. The reticuloendothelial system (RES) is made up of various tissue macrophages. Where are they? and what are they called?

26. Some macrophages are known as antigen-presenting (APCs). What other cells function as APCs?

27. How do lymphocytes differ from other white cells?

28. There are two oncology diagnoses associated with lymphocytosis (increased numbers of lymphocytes). What are they?

29. What is the response to antigen by T cells called?

30. T cells mature in the lymph nodes. True or False? Explain your answer.

31. In lymphocyte studies, what does "CD" represent? Give two examples.

32. Describe the various kinds of T cells and their functions.

33. Explain the anamnestic response. How does it relate to immunization?

34. The response to antigen by T cells is called cell-mediated immunity. What is humoral immunity?

35. The lymphatic system works in conjunction with the blood-vascular system. How do B cells demonstrate this?

36. Describe what happens in an autoimmune disease. Give two examples of such a disease.

CHAPTER **7**

Antigen, Antibody, and Complement

Introduction

White cells, antibody, and complement proteins make up the immune system. The combined efforts of these components help destroy antigen that enters the body and illicits an immune response.

Antigen and Immunogen

The term antigen (Ag) refers to any foreign matter that enters the body and meets either or both of the following criteria: (1) it can bind to antibody and/or (2) it can bind to a T or B cell receptor molecule. Technically, an antigen is a molecule, or a portion thereof, of proteins, carbohydrates, or lipids found on the surface of microorganisms, infected cells, tumor cells, and allogeneic cells. Antigen enters the body through various routes—the skin, mouth, bladder, nose, and blood, among others. Antigenic cells that are destined to be destroyed by the immune system are called target cells.

antigen:
binds antibody and/or
T or B cell receptor

target cells

In this book, for simplicity's sake, the term antigen also includes immunogen. The term immunogen refers to any substance that can generate an immune response. All immunogens are antigenic, which means that immunogens can bind antibody. Not all antigens are immunogens, however, because they do not necessarily initiate an immune response.

immunogen

The term pathogen is often confused or used interchangeably with the term antigen. Pathogen strictly refers to an antigen with the ability to cause a disease, and it is usually a microorganism or a toxin.

pathogen

115

Examples of Antigen

- Microorganisms, such as bacteria, viruses, parasites, fungi, and yeasts
- Allogeneic cells, which are cells from a genetically dissimilar individual
- Malignant (cancerous) cells
- Infected cells, cells inhabited by viruses, certain bacteria, and parasites

Recognition of Protein Antigen

CD4+ helper T cell
+
class II MHC
↓
immune response
(B cells and
cytotoxic T cells)

Protein molecules make up the majority of antigen and are the most potent, that is, they illicit the strongest immune response. They are not recognized directly by B cells or CD8+ cytotoxic T cells because these cells require the help of CD4+ helper T cells. As T cell-dependent antigen, protein antigen must be presented to CD4+ T lymphocytes by class II MHC molecules before an immune response can be generated.

Recognition of Lipid and Carbohydrate Antigens

lipid and carbohydrate
antigens:
T cell-independent
and recognized
directly by B cells

IgM antibody

Lipid and carbohydrate antigens can be recognized directly by B cells; they do not need the help of CD4+ helper T cells. B cells/plasma cells produce antibody in response. Examples of lipid and carbohydrate antigens are the outer capsule of some bacteria and other microorganisms. Lipid and carbohydrate antigens are T cell-independent antigens. IgM is the only antibody produced in response to T cell-independent antigens.

Antigenic Epitopes

antigenic epitope
binds to
↙   ↘
lymphocyte   antibody
receptor   molecule

The specific region of an antigen recognized by antibody or a lymphocyte receptor molecule is called the epitope. Every antigen has at least one epitope, and an epitope is unique to a given antigen. Each lymphocyte receptor and antibody molecule is specifically designed to bind to a particular antigen's epitope.

Antibody Molecules

Antibodies are protein molecules produced by B cells/ plasma cells and are always present in small amounts in blood and body tissues. There are five classes of antibody. Another name for antibody (Ab) is immunoglobulin. Antibody production in response to antigen is known as humoral immunity.

Antibody molecules are effective in destroying antigen only when they bind to the outer surface of micro-organisms, allogeneic cells, tumor cells, and toxins produced by microorganisms. Once microorganisms enter a cell, they are protected from antibody because antibody molecules cannot penetrate cell membranes.

Functions

Antibody has two major functions: (1) to opsonize (coat) antigen and (2) to activate the complement cascade.

The coating of an antigen by antibody and complement is called opsonization, a function that enhances the ability of phagocytic white cells to engulf and eat antigen. Opsonization provides the antigen with attachment points that allow phagocytic white cells to stick to antigen and engulf it. Surface molecules, called receptors, on white cells make possible the attachment of antigen opsonized by antibody and/or complement. The Fc receptor is the point on the phagocyte's membrane that binds antibody, and the C3 receptor is the point that binds complement. When antibody and/or complement attaches itself to a phagocyte receptor, they fit like pieces of a puzzle.

For an explanation of the complement cascade, see p. 123.

Antibody Synthesis

It was not until the 1950s that scientists learned how antibody is synthesized. Once B cells recognize antigen, they differentiate into plasma cells. These are specialized cells that produce an antibody specific for

protein molecules
produced by B cells/
plasma cells
immunoglobulin

humoral immunity

opsonization
complement activation

phagocyte receptors:
Fc binds antibody
C3 binds complement

the stimulating antigen. After antibody is released from a plasma cell, it circulates in plasma and lymphatic fluid seeking out antigen. The human body can provide a corresponding antibody for every antigen produced and for every one that can be produced, a truly remarkable capability.

All antibody molecules have the same basic molecular arrangement. Each molecule is made up of four chains of amino acids, two identical heavy chains and two identical light chains. The chains are held together by chemical bonds. Within each heavy and light chain are two separate and distinct regions, the variable and the constant. Each antibody molecule has two variable and two constant regions.

constant regions contain C3 and Fc receptors

The constant regions are where the C3 receptor for complement and the Fc receptor binding site are located. The variable regions are located at the Y ends of each heavy and light chain and are the points of antigen attachment. The amino acid arrangement in the variable regions are unique to each antibody, a characteristic that allows antibody to bind to the epitope of a specific antigen.

antibody variable regions bind antigen epitope

FIGURE 7.1 Antibody Molecule

This diagram depicts the four chains of amino acids that compose the polypetide structure of an antibody molecule. There are two identical chains that are heavy and two that are light. Each chain has a constant region and a variable region. The latter is unique to an antibody and allows the antibody to bind to a specific antigen's epitope.

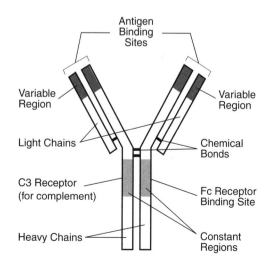

Primary Exposure Antibody is produced after the body's primary, or first, exposure to an antigen. Primary exposure is called sensitization, or immunization. After the initial exposure to antigen, antibody production takes approximately 14 days to reach full power. The time from antigen recognition to antibody production is referred to as the lag period. Several factors determine how long the lag period is, such as amount of antigen delivered, route of entry into the host, and the length of time the host can produce antibody.

The Anamnestic Response Reexposure to the same antigen constitutes a secondary, or anamnestic response. An anamnestic response produces antibody much faster, taking about 5 to 7 days. When an individual is exposed a second time, memory B cells produced as a result of primary immunization respond quickly to produce antibody. IgG antibody is produced in greatest amounts in an anamnestic response (see Classes, p. 120). The anamnestic response is more rapid than sensitization for the following reasons:

- Antibody is produced in larger quantities.
- Antibody responds to lower concentrations of antigen.
- Antibody has a higher affinity for antigen.

Antibody Destruction of Antigen

Antibody destroys antigen in many different ways. The following mechanisms are involved:

- Opsonization
- Lysis. Complement activation by antibody leads to development of the membrane attack complex (MAC), complement proteins that lyse the antigen's membrane.

- Antibody-dependent, cell-mediated cytotoxicity (ADCC). Cytotoxicity refers to the lysis by natural killer cells, macrophages, neutrophils, and eosinophils of target cells opsonized by antibody.

- Neutralization. In a neutralization process, antibody makes harmless the toxins released by microorganisms.

Classes of Antibody

IgG, IgM, IgD, IgA, IgE

isotypes

The five classes of antibody are IgG, IgM, IgD, IgA, and IgE. Some immunoglobulins have more than one type, called subtypes, or isotypes. Most antibody produced in the body is of the IgG or IgM class.

An antibody's class is determined by the amino acid arrangements of its heavy and light chains. All members of a given class have the same amino acid arrangement in the constant regions of their protein chains.

most potent antibody

serum concentration: 80%

anamnestic response

IgG Class   IgG is the most potent antibody in the immune system. It makes up about 80% of antibody that appears in serum. It is produced in the greatest amount in the anamnestic response and has the ability to diffuse into tissue spaces where it binds antigen.

IgG antibody is the only immunoglobulin that can cross the placenta from the mother into the fetus. IgG provides immunologic protection to the newborn until the newborn's immune system begins functioning. For example, maternal Rh antibody (anti-D) is an IgG-type antibody that crosses the placenta and attaches itself to Rh+ fetal red blood cells causing hemolytic disease of the newborn (HDN; see Ch. 13, ABO and Rh Blood Group Systems).

IgG is very effective at binding and destroying antigen. Its means of destruction are opsonization, activation of complement proteins, neutralization of viral and bacterial toxins, and immobilization of certain bacteria. IgG is also involved in antibody-dependent, cell-mediated cytotoxicity (lysis).

IgG Isotypes   The IgG antibody has four isotypes, each of which has a specific function. Several isotypes activate the complement system, which generates a stronger immune response.

- IgG_1 protects the body from bacteria, except those encased in a polysaccharide (sugar) coat. IgG_1 can bind complement.

- IgG_2 counters polysaccharide-coated organisms, attacking and destroying meningococcus, pneumococcus, and gonococcus bacteria. This class can bind complement, although poorly.

- IgG_3 has the greatest affinity for fixing complement proteins.

- IgG_4 does not bind complement proteins in the classical pathway, but it can bind complement proteins in the alternative pathway.

IgM Class IgM immunoblobulin is produced in large amounts in the early stages of the primary immune response to antigen. The serum concentration of IgM is 10 to 15% of circulating antibody. It is the first antibody that B cells/plasma cells produce against an antigen when it enters the blood. Being a large, complex molecule existing as five molecules linked together, IgM remains in the bloodstream because it cannot escape into body tissues.

serum concentration: 10 to 15%

first antibody produced by B cells/plasma cells

IgM is the first antibody produced by the fetus. Increased levels of IgM at birth indicate infection in the newborn. In the child and adult, increased levels of this immunoglobulin indicate a new infection or recent exposure to an antigen.

IgM has several functions. Its chief function is to activate the complement system. Due to its structure, IgM also has the ability to agglutinate (bring together) antigen. It is one of the main immunoglobulins expressed on the unstimulated (resting) B cell membrane, where it functions as a cell membrane receptor for antigen recognition.

complement activation

B cell membrane receptor

Anti-A and anti-B antibodies, which are naturally occurring antibodies against A and B antigens on red cells, are IgM antibodies. These antibodies are sometimes referred to as isohemagglutinins.

antibodies A and B/IgM

isohemagglutinins

IgD Class Little is known about IgD. It is found in small amounts in serum and body fluids and resides on the cell membrane of mature, unstimulated B cells. Researchers believe that IgD assists the B cell in reacting to helper CD4+ T^{H2} cell stimulation, thereby enhancing antibody production. IgD has little immunologic effect against antigen.

low serum concentration

little immunologic effect

IgA Class IgA immunoglobulin is the major antibody that exists in body fluids and mucus secreted by mucous membranes. It is found in such fluids as tears, breast milk, bronchiole secretions, and saliva. IgA binds and immobilizes antigen, thereby allowing mucin (the main ingredient of mucus) to remove the antigen-antibody complex. IgA is effective in preventing microorganisms from breaching the mucosal surface of organs, such as the lungs and intestine. It lacks the ability to activate complement proteins, but it can trigger cell-mediated immune reactions. Its serum concentration is 10 to 15% of antibody.

in body fluids and mucous membranes

serum concentration: 10 to 15%

IgA Isotypes There are two IgA isotypes.

- IgA_1 is found predominately in body fluids.

- IgA_2 is a secretory antibody that protects the mucous membranes lining the mouth, bladder, gut, nose, and vagina. It is the only immunoglobulin transported across the mucosal barrier.

IgE Class IgE is found in very low concentrations within plasma. It is measured in nanograms as opposed to milligrams by which the other antibodies are measured. The concentration of IgE increases in individuals having allergic reactions and parasitic infections, especially those caused by protozoa and parasitic worms (helminths).

low serum concentrations

IgE is the causative agent in asthma, hay fever, and many allergic reactions. When released, IgE binds to basophils and mast cells stimulating them to release histamine, which causes edema, sinus inflammation, itching, bronchiole constriction, and other symptoms.

allergic reactions

histamine

People with allergies produce IgE in excess. An allergic reaction is an abnormal immune response to a harmless antigen. A harmless antigen is called an allergen. For example, with hay fever, pollen is recognized by the body as foreign. An individual with an allergy is sensitive to the stimulating allergen.

allergen: harmless antigen

On reexposure to the sensitizing antigen or allergen, the IgE already bound to the basophil and mast cell membrane binds to the antigen. This event stimulates basophils and mast cells to release histamine and other active chemicals that precipitate allergic reactions.

histamine release by mast cells and basophils

IgE is involved in the most severe form of an allergic reaction, called anaphylaxis, also referred to as a type I hypersensitivity reaction or an immediate hypersensitivity reaction. Anaphylactic reactions occur only in hypersensitive individuals (those previously sensitized). They occur within seconds to minutes after an individual is reexposed to a sensitizing substance (see Ch. 9, The Immune System and Ch. 15, Transfusion Complications).

anaphylaxis/type I hypersensitivity reaction

The Complement System

The complement system consists of 25 to 30 soluble proteins that circulate in plasma in their inactive form. These proteins are vasoactive molecules that take part in the inflammatory response. They also opsonize and lyse antigen. Vasoactive refers to the effect molecules have on blood vessels, such as vascular permeability. Once activated, the complement system, like other body systems such as coagulation and clot lysis, occurs in a cascade that brings about a number of biologically significant events.

vasoactive

Complement Functions

The complement system has multiple functions in the immune response. It is involved in antigen destruction and the inflammatory response to tissue injury. Along with phagocytic white cells, complement proteins provide immune protection until antibody can reach full force, within 7 to 14 days. Complement proteins can work independently of antibody to destroy antigen, through opsonization and lysis, but they are most effective in destroying antigen when assisted by antibody.

inflammatory response

immune protection

opsonization
lysis

Complement proteins are activated by antigen-antibody complexes and foreign matter. The binding of complement to an antigen directly or to an antigen-antibody complex is referred to as complement

complement fixation/
binding

activated molecule C3
↓
C3a
↓
inflammation
and C3b
↓
opsonization

fixation. Unlike antibody, the amount of complement in plasma is not increased when the body is reexposed to the same antigen.

The central component of the complement system is the molecule C3. When C3 is activated it splits into two fragments: C3a and C3b. C3a is an anaphylatoxin and is responsible for causing inflammation. C3b is the opsonizing fragment that enhances phagocytosis. The C3b fragment attaches to the C3 receptor on the white cell membrane.

If complement proteins and phagocytic white cells cannot completely destroy invading antigen, other immune functions are initiated. T and B cells become active and amplify the immune response by producing antibody and/or cytotoxic T cells.

Complement Proteins

immune functions:

inflammation

Complement proteins work within the immune system in the following ways:

- They cause inflammation. One of the first responses to tissue injury is inflammation, which induces pain, swelling, heat, and redness. The degree of severity depends on the cause of the inflammation, the health of the individual, and the area of the body affected.

chemotactic factors

- They function as chemotactic factors to attract white cells to the area of antigenic invasion.

vascular permeability

- They increase vascular permeability, which enhances the ability of white cells to enter the infected area.

opsonization

- They assist macrophages and neutrophils by opsonizing antigens to promote phagocytosis.

MAC formation

- They bind directly to antigen and form the membrane attack complex (MAC). The MAC lyses antigen or the infected cell (see p. 127).

adherence

- They cause adherence of antigen-antibody complexes to surfaces, such as capillary endothelium, whereupon the complexes can be phagocytized.

complement inhibitors

When complement activity is no longer needed, the liver and spleen release chemical factors called inhibitors.

These inhibitors "turn off" the action of complement proteins so they will not damage normal tissue.

Complement Pathways

Complement proteins function in a sequence of chemical chain reactions that bring about increased vascular permeability, opsonization, and lysis. Complement system proteins are activated through either the classical or alternative pathway. Different antigens activate the proteins in the pathways.

The Classical Pathway   The classical pathway is triggered by antigen opsonized by either IgM or IgG. Antigen-antibody complexes that activate this pathway are usually antigens bound by either IgM or IgG. Proteins of the classical pathway are designated by a letter and number, C1 to C9. Added a and b subscripts, such as C1a and C1b, indicate that the complement protein has been cleaved (split) into its active components.

activated by IgM or IgG antigen-antibody complexes

Three activated complement proteins of the classical pathway can be potent causes of anaphylactoid reactions (see Ch. 15, Transfusion Complications). Activated protein components C3a, C4a, and C5a are called anaphylatoxins. C5a is the most potent.

activated proteins C3a, C4a, and C5a (anaphylatoxins)
↓
mast cells and basophils
↓
histamine release

Anaphylatoxins, much like IgE, stimulate mast cells and basophils to release histamine, a molecule that can cause capillary leakage, edema, smooth muscle contraction, bronchiole constriction, feeling of doom, and tachycardia, as well as other symptoms. Anaphylatoxins are strongly chemoctactic agents and function in the inflammatory response to antigen and tissue injury. When anaphylotoxins cause the reaction, it is called anaphylactoid rather than anaphylactic, a reaction that requires the presence of IgE.

anaphylactoid reaction: no IgE

The Alternative Pathway   The alternative pathway is triggered by IgA, certain isotypes of IgG, some toxins produced by microorganisms, polysaccharides, and lipopolysaccharides found on the outer membrane of certain microorganisms. Antibody and macrophages are

activated by IgA, IgG isotypes, toxins

prevented from directly binding and phagocytizing these microorganisms, but once complement opsonizes these microorganisms, phagocytosis can occur.

In the alternative pathway, complement proteins are usually designated by letters only. For example, they are referred to as factors (proteins) B, D, H, I, and P (properdin).

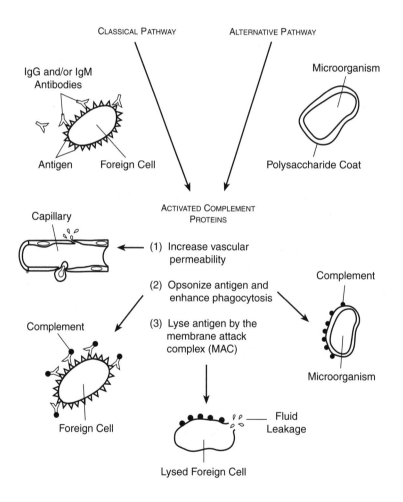

FIGURE 7.2 Complement System

This schematic representation of the complement system shows the functions of the complement proteins in the classical and alternative pathways.

The Membrane Attack Complex

The membrane attack complex (MAC) is a group of five complement enzymes (C5, C6, C7, C8, and C9) with the ability to bind to the surface of any antigen and lyse it. The MAC is initiated by either the alternative or the classical pathway. Once MAC enzymes are bound to an antigen, they lyse holes in the antigen's outer membrane causing fluid leakage that ultimately destroys the antigen.

MAC:
complement enzymes
↓
antigen lysis

Defects and Deficiencies of Complement Proteins

Some individuals are genetically deficient of one or more of the complement components of the classical or alternative pathways or the MAC. Deficiencies or defects in complement proteins result in frequent infections. For example, with hereditary angioedema, a defective chemical inhibitor blocks the classical pathway and causes tissue and vascular edema (angiodema) to develop. Cleavage products released by the C2 protein component of the classical pathway are responsible. With paroxysmal nocturnal hemoglobinuria, red cell membranes are fragile and easily lysed by complement. The fragility of red cells is due to a deficiency of certain proteins that regulate complement activation. Physicians are not sure why most red cell lysis occurs at night.

Complement Activation in the Absence of Antigen

For reasons not entirely clear, the complement system can be activated at times when antigen is not present. Platelets that have been agglutinated (clumped) by immunoglobulins, foreign surfaces, or enzymes released from damaged tissues can activate complement proteins. Complement activation can also occur as the result of medical procedures in which an individual's blood is exposed to foreign surfaces. For example, the complement system can be activated by tubing used in hemodialysis and open heart surgery and by plastic containers used to collect autologous blood lost either intra- or postoperatively.

agglutinated platelets

medical procedures

complement activation
by foreign surfaces
↓
destruction of
blood cells

When the complement system is activated by foreign surfaces, complement proteins attack an individual's own cells, such as red cells, white cells, and platelets. Complement proteins attach themselves to cell membranes, and cells are either phagocytized or lysed. If complement proteins bind red cells, hemolysis (destruction) results, a potentially lethal situation. If hemolysis becomes widespread and a large number of red cells is destroyed, fewer red cells remain to transport oxygen to body tissues. When white and red cells and platelets are lysed, they are rendered nonfunctional.

■ **QUESTIONS** ■

1. Are the terms antigen, immunogen, and pathogen interchangeable? Explain.

2. Define target cells.

3. List four categories of antigen.

4. Protein molecules make up the majority of antigen and are the most potent. Before they can generate an immune response what must happen?

5. Lipid and carbohydrate antigens are T cell-independent antigens. What does this mean?

6. Define epitope.

7. When is an invading microorganism safe from the body's immune system?

8. Antibody has two major functions. Explain them.

9. Phagocytic cells have both Fc and C3 receptors. How is one different from the other?

10. The human body can provide a corresponding antibody for every antigen produced and for every one that can be produced. True or False?

11. Describe the part of an antibody molecule that is unique to each antibody. What is its function?

12. Which is more rapid, the anamnestic response or primary (sensitization)? Why?

13. Enumerate four mechanisms involved in antibody destruction of antigen.

14. There are five classes of antibody (immunoglobulin): IgG, IgM, IgD, IgA, and IgE. How are these classes determined?

15. IgG is the only antibody that provides immunologic protection for the newborn. Why is this so?

16. What do increased levels of IgM at birth indicate?

17. IgA immunoglobulin is the major antibody in body fluids and mucus. What fluids are involved?

18. Describe an allergic reaction and the role of IgE in it.

19. When do anaphylactic reactions occur?

20. When are complement proteins most effective in destroying antigen?

21. The central component of the complement system is C3. How does this molecule operate?

22. If complement proteins and phagocytic white cells are unable to destroy invading antigen, what other recourse does the body have?

23. Complement proteins work in many ways. Enumerate at least five of their functions.

24. Complement proteins react in a chemical chain reaction. True or False?

25. Define anaphylatoxins. Describe their role in the classical pathway of the complement system.

26. What is the long-term effect of complement protein deficiencies or defects?

27. How could an individual on dialysis be affected by complement activation in the absence of antigen?

CHAPTER 8

The Major Histocompatibility Complex Molecules

Introduction

Major histocompatibility complex (MHC) molecules are cell surface glycoproteins that present a piece of protein antigen, called an antigenic peptide, to T cells. MHC molecules allow T cells to recognize protein antigen, which they are unable to recognize on their own. Once a T cell recognizes protein antigen, it can then direct the destruction of that antigen. MHC molecules are found on almost all body cells. In blood, they are found on white cells and platelets; however, they are not present on red cells.

allow protein antigen recognition by T cells

found on:
most body cells
white cells
platelets

MHC molecules have several names, including tissue antigens, major histocompatibility antigens, transplant antigens, and human leukocyte antigens (HLA). All mammals have MHC molecules. In humans, MHC molecules are referred to as HLA.

HLA

Like fingerprints, HLA are unique to every individual, the exception being identical twins, who have the same HLA. HLA cause humans to be immunologically different from one another. Differences in HLA between donor and recipient prompt vigorous formation of antibody and the activation of cytotoxic T cells against donor cells bearing foreign HLA. Graft rejection follows this strong immune response.

Alloimmunization

Immunization, antigen, and antibody are often used as shorthand for the terms alloimmunization, alloantigen, and alloantibody.

alloimmunization
alloantigen
alloantibody **131**

alloimmunization
alloantigen

alloantibody

Alloimmunization is the production of alloantibody following exposure to alloantigen. Alloantibody also develops in females following pregnancy. Alloantigens are molecules in certain individuals that generate the formation of alloantibodies in other members of the same species. In humans, alloantigens include HLA and the red cell antigens A and B (see Ch. 13, The ABO and Rh Blood Group Systems), among others. Alloantigen causes an immune response in organ and bone marrow transplant recipients that leads to graft rejection. Isoantigen is another term for alloantigen, and isoantibody is a term that can be used for alloantibody.

isoantigen
isoantibody

Classes of MHC Molecules

There are three classes of MHC molecules, class I, II, and III. In this book, class I and II molecules are addressed because they are essential for presentation of antigenic peptides to T cells for generation of the immune response. Class III molecules are involved with the production of complement proteins and certain cytokines, such as tumor necrosis factors (TNFs).

MHC class I restriction

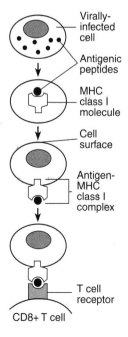

Virally-infected cell

Antigenic peptides

MHC class I molecule

Cell surface

Antigen-MHC class I complex

T cell receptor

CD8+ T cell

Class I and II MHC molecules are distinguished from one another in the following ways:

- They differ in their molecular structure.
- They are found on different body cells.
- They present different types of antigen to either CD4+ or CD8+ T cells.

Class I MHC Molecules

Class I MHC molecules are required for the recognition and destruction of cells infected by viruses and certain intracellular bacteria, such as those that cause leprosy and tuberculosis. These intracellular microorganisms produce antigenic peptides that bind to class I MHC molecules to form complexes. An antigen-MHC complex migrates to the cell surface for presentation to and recognition by a CD8 + cytotoxic T cell. CD8 + T cells can recognize only antigenic peptides bound to MHC class I molecules and are, therefore, referred to as being MHC class I restricted.

When donor cells bearing class I molecules are transplanted, they strongly stimulate antibody production and cytotoxic T cell activation by the recipient. Antibody production and cytotoxic T cell activation lead to destruction of donor cells by lysis.

The most powerful immune response is directed against MHC class I molecules coded for by genes at the A and B loci on chromosome 6.

Class II Molecules

Class II MHC molecules are essential for CD4+ T cell recognition of an antigenic peptide. Without class II MHC, CD4+ helper T cells would be unable to generate an immune response to protein antigen. CD4+ helper T cells must have protein antigen presented to them by class II molecules on the surface of antigen-presenting cells (APCs), such as B cells, monocytes, macrophages, activated T cells, dendritic cells, and endothelial cells. Antigen-presenting cells phagocytize exogenous antigens (extracellular microorganisms) and their toxins. The antigenic peptide is bound to a class II MHC molecule. This complex migrates to the cell surface where it presents antigen to CD4+ helper T cells. These cells can recognize only antigenic peptides attached to MHC class II molecules. CD4+ T cells are, therefore, referred to as being MHC class II restricted.

The most powerful immune response is directed against MHC class II molecules coded for by genes at the DR locus on chromosome 6.

MHC class II restriction

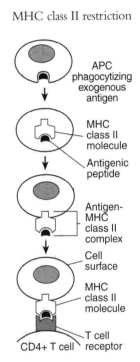

APC phagocytizing exogenous antigen

MHC class II molecule

Antigenic peptide

Antigen-MHC class II complex

Cell surface

MHC class II molecule

CD4+ T cell   T cell receptor

Human Leukocyte Antigens

Major histocompatibility complex molecules are referred to as HLA (human leukocyte antigens) because (1) they were discovered on leukocyte membranes, and (2) they induce alloantibody formation and CD8+ cytotoxic T cell activity in the recipient.

HLA in Blood Transfusion

Blood transfusion recipients become alloimmunized to donor HLA following transfusion. For example, patients receiving a platelet transfusion develop allo-antibodies to HLA on donor platelets and any leukocytes in the unit. During a subsequent transfusion, HLA alloantibodies formed during primary immunization can attach themselves to transfused platelets bearing complementary HLA. The result is loss of platelet function, which is called platelet refractoriness.

platelet refractoriness

HLA alloantigens and alloantibodies are implicated in the following transfusion reactions: febrile nonhemo-lytic transfusion reactions (FNHTRs), platelet refrac-toriness, transfusion-related acute lung injury (TRALI), and transfusion-associated graft-versus-host disease (TAGVHD; see Ch. 15, Transfusion Complications).

The use of leukocyte-reduction filters can help prevent alloimmunization to HLA by removing white cells (see Ch. 15, Transfusion Reactions). A blood transfusion recipient needing HLA-compatible blood components, such as platelets, obtains them from an HLA-compatible donor by apheresis (see Ch. 18, Apheresis).

HLA in Solid Organ Transplantation

recipient CD4+ T cells
↓
CD8+ cytotoxic T cells
↓
lysis of donor tissue
↓
graft rejection

Allogeneic organ transplantation (kidney, heart, liver, and lungs, among others) is becoming a common therapy for certain congenital and acquired conditions and diseases. The major obstacle to successful organ transplantation is the reaction generated by the recipient's acquired immune system against donor tissue, that is, cells bearing foreign HLA. In allogeneic organ transplants, graft rejection occurs when recipient CD4+ helper T cells recognize HLA on donor graft tissue as foreign. Recipient CD4+ T cells then activate CD8+ cytotoxic T cells, which lyse donor tissue. Graft rejection follows.

HLA alloantibodies usually are not involved in solid organ graft rejection unless the recipient has a high titer of HLA alloantibodies. When the titer is sufficiently high, HLA alloantibodies bind donor cells, which stimulates complement activation. Cell lysis results. Both complement and alloantibodies are responsible for graft rejection.

An HLA match between donor and recipient increases the likelihood of successful organ transplantation, but rejection is still possible. Precise HLA matches can be found only in donors who are siblings or an identical twin. Even in these cases, rejection can occur due to minor differences in histocompatibility, although at a much slower rate. The reasons are (1) HLA typing is imprecise, and (2) an HLA-identical match usually is not a gene match. HLA similarity between donor and recipient is referred to as histocompatibility, whereas HLA dissimilarity is called histoincompatibility

histocompatibility
histoincompatibility

All graft recipients, with the exception of identical twins, need to be immunosuppressed in order to prevent graft rejection. Although HLA matching is an essential procedure, improvements in immunosuppressive therapy are chiefly responsible for the success of solid organ transplantations.

immunosuppressive
therapy

HLA in Bone Marrow Transplantation

HLA are the most problematic antigens involved in the success or failure of a bone marrow transplant (BMT). Whether a BMT recipient accepts or rejects the graft or develops graft-versus-host disease (GVHD) is directly related to the degree of HLA similarity existing between donor and recipient. Bone marrow transplant recipients will violently reject donor marrow that is not an HLA match (see Ch. 20, Bone Marrow Transplantation).

Genetics of the MHC Molecules

Major histocompatibility molecules are produced by a group of genes very close together on chromosome 6. Genes close together on a chromosome are called linked genes, which usually are inherited as a block of genes called a haplotype.

chromosome 6

linked genes
haplotype

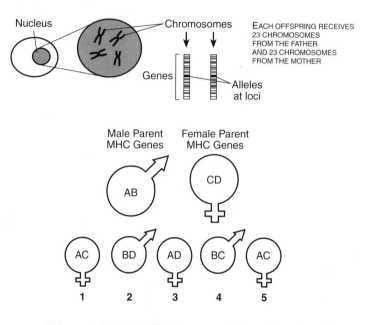

FIGURE 8.1 Major Histocompatibility Complex Genes
This schematic diagram shows the possible parental HLA haplotype arrangements in 5 offspring.

Offspring 1 and 2 share no HLA haplotype.
Offspring 1 and 3 share one HLA haplotype.
Offspring 1 and 4 share one HLA haplotype.
Offspring 1 and 5 share two HLA haplotypes and are a match.

Even with a match, there are minor HLA differences between offspring.

Individuals inherit two genes for MHC molecules, one from the mother and one from the father. Offspring can receive either one of the two parental haplotypes (50% x 50% = .25). Siblings, therefore, have a 25% (0.25) chance of sharing the same MHC genes. When an organ donor is required, siblings are the first candidates examined because they are the most likely to be an HLA match. Siblings may or may not share the same HLA, however (see Figure 8.1). Identical twins always share the same HLA genes and are referred to as syngeneic. There is little likelihood of finding an HLA-matched donor within the general public.

Most genes are expressed as either dominant or recessive. If an individual has two dominant genes or two recessive genes for a particular trait, he or she is homozygous for that trait. If one gene is dominant and the other recessive, the individual is heterozygous for that trait. Pairs of genes that code for the same trait are called alleles. Unlike the majority of genes, MHC genes are codominant, which means that neither allele is dominant nor recessive. Instead, each allele shares equal expression in the MHC molecules produced. Scientists believe that there are approximately 100 million alleles for MHC, which makes MHC the most polymorphic genes known in humans. The polymorphism associated with MHC makes it difficult to find an MHC match within the general population.

alleles

codominant genes

polymorphic genes

Genetic Loci of the MHC

Class I MHC genes are found at the A, B, and C loci. Class I MHC molecules are designated by a letter that represents their locus and number, such as A1, B3, and Cw3. Class II MHC genes are located in the D region. The D locus is further subdivided into the DP, DQ, and DR loci. Class II MHC molecules are designated by letters along with a number that represent their locus, for example, DR4, DQ3, and DPw5.

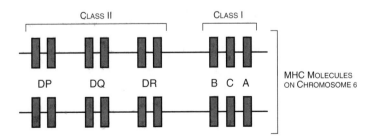

FIGURE 8.2 Chromosome 6 Showing MHC Loci
This schematic diagram shows the relationship of class I and class II MHC molecules on chromosome 6.

Identification of HLA

Transplantation of organs and bone marrow is used to treat a variety of hematologic, immunologic, and solid organ diseases, such as breast cancer. The transplant team identifies the best donor-recipient match through histocompatibility testing, antibody screening, and cross matching. Histocompatibility testing, also called tissue typing, identifies class I and II HLA on the cells of the recipient and the prospective donor. Serologic, cellular, and molecular (DNA) assays are types of histocompatibility tests that identify HLA.

histocompatibility
testing/tissue typing

Histocompatibility Tests

identification of class I
and some class II HLA
and HLA antibodies

serologically defined
antigens

Serologic Assays   Serologic assays identify class I and certain class II HLA and antibodies to HLA. Once recipient HLA are identified, the physician knows the HLA to look for in a prospective donor that will constitute a match. The lymphocytotoxicity test is a serologic assay that identifies HLA-A, HLA-B, and HLA-C class I as well as class II HLA-DR, and HLA-DQ. Because these HLA are identified using serum, they are called serologically defined antigens.

identification of HLA
similarity between
donor and recipient

cellular defined
antigens

MLC/MLR

Cellular Assays   Cellular assays do not identify specific HLA. They do, however, identify the degree of similarity between donor and recipient HLA class II DP, DQ, and DR. Class II HLA are called cellular defined antigens because lymphocytes are used to identify them. The tests are called the mixed lymphocyte culture (MLC) or the mixed lymphocyte reaction (MLR).

The degree of similarity between donor and recipient is indicated by the amount of proliferation of recipient lymphocytes caused by donor HLA. The greater the difference between donor and recipient HLA, the more cellular proliferation there is. If no proliferation of lymphocytes occurs, strong similarity between donor and recipient HLA is indicated. This donor can be used for this recipient.

Molecular Testing   Molecular testing techniques utilize fragments of DNA to identify the HLA gene itself. Molecular assays are very specific and highly sensitive. At the present time, only class II MHC molecules are determined by molecular methods. Molecular testing is very complex and describing them is beyond the scope of this book.

identification of class II HLA by DNA

Antibody Screening

Antibody screening examines recipient serum for preformed antibodies to HLA. Preformed antibodies form following blood transfusion and organ transplantation. In women, HLA antibodies can form following pregnancy. Preformed HLA antibodies in the recipient can contraindicate a transplant procedure.

identification of preformed antibodies to HLA

The amount of alloimmunization in the recipient is determined by mixing recipient serum (containing antibodies) in a panel of cells containing lymphocytes with known HLA. The total percentage of lymphocytes destroyed by the recipient's antibodies is called the panel reactive antibody (PRA). A high PRA indicates extensive alloimmunization. Individuals with a high PRA will have a difficult time locating a donor within the general population.

PRA

Cross Matching

Cross matching determines if the recipient is alloimmunized to donor HLA. Recipient serum is mixed with prospective donor lymphocytes. If the recipient has preformed antibodies against donor HLA, organ and bone marrow transplantation from this donor is contraindicated. The antibodies will provoke a strong immune response leading to graft rejection.

determination of alloimmunization of recipient to donor HLA

▪ QUESTIONS ▪

1. What is the relationship between major histocompatibility complex (MHC) molecules and T cells?

2. In the blood, what percentage of MHC molecules is found on red cells?

3. Explain how human leukocyte antigens (HLA) were named.

4. Like fingerprints, HLA are unique, except for what individuals?

5. Explain alloimmunization and compare it with immunization.

6. Identify the three major classes of MHC molecules.

7. Contrast class I and class II MHC molecules.

8. Identify one function of class III MHC molecules.

9. Leprosy and tuberculosis are two long-standing and devastating human diseases. How are they affected by MHC molecules?

10. List four transfusion reactions in which HLA are implicated.

11. Leukocyte-reduction filters are used with some blood transfusions. Explain why.

12. Define human leukocyte antigens (HLA).

13. What kind of blood transfusion can cause platelet refractoriness?

14. Allogeneic organ transplantation is becoming a common therapy for certain congenital and acquired conditions and diseases. Describe the sequence leading to graft rejection as it relates to foreign HLA.

15. Precise HLA matches can be found only in donors who are siblings or an identical twin. True or False?

16. Explain histocompatibility and also histoincompatibility.

17. Liver and other solid organ transplantations are becoming more common and more successful. What is mainly responsible for this increasing success?

18. A successful bone marrow transplantation (BMT) depends on many factors. Identify one.

19. Siblings, especially identical twins, are the most likely to provide an MHC match. It is very difficult to find an MHC match within the general population. Explain why.

20. The transplant team identifies the best donor recipient match for transplantation surgery. How does it accomplish this important task?

21. Clarify the goal of the lymphocytotoxicity test.

22. Define mixed lymphocyte culture. What is its role in finding a good donor-recipient match?

23. How is DNA involved in producing a good donor-recipient match?

24. What is a panel reactive antibody (PRA)? and what does it indicate?

25. When a recipient has preformed antibodies against donor HLA, what happens? How is this prevented?

26. Explain the premise of cross matching for HLA.

CHAPTER 9

The Immune System

Introduction

The immune system protects the individual against foreign matter that breaches either the physical or chemical barriers of the body causing infection and disease. A wide variety of microorganisms and foreign substances bombard the body constantly. Even the smallest splinter harbors antigen like bacteria, fungi, viruses, and other microorganisms that can be harmful. The immune system perceives microorganisms, allogeneic cells, tumor cells, and infected cells as antigen and, therefore, targets them for destruction. Ultimately, foreign matter is destroyed by the combined efforts of the immune system. When the immune system breaks down or is absent, disorders and diseases occur that may cause death.

The immune system is not a fixed system of channels like the circulatory system, nor is it an electrical network like the nervous system. White cells, antibody, and complement of the immune system move freely throughout the body, penetrating fluids and tissues. The immune system has the complicated task of recognizing and destroying harmful invaders without damaging the body's own tissues. It is one of the most difficult systems of the body to understand. Highly complex cellular and chemical interactions take place continuously. Furthermore, discoveries about the immune system happen so rapidly that immunologists disagree among themselves about how this system works.

Innate and Acquired Immunity

The immune system is considered as two separate but closely connected branches: the innate (nonspecific) and the acquired (specific). Both branches work together to destroy antigen.

Innate Immunity

Humans are born with innate immunity; therefore, this branch is called inborn or natural. Innate immune components—complement, neutrophils, monocytes, and tissue macrophages—act within minutes to destroy microorganisms and toxins by phagocytosis. Innate immunity is effective against extracellular foreign matter and microorganisms. It offers the first line of defense against antigenic invaders, such as bacteria, that penetrate the body through the (1) skin; (2) mucous membranes of the mouth, intestine, bladder, vagina, and nose; (3) ciliated epithelia of the respiratory system; and (4) acids and chemicals of the gastrointestinal tract.

When microorganisms penetrate the body's physical and chemical barriers, the inflammatory response is generated by myeloid white cells, complement, and cytokines released by lymphocytes and macrophages. At times in antigen invasion, inflammation is sufficient to overcome the antigenic invasion and prevent tissue injury. Signs of inflammation include: edema, soreness, heat, and redness at the site of antigen invasion.

Although capable of defeating most antigen, the innate immune system is powerless against certain antigen, such as infected cells, malignant cells, and allogeneic cells. These antigen must be destroyed by cytotoxic T cells and antibody of acquired immunity.

Acquired Immunity

Acquired immunity is a specialized form of immunity carried out by T and B lymphocytes in response to antigen. As the name suggests, acquired immunity is obtained and developed as one is exposed to antigen.

Margin notes:

inborn or natural complement, neutrophils, monocytes, tissue macrophages

first line of defense against extracellular antigen

inflammatory response

T and B cell response to antigen
obtained and developed on exposure to antigen

The greater variety of antigen to which one is exposed, the more developed acquired immunity becomes. Acquired immunity takes several days to reach full potential and, therefore, is not immediate.

Characteristics of Acquired Immunity

The main characteristics of acquired immunity are:

- Specificity: Immune reactions are specific for the offending antigen.
- Diversity: Lymphocytes have the ability to respond to a variety of antigen.
- Memory: Lymphocytes have the ability to remember antigen they have encountered previously.
- Self-regulation: Lymphocytes have the ability to shut down their activity after antigen is destroyed.
- Self-tolerance: Lymphocytes have the ability to distinguish self-tissue from nonself tissue.

Role of Cytokines in Immunity

The term cytokines encompasses a broad class of glycoproteins that have diverse functions within the body. Cytokines have major roles in hematopoiesis (blood cell production), the immune response, inflammation, and wound healing. Cytokines are released by macrophages and lymphocytes and have specific names, depending on the white cells that secrete them. Those released from macrophages are referred to as monokines, and those released from lymphocytes are called lymphokines.

fuction in:
hematopoiesis and
immune response
macrophages and
lymphocytes
↓
cytokine release
monokines
lymphokines

Cytokines allow white cells to communicate among themselves and with other cells in response to inflammation and infection. Cytokines that take part in cellular communication among the various white cells are referred to as interleukins (ILs). Other significant cytokines are interferons (INFs) and tumor necrosis factors (TNFs). INFs help provide immunity against viruses, and TNFs help provide immunity against tumor cells. Cytokines may work together or against one another to bring about their desired effect.

cytokines:
ILs–white cell
communication
INFs–immunity
against viruses
TNFs–immunity
against tumor cells

Cell-mediated and Humoral Immunity

Cell-Mediated Immunity   T cells direct cell-mediated immunity. When T cells respond to antigen, the response is referred to as cell-mediated. Helper T cells and cytotoxic T cells have specific roles in immunity leading to antigen destruction. T cells are also responsible for some types of autoimmune diseases and graft rejection.

T cell response to antigen

Humoral Immunity   The production of antibody by B cells/plasma cells in response to antigen is called humoral immunity. B cells encounter antigen and produce antibody in secondary lymphatic tissue, such as the lymph nodes and the spleen. Once plasma cells release antibody, antibody can leave the lymphatic system and enter the circulatory system where it encounters antigen that might have escaped into the bloodstream. When antibody is produced in response to antigen, the immune response is said to be antibody-mediated.

production of antibody by B cells/plasma cells in response to antigen

antibody-mediated

The Immune Response

The immune system is activated and an immune response initiated when antigen stimulates T and B cells. The combined efforts of the immune system—T cell activation along with antibody production by B cells—constitute the immune response. The body's ability to generate an immune response is called immunocompetence, that is, the immune system is intact and functioning. When the body cannot generate an immune response, immunoincompetence results. Immunoincompetence is the absence of a competent immune system. Another term for immunoincompetence is anergy. Immunoincompetence is due to either genetic or acquired defects or to suppression of the immune system by drugs and radiation.

immune response:
antigen
↓
antibody production and T cell activation

immunocompetence

immunoincompetence/ anergy

Three Phases of the Immune Response

The immune response occurs in three steps, or phases. In the first step, called the cognitive phase, the antigen-

cognitive phase:
antigen-MHC complex binds T cell receptors

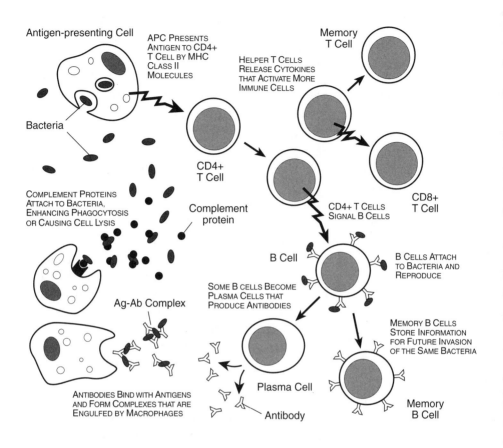

FIGURE 9.1 The Immune Response to Exogenous Antigen

Following phagocytosis, CD4+ helper T cells direct the immune response to antigen through cell–mediated immunity.

MHC complex binds to the T cell receptor. In the second step, or activator phase, T cells respond to bound antigen and release cytokines that cause the proliferation of T and B cells. Once there are sufficient numbers, T and B cells mount an attack against the antigen that stimulated them. The third step, called the effector phase, brings about antigen destruction. In this phase, granulocytes, macrophages, and complement are activated to opsonize and engulf antigen.

activator phase:
T cells release cytokines
↓
T and B cell proliferation

effector phase:
antigen destruction

Targets of the Immune Response

Microorganisms

exogenous antigen
exotoxins

endotoxins

Microorganisms that do their damage outside body cells by the release of toxins are called exogenous antigen. There are two types of toxins: (1) exotoxins, which are released from bacterial membranes, and (2) endotoxins, which are produced within bacterial cells and released when the bacteria is destroyed.

CD4+ helper T cell
antigen destruction:
APCs phagocytize
antigen

antigen-MHC class II
complex
↓
CD4+ helper T cell
recognition
↓
cytokine release
↓
opsonization by
complement and
antibody
↓
phagocytosis

Microorganisms include the majority of bacteria, protozoa, fungi, and parasites. Destruction of these antigens requires the assistance of white cells, such as antigen-presenting cells (APCs), CD4+ helper T cells, B cells/plasma cells, and macrophages. Antigen-presenting cells (APCs) phagocytize antigen. The phagocytized antigen is digested into small fragments, called antigenic peptides, which attach themselves to class II MHC molecules. The antigen-MHC complex migrates to the cell membrane where it flags CD4+ helper T cells. Once the complex is recognized by CD4+ T cells, the helper T cells release cytokines that stimulate complement activation and the production of antibody release by B cells. Complement and antibody opsonize antigen, which is then phagocytized by macrophages.

Infected Cells

antigen destruction
by CD8+ cytotoxic
T cells:
viral peptide-MHC
class I complex
↓
CD8+ cytotxic T cell
recognition
↓
cell lysis

Viruses are nonliving microorganisms. When viruses enter the body, they induce activation of antibody and complement, which usually is not sufficient to destroy them. Viruses attack cells from the inside. To make copies of themselves, viruses must enter cells, and once inside, they take over cell function. When viruses enter a cell, the cell is considered infected. Intracellular microorganisms cannot be destroyed by antibody or complement; once inside the cell, they cannot be opsonized.

An infected cell produces viral peptides that form a complex with class I MHC molecules. The MHC-antigen complex migrates to the cell membrane.

CD8+ cytotoxic T cells recognize this viral peptide-MHC class I complex and lyse the infected cell.

Certain bacteria, parasites, and fungi can also attack cells internally. On entering the cell, these micro-organisms are considered endogenous antigen.

endogenous antigen

Allogeneic Cells

Allogeneic cells in transplanted organs and transfused blood components generate an immune response in the recipient because they express donor HLA that is foreign to the recipient. Cells from an identical twin are not considered allogeneic because they have the same HLA molecules; these cells are syngeneic. Allogeneic cells stimulate the recipient's cell-mediated and humoral immune responses. Once the recipient's immune system recognizes allogeneic cells, it destroys them by lysis.

destruction of allogeneic and malignant cells: cell-mediated and humoral immunity response
↓
cell lysis

Malignant Cells

Malignant cells generate tumor proteins within themselves that an individual's immune system recognizes as foreign. Tumor cells elicit humoral and cell-mediated immune responses. These cells can be destroyed by the following means:

- Cytokines, such as tumor necrosis factors (TNFs)
- Antibody produced against them
- Cytotoxic T cells
- Killer cells through antibody-dependent, cell-mediated cytotoxicity (ADCC)
- Macrophages
- A combination of all listed

Role of the Lymphatic System in Immunity

The lymphatic system, also known as the lymphoid system, has important physiologic functions within the body. The lymphatic system consists of lymphatic

lymphoid system

channels, organs, nodes, and ducts throughout the body that assist in antigen destruction (see Ch. 2, The Circulatory System, Figure 2.5, p. 22).

Primary and Secondary Lymphatic Tissue

primary lymphatic tissue:
thymus gland and bone marrow

Lymphatic tissue is divided into primary and secondary tissue. Lymphocytes mature within primary lymphatic tissue, with the thymus gland as the site of T cell development and the bone marrow as the site of B cell development.

secondary lymphatic tissue:
lymphatic organs and lymph nodes

antibody production

Secondary lymphatic tissue includes (1) lymphatic organs, such as the spleen, tonsils, mucosa-associated lymphatic tissue (MALT), and (2) lymph nodes. Lymphatic channels carry antigen from their point of entry into the body to secondary lymphatic organs. Antibody production begins in the secondary lymphatic organs before antigen has a chance to enter the blood and spread throughout the body. T and B cells primarily reside in the secondary lymphatic organs and respond to antigen there.

The Spleen   The largest secondary lymphatic organ is the spleen. Weighing about 150 g (1/4 lb), it lies in the upper left corner of the abdomen under the ribs. Blood enters the spleen through the splenic artery. It flows through arterioles surrounded by lymphatic tissue heavily endowed with T cells and macrophages. As blood filters through the spleen,

T cells, macrophages
↓
antigen destruction

T cells and macrophages survey it for antigen so that they can destroy the antigen before it has a chance to enter the blood and spread throughout the body. Filtered blood exits the spleen through the splenic vein.

Lymph Nodes   Structures called lymph nodes are found at intervals along lymphatic channels throughout the body. Lymph nodes are masses of lymphatic tissue

T and B cells, APCs
↓
antigen destruction in lymph fluid

containing T and B lymphocytes and APCs. Lymph nodes act as filtering stations to trap antigen found circulating in lymph fluid. Lymph nodes swell in the area of antigen invasion, a condition called lymphadenopathy. Swelling is due to proliferation of B cells/plasma cells as they produce antibodies within the lymph nodes.

lymphadenopathy

Human Intervention: Vaccination and Antiserum

Vaccination

The medical therapy used to stimulate an individual's acquired immune system is called vaccination. The vaccine is composed of weakened (attenuated) fragments of pathogenic microorganisms and administered by injection or by mouth. In response to the vaccine (antigen), the body becomes sensitized and produces antibody and memory T and B cells. If the individual becomes infected by the organism, the antibody and memory cells are able to destroy the organism before it has a chance to take hold. Antibody generated in response to vaccination is called active immunity. Active immunity is when the antibody is produced within the individual.

stimulation of acquired immune system

production of antibody and memory T and B cells

active immunity

Vaccine solutions, such as the polio vaccine or hepatitis B vaccine, are prepared by pharmaceutical companies. A vaccine is usually administered in 2 or 3 doses by mouth or by injection, depending on the vaccine.

Antiserum

For individuals unable to defeat pathogenic organisms on their own, a form of therapy called passive immunity is available. Passive immunity occurs when antibody used to fight infection is produced within another individual or animal. An individual receives a concentrated solution of antibody in serum removed from a human or animal previously exposed to an infectious microorganism. The generic terms used for antibody given in passive immunity are gammaglobulin or antiserum. Examples of gammaglobulin include: hepatitis B immune serum globulin, Rh immune globulin, and tetanus toxoid, among others.

passive immunity

antiserum to a specific microorganism

gammaglobulin or antiserum

Disorders of Immunity

hypersensitivity reactions
autoimmune diseases
immune deficiency
disorders

There are times when the immune system is absent, deficient, or defective. Diseases or defective immune responses result. Disorders of the immune system are divided into (1) hypersensitivity, or allergic, reactions (p. 152), (2) autoimmune diseases (p. 157), and (3) immune deficiency disorders (p. 158).

(1) Hypersensitivity Reactions

Hypersensitivity reactions are abnormal or inappropriate immune responses that cause tissue damage and disease. They occur only in individuals previously sensitized to an allergen (antigen). Such persons are referred to as hypersensitive because they are extremely sensitive to the offending allergen. Many different allergens can cause hypersensitivity reactions. An allergen is a harmless substance that some individuals' immune systems perceive as foreign.

allergen

Hypersensitivity reactions vary. They can be mild and uncomfortable, as in the case of itching caused by poison ivy. They can also be serious and life-threatening, as in the case of sometimes fatal anaphylactic reactions. Hypersensitivity reactions include: type I, type II, type III, and type IV.

Type I Hypersensitivity Reactions   A type I reaction is an immediate, fast-acting, immune-mediated response commonly known as an allergic or anaphylactic reaction. Type I reactions are a true medical emergency because the individual can die if immediate medical attention is not available. The term anaphylactic is used for the most serious reaction.

allergic or anaphylactic
reaction

first exposure:
IgE antibody binds
basophils and mast cells

second exposure:
allergen binds
previously formed IgE
↓
histamine release
↓
anaphylactic reaction

In the sensitizing event, an individual develops IgE antibody, which has a strong affinity for basophils and mast cells and binds to them. When the individual is subsequently exposed to the same allergen, the allergen attaches to previously formed IgE causing basophils and mast cells to release histamine and other potent molecules. An immediate anaphylactic reaction occurs.

Type I hypersensitivity reactions can be caused by the following: foods, such as shellfish, peanuts, eggs, milk, beans; insect venoms, such as those from honeybees or yellow jackets; snake venoms; drugs, such as hormones, vaccines, toxoids, dextran, some antibiotics; and some diagnostic agents, such as iodine.

Histamine release in type I reactions affects several organ systems. Effects include bronchiole constriction, capillary leakage, increased secretions from mucosal surfaces, hemorrhage, laryngeal edema, and myocardial ischemia, among others. When capillary leakage is severe, shock can occur. This is called anaphylactic shock.

anaphylactic shock

The Anaphylactoid Reaction   A reaction very similar to the anaphylactic reaction is the anaphylactoid reaction. It can occur following the release of any one of three complement proteins: C3a, C4a, and C5a. These proteins are called anaphylatoxins. They cause mast cells and basophils to release histamine and other molecules that produce anaphylacticlike signs. Anaphylactoid reactions are not mediated by antibody, however, which means that IgE is not produced.

anaphylatoxins/
complement proteins
↓
histamine release

no production of IgE

Type II Hypersensitivity

Type II hypersensitivity refers to antibody-mediated reactions. Antibody binds to antigen on cell membranes, such as A and B antigens found on the red cell membrane. Antigen involved in type II reactions can be naturally occurring, such as A and B red cell antigens, or exogenous antigens, such as toxins, that attach themselves to cell membranes. In either case, antibody bound to these antigens leads to the target cell's destruction, usually by lysis.

antibody-mediated
reactions

Type II reactions occur by one of the following:

- Antigen-antibody complexes bind complement proteins leading to opsonization and cell lysis. Type II reactions occur, for example, in recipients who receive blood transfusions with incompatible red cells. Once complement proteins bind to the antigen-antibody complex, the complex lyses donor red cells.

antigen-antibody
complexes bind
complement
↓
opsonization and
cell lysis

ADCC:
IgG or IgM
opsonize cells
↓
cell lysis

- Antibody-dependent, cell-mediated cytotoxicity (ADCC) refers to type II reactions in which IgG or IgM opsonize target cells. Opsonized cells are then lysed by IgG or IgM and certain white cells, such as natural killer cells and macrophages. An example of an ADCC reaction occurs in hemolytic disease of the newborn (see Ch. 13, ABO and Rh Blood Group Systems).

antireceptor antibody
binds to cell surface
receptors

- Antireceptor antibody is antibody that forms against cell surface receptors on body cells. Antireceptor antibody binds to cell surface receptors thus blocking their function. For example, in myasthenia gravis, antibody is directed against acetylcholine receptors at nerve synapses. Acetylcholine receptors function to transmit nerve impulses to muscles. Antibody binds to these receptors, blocking their ability to transmit nerve impulses.

Type II hypersensitivity reactions include: transfusion reactions, hemolytic disease of the newborn, some types of hemolytic anemias, immune thrombocytopenia, some drug reactions, and hyperacute allograft rejection.

Type III Hypersensitivity

antigen–antibody
complexes
↓
chemical activation
↓
destruction of tissue

Type III hypersensitivity reactions are reactions in which antigen-antibody complexes deposit themselves in body tissues. These complexes have the ability to activate cytokines and complement that destroy tissue. Not all immune complexes cause type III reactions, however.

There are many possible causes of type III reactions. Bacteria, viruses, parasites, drugs such as heroin, and tumor antigens can precipitate a type III response.

Type III reactions include: rheumatic fever, serum sickness (inflammation in response to administration of antitoxins), rheumatoid arthritis, polyarteritis (disease of small arteries), and cryoglobulinemia (abnormal proteins that aggregate at low temperatures). With each condition, a specific antigen binds with the antibody that stimulates the release of complement. Complement and cytokines damage body tissue, such as the joint cartilage with rheumatoid arthritis.

Type IV Hypersensitivity Reactions

Type IV hypersensitivity reactions are mediated by T cells. Sensitized helper T cells recognize foreign antigen and stimulate cytotoxic T cells to destroy target cells. Type IV hypersensitivity reactions can cause tissue damage when helper T cells release cytokines that attract macrophages. Cytokines, macrophages, and cytotoxic T cells all play a role in tissue damage.

Type IV hypersensitivity reactions do not occur immediately following an individual's exposure to an antigen, but usually happen within 1 to 2 weeks. They are, therefore, referred to as delayed-type hypersensitivity (DTH) reactions. These reactions can be caused by intracellular microorganisms, such as mycobacteria, fungi, and parasites, or by allogeneic cells.

Type IV hypersensitivity include: contact dermatitis (poison ivy), graft-versus-host disease, graft rejection, tuberculosis, and sarcoidosis, which is a disease that can affect the liver, lungs, skin, and lymph nodes.

Graft Rejection

Rejection of donor organs is a major problem for transplant specialists. Recipients will reject most transplanted organs and tissues unless they receive immunosuppressive drugs.

Graft rejection is a complex process. The principle cause of allograft rejection is usually a cell-mediated immune response. But antibodies within the recipient can also be the cause. Differences between the HLA molecules of the host and grafted tissue activate the host's CD4+ helper and CD8+ cytotoxic T cells. These cells attack donor tissue bearing foreign HLA molecules. Host cytotoxic T cells lyse the transplanted cells, promoting tissue necrosis and destruction of the graft.

T cell-mediated
reactions
sensitized helper
T cells
↓
cytotoxic T cell
stimulation and
cytokine release and
macrophage activity
↓
tissue damage

DTH

causes:
cell-mediated
immune response and
recipient antibodies

Classic signs of graft rejection are tenderness and swelling at the site of implant. There is also a decrease in the graft's function, such as decreased urine production following kidney transplant.

Mechanisms of Solid Organ Graft Rejection

Solid organ graft rejection occurs through one of the following mechanisms:

- Hyperacute rejection, which is antibody-mediated
- Acute rejection, which is both antibody- and cell-mediated
- Chronic rejection, which is T cell-mediated

anti-A, anti-B antibodies attack donor tissue

Hyperacute Graft Rejection   In hyperacute rejection, preformed antibodies (either anti-A, anti-B, or anti-HLA antibodies) in the recipient attack donor tissue and cause an immediate graft rejection within

within minutes to hours
antibody-antigen complex
↓
complement activation

minutes to hours after the transplant. Antibody that forms a complex with antigen activates complement. Complement release causes tissue swelling, hemorrhage, thrombosis, endothelial damage, and tissue necrosis. These conditions in combination with one another lead to graft rejection. There is no effective therapy for hyperacute rejection.

Acute Graft Rejection   The most common cause of graft rejection is the acute reaction. Usually the graft

within 2 to 3 weeks

is rejected within 2 to 3 weeks following transplant. It most often occurs when the donor and recipient are an HLA-mismatch or when the recipient is receiving insufficient immunosuppressive therapy.

causes:
cell-mediated reaction
antibody production

Acute rejection is caused by both cell-mediated events and antibody production against donor HLA that begin several days following transplant. Acute rejection can be treated with increased amounts of immunosuppressive drugs.

after months

Chronic Graft Rejection   Chronic rejection occurs months following solid organ transplant, after the organ has been carrying out its function. This

T cell-mediated reaction

type of rejection is a T cell-mediated immune response. Usually with chronic graft rejection, there is a slow progressive failure of the organ. Immuno-suppressive therapy is useless and little can be done to save the graft.

Graft-versus-Host Disease

When allogeneic cells are transplanted into an immunoincompetent individual, viable donor CD4+ helper and CD8+ cytotoxic T cells attack the tissue of the recipient bearing both class I and II HLA molecules. Donor cytotoxic T cells destroy recipient tissues via lysis. Tissue destruction is called graft-versus-host disease (GVHD) and is an example of a cell-mediated type IV hypersensitivity reaction.

cause: viable T cells attack recipient tissue

cell-mediated type IV hypersensitivity reaction

In GVHD, recipient tissues most affected are the skin, liver, lymphatic tissue, and intestine. Skin rash, diarrhea, liver failure, weight loss, and often death can ensue (see Ch. 20, Bone Marrow Transplantation).

(2) Autoimmune Diseases

Autoimmune diseases or disorders are reactions in which individuals produce an abnormal immune response against their own cells. Such disorders arise when the body fails to recognize its own tissue; it perceives them as foreign and loss of self-tolerance occurs. Self-tolerance is the ability of the body to recognize its own cells and endure them without destroying them.

abnormal immune response

loss of self-tolerance self-tolerance

Autoimmune disorders can be very specific in that they destroy a specific cell type, as in rheumatoid arthritis, or they can attack almost every cell in the body, as in lupus erythematosus. With rheumatoid arthritis, the body reacts by inflaming cartilage tissue in joints of the skeletal system. Lupus erythematosus is an inflammatory disease of connective tissue throughout the body. It affects skin, joints, kidneys, and mucous membranes.

There is a growing list of disease states attributable to autoimmune disorders—some types of hemolytic anemia, arthritis, multiple sclerosis, insulin-dependent diabetes mellitus, and scleroderma, among others.

Mechanisms Involved in Loss of Self-Tolerance   Many mechanisms cause the loss of self-tolerance, and possibly more than one may be involved in a given autoimmune disorder. Mechanisms causing autoimmunity include: breakdown of helper T cell function, microbial antigens (microorganisms), antibodies against self-tissue, defective suppressor T cell function, and genetic anomalies.

(3) Immune Deficiency Disorders

Immune deficiency disorders are defects in one's own immune system. When they are caused by congenital defects, they are called primary immunodeficiency disorders. When they are acquired disorders, they are called secondary immunodeficiency disorders. Both primary and secondary immunodeficiency disorders can cause serious and repeated infections that can be fatal.

Primary Immunodeficiency Disorders   These disorders usually affect a specific type of immune cell, such as T or B cells, complement proteins, or myeloid white cells. If a lymphocyte, complement protein, or myeloid white cell is defective, the immune system cannot respond normally to certain types of antigen.

There are many primary immunodeficiency disorders. The following are examples:

- IgA deficiency results from defective B cells that do not produce IgA.
- Agammaglobulinemia, a deficiency of all immunoglobulins, results from defective B cells.
- Thymic hypoplasia results in diminished production of T cells by the thymus.
- Severe combined immunodeficiency syndrome (SCIDS) results from defective T and B cells.
- Congenital deficiencies of the complement system proteins result from defective or absent complement proteins. Examples include hereditary angioedema and absence of the C3 complement inhibitor.
- Phagocytic dysfunctions result from defects in digestive enzymes that destroy phagocytized antigen.

Margin notes: congenital: primary immunodeficiency disorders; acquired: secondary immunodeficiency disorders; IgA deficiency; agammaglobulinemia; thymic hypoplasia; SCIDS; congenital deficiencies of complement; phagocytic dysfunctions

Individuals with primary immunodeficiency disorders experience many types of recurrent bacterial, fungal, viral, and protozoan infections.

Secondary Immunodeficiency Disorders   The loss of certain immune cells, such as T and B cells, are called secondary immunodeficiency disorders. They result from disease, radiation, chemotherapy, or immunosuppression that block or prevent the immune response. The body lacks the ability to destroy antigen.

loss of immune cells

An example of an acquired immune disorder is AIDS. Leukemia, a cancer of white cells, can also cause secondary immunodeficiency disorders because abnormal white cells are produced. Secondary immune disorders can be caused by immunosuppressive drugs following organ transplantation.

▪ QUESTIONS ▪

1. Why do immunologists disagree among themselves about the immune system?

2. How can foreign matter, including microorganisms such as bacteria and viruses, attack the human body as antigenic invaders?

3. What do edema, soreness, heat, and redness at the site of antigen invasion indicate?

4. True or False?. The greater variety of antigen to which one is exposed, the more developed acquired immunity becomes.

5. Identify five characteristics of acquired immunity.

6. Define cytokines and explain the difference between monokines and lymphokines.

7. List three types of cytokines along with their major functions.

8. T cells and B cells play an important role in the immune response. What is the major difference in their roles?

9. What is another term for immunoincompetence? What does it mean?

10. Describe the three phases of the immune response.

11. Explain the two types of toxins in the immune response.

12. Unlike bacteria, viruses cannot be destroyed by antibody and complement. Why is this so?

13. Malignant cells can be destroyed by a variety of elements within the immune response. List four of these.

14. What do the spleen, the tonsils, mucosa-associated lymphatic tissue (MALT), and lymph nodes have in common?

15. Where can T cells and macrophages destroy antigen before it has a chance to enter the spleen and spread throughout the body?

16. Explain vaccination: how it works and how it is administered.

17. Discuss the difference between active and passive immunity.

18. There are three major categories of disorders of the immune system. List them.

19. What type of immune disorder is anaphylaxis? Explain its symptoms.

20. Explain ADCC and give an example of its occurrence.

21. Rheumatic fever, once very common, is what type of immune disorder?

22. What category of immune disorder covers graft rejection?

23. Identify the three mechanisms of solid organ graft rejection.

24. What occurs at the cellular level in graft-versus-host disease (GVHD)?

25. Self-tolerance is the abilty of the body to recognize its own cells without destroying them. What happens when this ability is lost?

26. The list of disease states attributable to autoimmune disorders is growing. Identify three.

27. Explain the difference between primary and secondary immunodeficiency disorders.

CHAPTER 10

Plasma

Introduction

Plasma is the liquid portion of blood in which blood cells are suspended. The main function of plasma is to transport blood cells and solutes to and from tissue cells. Within plasma are particles called solutes, which dissolve in a liquid, or solvent. Solutes provide tissue cells with nutrients and other vital substances. Examples of solutes dissolved in plasma are: proteins, carbohydrates, lipids, vitamins, electrolytes (salts), and hormones. Solutes make up about 10% of the plasma volume and have many functions in maintaining homeostasis (constant equilibrium) within the body. The two major types of solutes are protein and nonprotein molecules. Most plasma solutes, except for large molecular weight proteins and lipids, are in constant communication with body cells via interstitial fluid.

protein and nonprotein solutes: 10% of plasma volume

Plasma is composed mostly of water (H_2O). Approximately 4% of an individual's total body weight (40 to 45 mL/kg) is plasma. Normally plasma is straw colored, but it can appear reddish, cloudy, or milky depending on the condition and health of an individual. The viscous, sticky consistency of plasma is mainly due to proteins dissolved within it.

mostly H_2O

Plasma not only transports solutes but removes waste products of cellular metabolism to various organs, such as the lungs, skin, and kidneys, for excretion. Because plasma travels throughout the body it provides a window to the chemical environment of the body. By analyzing plasma or serum medical professionals can gain much valuable information about what is happening in the body.

transports solutes and removes waste products of cellular metabolism

163

serum:
plasma minus
fibrinogen

The term serum is sometimes used interchangeably with plasma, but the fluids are not the same. When a tube of blood is allowed to stand, the formed elements and coagulation factors in the sample clot on the bottom of the tube while the serum, a straw-colored fluid, rises to the top. Serum is plasma minus fibrinogen. Serum is used for some blood tests, such as serology tests, routine blood bank tests, and chemistry tests.

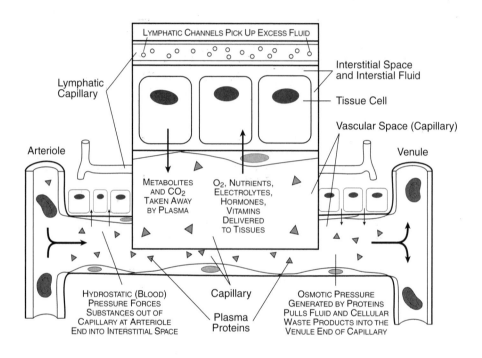

FIGURE 10.1 Movement of Plasma, Solutes, and Gases

This illustration depicts the movement of fluid and solutes between capillary networks and tissue cells. Hydrostatic pressure at the arterial end of a capillary forces fluids and solutes, such as electrolytes and hormones, to move from plasma into interstitial spaces, allowing tissue cells to take up these substances for cellular metabolism. Protein solutes remain in plasma and are responsible for maintaining osmotic pressure. This pressure draws fluid and waste products of cellular metabolism from interstitial spaces into the venous end of a capillary. The lymphatic system picks up any excess fluid from interstitial spaces that capillaries do not take up. This back and forth movement of fluid, solutes, and gases between interstitial spaces and capillaries occurs simultaneously.

Blood Volume

Many organ systems of the body, including the heart, brain, and kidneys, depend on a constant blood volume in order to function properly. When an adequate blood volume is not maintained an individual can develop serious problems that can cause death. Plasma proteins are essential in helping to maintain a constant blood volume throughout the body because they exert osmotic pressure in the vasculature. Congestive heart failure and pulmonary edema are complications associated with fluid imbalances.

Mechanisms that maintain balanced blood volume throughout the body are:

(1) Vascular integrity, which refers to intact vessels,

(2) Osmotic pressure, and

(3) Lymphatic vessels, which return interstitial fluid to the vascular system.

Plasma Proteins

Proteins are the most abundant solutes in plasma, making up about 7% of the total solutes. The concentration of proteins within the blood is about 6.5 to 8 g/dL (65 to 80 g/L). The majority of plasma proteins are produced in the liver.

7% of total solutes
blood concentration:
6.5 to 8 g/dL

Plasma proteins have many functions:

functions:

- They maintain osmotic pressure and fluid volume in the body.

osmotic pressure,
fluid volume

- They act as transport molecules that carry hormones, vitamins, and other substances used by cells.

transport molecules

- They play a role in immunity as complement and immunoglobulins (Ch. 9, The Immune System).

immunity

- They make up the clotting proteins (Ch. 12, Coagulation).

clotting proteins

- They act as enzymes for numerous chemical reactions that take place within the body.

enzymatic

bind drugs, toxins

regulate blood pH

provide nutrition

- They bind to drugs and toxins and transport them to the liver for detoxification.
- They act as buffers to help regulate blood pH (acid-base balance).
- They provide nutrition when protein intake is inadequate.

Albumin, Globulins, and Fibrinogen

There are three main classes of proteins in plasma: albumin, globulins, and the clotting protein fibrinogen. The majority of plasma proteins are synthesized in the liver. If the liver is diseased from such conditions as cirrhosis, hepatitis, or liver failure, production of proteins is severely restricted.

The percentages of albumin and globulins in circulation are:

- Albumin, 60%
- Globulins, 40%
  - Alpha-1 globulins, 4%
  - Alpha-2 globulins, 8%
  - Beta globulins, 12%
  - Immunoglobulins, 16%

Albumin

Albumin is essential for the body to maintain blood volume. This solute accounts for about 60% of the total proteins made in the liver. Its main functions are to maintain osmotic pressure between blood and body tissues and to act as a major transport (carrier) protein of other molecules, such as hormones and lipids, within plasma.

A decrease or lack of albumin can seriously affect the body's ability to maintain osmotic pressure and transport substances within the blood. An albumin deficiency can promote edema, which is tissue swelling due to a retention of fluid in interstitial spaces. Normal levels of albumin in plasma can be depleted by nephrotic syndrome, a type of kidney disease; liver disease; protein-losing enteropathy, a type of intestinal disease; and severe burns, a condition in which plasma leaks from the burned surface. Individuals with these conditions are observed closely for fluid imbalances.

Pharmaceutical companies process albumin from plasma to be used in transfusion therapy for patients with large volumes of blood loss. In the preparation process, albumin is heat pasteurized and has little, if any, chance of spreading viral diseases, such as AIDS and hepatitis.

Globulins

The globulins include: AT-III (antithrombin III), complement proteins, immunoglobulins (antibodies), and the many enzymes that exist in plasma. Globulin is a generic term that refers to all proteins in plasma— excluding albumin and fibrinogen. There are four types of globulin proteins: alpha-1 globulins, alpha-2 globulins, beta-1 globulins, and immunoglobulins.

AT-III, complement proteins, immunoglobulins, enzymes

Globulins have many functions:

functions:

- They act as enzymes in many metabolic processes.

enzymatic

- They are responsible for humoral immunity (the immunoglobulins).

humoral immunity

- They transport heme to bone marrow where it is recycled to produce new hemoglobin.

transport of heme

- They transport hormones to their target organs.

transport of hormones

- They transport metals such as copper and iron.

transport of metals

Immunoglobulins This group of globulins is produced by B cells (plasma cells) and plays a major role in defending the body against infection. The majority of immunoglobulins within blood are of the IgG class. Immunoglobulins are also referred to as gammaglobulins (see Ch. 7, Antigen, Antibody, and Complement).

majority: IgG gammaglobulins

Fibrinogen

Fibrinogen is the inactive form of fibrin. It is the clotting protein that stabilizes the platelet plug (see Ch. 12, Coagulation).

Protein Abnormalities

plasma protein
deficiencies

Hypoproteinemia This term refers to plasma protein deficiencies. Causes of hypoproteinemia include: decreased intake of proteins, such as occurs in malnutrition; decreased production, such as occurs in cirrhosis; decreased absorption of proteins, such as occurs in malabsorption syndrome; excretion of proteins, such as occurs with nephrotic syndrome; and hemodilution of blood in surgery.

Plasma protein deficiencies interfere with (1) acid-base balance, (2) clotting mechanisms, (3) enzyme-dependent reactions, (4) fluid balance, and (5) transport of substances, such as hormones and nutrients, to body tissues and organs. Individuals with protein deficiencies may be unable to generate sufficient osmotic pressure to pull fluid from the interstitial space back into the blood and therefore develop edema. (For information on fibrinogen abnormalities see Chapter 12, Coagulation.)

increased plasma
proteins

Hyperproteinemia This term refers to increased plasma proteins. Hyperproteinemia is due to conditions such as multiple myeloma, which is the abnormal production of paraproteins, and dehydration (loss of water from the body), among others. A paraprotein is an abnormal immunoglobulin produced in response to certain malignancies of the spleen, liver, and bone marrow.

excess of
immunoglobulins

Hyperviscosity Individuals with an excess of immunoglobulins (paraproteins) in the plasma experience hyperviscosity. Plasma becomes thick and blood flow is slowed. These conditions increase the likeli-hood of clot formation in the microvasculature. Hyperviscosity is caused by diseases such as multiple myeloma (B cell tumor) and Waldenström's macro-globulinemia in which large, molecular weight globulins are produced. Treatment of hyperviscosity consists of plasmapheresis, which is the removal of plasma from the individual, and suppressing the synthesis of paraproteins.

Nonprotein Plasma Solutes

Nonprotein solutes make up 1 to 3% of all solutes in plasma. They are as important as the protein solutes because the body cannot survive without them. As they circulate constantly between blood and body tissues, nonprotein solutes serve many vital functions. Most nonprotein solutes must be taken in with the diet because the majority are not synthesized within the body. Electrolytes, lipids, carbohydrates, and vitamins are nonprotein plasma components. Vitamins are a broad class of molecules necessary for normal physiology. Lipids (fats) and carbohydrates, of which glucose is the most important, are essential energy sources.

1 to 3% of all solutes

electrolytes, lipids, carbohydrates, vitamins

Electrolytes

Electrolytes are one of the most important nonprotein solutes found in plasma. Normal concentrations of electrolytes are essential for physiologic processes, primarily nerve conduction, muscle contraction, blood clotting, fluid balance, and acid–base regulation. Electrolytes and bicarbonate help maintain the pH of blood compatible with life. The acid–base balance of blood is essential for normal physiology (see Blood Test 62).

pH and acid–base balance

Electrolyte disturbances have profound effects on the body. For example, if the plasma concentration of an electrolyte is increased or decreased, fluid shifts, abnormal heart rhythms, clotting disorders, abnormal nerve conduction, and other problems can occur.

electrolyte disturbances

The main electrolytes and their normal concentrations in plasma are:

Calcium ions (Ca^{++})	8.5 to 10.5 mmol/L*
Chloride ions (Cl^-)	98 to 111 mmol/L
Potassium ions (K^+)	3.5 to 5.2 mmol/L
Sodium ions (Na^+)	138 to 148 mmol/L
Magnesium ions (Mg^{++})	0.7 to 1 mmol/L

* mmol/L is millimoles per liter of solution, a millimole being 1/1000 of a mole. The term mole is a number such that one mole of a substance has a mass equal to its molecular weight expressed in grams

The different electrolytes have specific functions:

- Ca^{++}, K^+, and Na^+ are necessary for promoting normal impulse conduction in nerve and muscle fibers.

- Ca^{++} is essential for clotting blood and maintaining cardiac rhythm.

- K^+ is essential for maintaining cardiac rhythm.

- Cl^- is necessary for replacing bicarbonate ions (HCO_3^-) taken up by red cells, a process known as the chloride shift (see Ch. 5, Oxygen and Carbon Dioxide Transport).

- Na^+ and Cl^- are necessary for maintaining fluid balance between blood and body tissues. If concentrations of Na^+ and Cl^- are too high or too low, fluid balance in the body shifts, with blood or tissues either retaining or losing too much fluid.

- Mg^{++} is vital for promoting normal neuromuscular function.

Bicarbonate   Although bicarbonate (HCO_3^-) is not an electrolyte, it does assist in maintaining acid–base balance within the body by acting as a buffer that helps control the acidity or alkalinity of the blood. Bicarbonate helps to maintain the pH of blood between 7.35 to 7.45, which equals a H^+ concentration of about 40 nmol/L.* The concentration of bicarbonate ions in plasma is 22 to 26 mEq/L.

buffer

pH scale

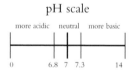

more acidic   neutral   more basic

0   6.8 7 7.3   14

* nmol/L nanomoles per liter of solution, a nanomole being one one billionth of a mole (1/1,000,000,000).

Carbohydrates and Lipids

The concentration of carbohydrate (glucose) and lipids within plasma are:

- Glucose, 72 to 137 mg/dL (fasting)
- Cholesterol, less than 200 mg/dL
- Lipoprotein, less than 50 mg/dL

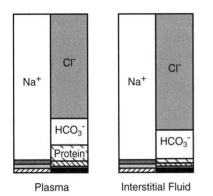

FIGURE 10.2 Solutes in Plasma and Interstitial Fluid

This schematic diagram shows the relative amounts of solutes found in plasma and interstitial fluid. Except for the large molecular weight plasma proteins, plasma and interstitial fluid have basically the same concentration of solutes.

Plasma   Interstitial Fluid

Mechanisms of Fluid Movement

The movement of water and plasma solutes from plasma into the tissues and vice versa is controlled by several mechanisms that include: filtration, reabsorption, hydrostatic pressure, and osmotic pressure. The movement of water and substances between the blood and tissues is analogous to the ebb and flow of the tide. The "tidal flow" is assisted by the porous nature of the capillary.

filtration, reabsorption, hydrostatic pressure, osmotic pressure

Filtration

Tissue cells require water and solutes (nutrients) in plasma to carry out their metabolic reactions. Water and dissolved solutes filter through the very porous capillary membranes into the interstitial spaces. Once water and solutes move out of the plasma into the tissue spaces they are called interstitial fluid. Plasma and interstitial fluid are very similar except that plasma retains proteins, which cannot leave the capillary because capillary pores are smaller than proteins. The smaller proteins, such as albumin, can pass through the pores and are found in interstitial fluid. Tissue cells extract nutrients and water from the interstitial fluid that the cells use to carry out their functions.

interstitial fluid

Reabsorption

Metabolic processes take place constantly and therefore waste products are continuously produced by tissue

metabolic processes
↓
waste products
↓
reabsorption of interstitial fluid into vascular system
↓
excretion

cells. The waste products must be removed from the tissues or they will cause fluid and acid-base imbalances. Reabsorption is an ongoing function in the removal of waste products. Tissue cells excrete waste products into the interstitial fluid, which is then reabsorbed into the vascular and lymphatic capillaries and returned to the vascular system for transport to various organs for excretion. Fluid and solutes that leave the capillary must ultimately be returned to the circulatory system to maintain blood volume.

Hydrostatic Pressure

capillary blood pressure: about 35 mm Hg

Blood entering the capillary has a pressure imparted to it from the force of the heart contracting. This is called hydrostatic pressure, or capillary blood pressure, and is about 35 mm Hg. The hydrostatic pressure forces water and solutes to filter through capillary pores into the interstitial spaces.

Osmotic Pressure

about 35 mm Hg

As fluid filters from plasma through the capillary pores into the interstitial space the increased concentration of proteins in the capillary creates osmotic pressure. This pressure is about 35 mm Hg and determined by the concentration of proteins in the capillary blood. The osmotic pressure acts like a magnet and pulls interstitial fluid from the interstitial space back into the capillary.

FIGURE 10.3 Principle of Osmosis

Osmosis characterizes the movement of water across a semipermeable membrane from an area of lower solute concentration to one of greater solute concentration. The movement of water stops when the concentrations are approximately equal. In the body, osmotic pressure exerted by protein solutes is responsible for the return of interstitial fluid (water) into the vascular space via capillary pores.

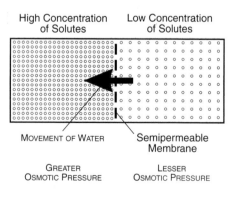

High Concentration of Solutes   Low Concentration of Solutes

MOVEMENT OF WATER   Semipermeable Membrane

GREATER OSMOTIC PRESSURE   LESSER OSMOTIC PRESSURE

Interstitial fluid that is not pulled into the capillary by osmotic pressure is returned to the circulatory system by the lymphatic channels. If fluid remained in the interstitial space, edema would develop. Any conditions that affect hydrostatic pressure or osmotic pressure create tissue edema.

Edema

Swelling of tissue spaces caused by the retention of fluid is called edema. Causes of edema include: increased hydrostatic pressure from venous blockage or from arteriole constriction; decreased concentration of proteins in the plasma from starvation, dietary deficiency, liver disease, and kidney disease; increased capillary permeability such as occurs following burns, allergic reactions, and inflammation; and the obstruction of lymphatic channels, such as destruction due to surgical procedures.

■   **QUESTIONS**   ■

1. Describe the function of plasma in the physiology of the body.

2. Identify six of the solutes dissolved in plasma that make up about 10% of its volume.

3. The two main types of solutes are protein and nonprotein molecules. True or False?

4. Most plasma solutes are in constant communication with body cells. There are two exceptions. What are they?

5. What does plasma look like?

6. Why is plasma of particular importance to medical professionals?

7. What is serum? and how is it different from plasma?

8. What three mechanisms help maintain a balanced blood volume throughout the body?

9. Identify two major clinical complications associated with fluid imbalances.

10. How are plasma proteins important in the maintenance of blood volume in the body?

11. What are the three main classes of proteins found in plasma?

12. Classify the main functions associated with the three classes of protein in plasma.

13. Identify five causes of protein deficiency.

14. What kinds of problems can protein deficiency cause?

15. Define paraprotein.

16. Electrolyte disturbances have profound effects on the body. Give four examples.

17. What causes hyperviscosity of the blood and how is it treated?

18. What do electrolytes, lipids, carbohydrates, and vitamins have in common?

19. List the five main electrolytes in the blood.

20. Why are normal concentrations of electrolytes in plasma important in human physiology?

21. What is the role of bicarbonate in the blood?

22. When does filtration occur in the body? and how is plasma different from interstitial fluid?

23. When does reabsorption occur? and why is it important?

24. Contrast hydrostatic pressure with osmotic pressure.

CHAPTER 11

Platelets

Introduction

Platelets are called thrombocytes. They are small, colorless, enucleated (lacking a nucleus) bodies found in blood. These formed elements play a vital role in preventing blood loss from damaged blood vessels, a function known as hemostasis. When endothelium, the inner lining of a blood vessel, is traumatized and blood loss occurs, platelets cover the injured site forming a platelet plug. This plug helps to reduce further blood loss until the process called coagulation establishes a fibrin clot.

thrombocytes

hemostasis

coagulation

Platelets contain numerous organelles (bodies), such as alpha granules, dense bodies, microtubules, and filaments. Alpha granules and dense bodies contain molecules that play vital roles in hemostasis, inflammation, and wound healing. Examples of these molecules are adenosine diphosphate (ADP), von Willebrand factor (vWF), serotonin, and fibronectin. Microtubules and filaments are essential in maintaining platelet shape and assisting in clot retraction.

platelet organelles:
alpha granules
dense bodies
ADP
vWF
microtubules
filaments

Platelets develop in the bone marrow from megakaryocytes, which are large cells that undergo fragmentation of their cytoplasm to form platelets. A megakaryocyte is between 35 to 150μ in diameter. Platelet production is predominantly under the control of a glycoprotein hormone called thrombopoietin.

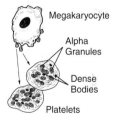

Megakaryocyte

Alpha Granules

Dense Bodies

Platelets

thrombopoietin

Shape, Life Span, and Location

Platelets range in size from 2 to 4μ. When forming a platelet plug they change from a flattened to a

177

spherical shape. They also extend long pseudopods and develop spikelike structures on their outer membrane. All structural changes of platelets aid in their adhesion to damaged endothelium.

life span:
9 to 12 days

Platelets have a life span of 9 to 12 days. Young platelets are thought to be the most effective in achieving and maintaining a platelet plug. Old, damaged, and nonfunctional platelets are removed from the circulatory system by macrophages in the spleen and liver.

sequestration

Once platelets are released from bone marrow into the circulatory system, they migrate to the spleen where they spend time before returning to the bloodstream. The retention of platelets in the spleen is called sequestration. About one third of platelets are sequestered in the spleen at any one time.

Numbers

150,000 to 450,000 per microliter

The normal platelet count in all individuals ranges from 150 to 450 x 10^3/uL, (150 to 450 x 10^9/L). The average count is 250 x 10^9/L.

Thrombocytosis and Thrombocytopenia

thrombocytosis:
platelet increase
thrombocytopenia:
platelet decrease

An increase in the number of platelets above 450 x 10^9/L is called thrombocytosis, also called thrombocythemia, and a decrease in the platelet count below 150 x 10^9/L is called thrombocytopenia. Both disorders can result from congenital or acquired defects, such as thrombasthenia (platelets function abnormally), gray platelet syndrome (platelets cannot adhere to endothelium), chronic infections, malignancies, and blood diseases, such as iron deficiency anemia.

Hemostasis

prevention of blood loss

vascular integrity

Hemostasis refers to the prevention of blood loss from the body. Normally, blood is not lost from the closed, intact vascular system. Vascular integrity exists when there are no mechanical breaks in blood vessel walls.

When trauma is inflicted on a blood vessel, the body relies on its hemostatic mechanisms to inhibit blood loss and restore endothelial tissue.

Hemostasis is one of the most important physiological events that occurs in the body. An understanding of hemostasis and its highly complex chemical reactions is derived from clinical research on individuals with bleeding disorders and in vitro (outside the body) experiments performed in the laboratory.

VASCULAR DAMAGE AND LOSS OF VASCULAR INTEGRITY

Denuded (Damaged) Endothelium

Normal Endothelial Lining

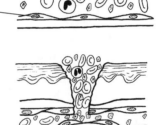

1. VASCULAR CONSTRICTION REDUCES BLOOD FLOW.

2. PLATELETS FORM A TEMPORARY PLUG OVER THE AREA OF DAMAGE. COAGULATION FACTORS BECOME ACTIVATED THEREBY INITIATING THE FORMATION OF A FIBRIN CLOT WITHIN THE COAGULATION CASCADE.

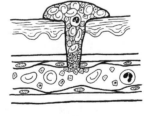

3. THE COAGULATION CASCADE IS COMPLETED AND FIBRIN IS DEPOSITED. STABLIZATION OF THE FIBRIN CLOT OCCURS. FIBRIN THREADS FORM A MESHWORK OVER THE PLATELET PLUG.

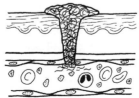

FIGURE 11.1 Steps in Hemostasis and Coagulation

Hemostatic Processes

Processes preventing blood loss include: (1) vascular spasm, (2) platelet plug formation, (3) coagulation protein activation, leading to clot formation and finally, (4) clot lysis, the breakdown of a fibrin clot. These steps occur in the sequence given, and each is essential for normal hemostasis. A defect in any step leads to continued blood loss.

immediate hemostatic responses: vasoconstriction

The most immediate hemostatic response to blood vessel injury is vascular spasm, also called vasoconstriction. Smooth muscle fibers and elastic tissue within walls of blood vessels cause the vessel to constrict, thereby slowing blood flow and allowing the platelets to attach to the damaged endothelium.

Other events occur simultaneously with vascular spasm and assist in the prevention of blood loss. They are the following:

edema

- Tissue spaces swell as the result of increased fluid leakage from the damaged vessel.

chemical release

- Endothelial cells of blood vessel walls release molecules (serotonin, adenosine diphosphate, von Willebrand factor, and fibronectin, and others) that assist platelet aggregation.

shunting of blood flow

- Blood flow is shunted or redirected to nearby vessels.

temporary platelet plug formation

Following vascular spasm, platelets form a temporary plug at the site of injury. This plug provides an effective barrier against further blood loss until a fibrin clot can form.

Hemostasis via platelet plug and fibrin clot formation is effective in small to medium size arteries and veins. Larger size vessels require surgical intervention (sutures) to stop bleeding. Capillaries can usually arrest bleeding with a platelet plug only.

Vascular Endothelium

Normal, intact vascular endothelium does not support platelet adhesion or fibrin clot formation. Only damaged endothelium exposes molecules that activate blood coagulation. When vascular damage does occur, the endothelial lining plays an active and important role in hemostasis. Vessel walls release molecules that (1) attach themselves to activated platelets, (2) assist in fibrin clot formation, and (3) are involved with clot dissolution. Endothelial cells produce anticoagulants, such as antithrombin III (AT-III) and thrombomodulin; vasodilators; clot inhibitors, such as the prostaglandin PGI_2; and fibrinolytics that lyse fibrin clots, such as tissue plasminogen activator (tPA). For clot lysis, see Ch. 12, Coagulation.

anticoagulants: AT-III, thrombomodulin

vasodilators and clot inhibitors

fibrinolytics: tPA

Steps in Platelet Plug Formation

The role of platelets in coagulation begins with the formation of the platelet plug. There are five steps involved in platelet plug formation.

(1) The first step involves contact between platelets and damaged endothelium. The damaged endothelial surface releases molecules, (von Willebrand factor, serotonin, fibronectin, ADP, and others) that attach to platelet membrane receptors allowing the platelets to adhere to the damaged endothelium. These molecules appear only on damaged tissue.

contact

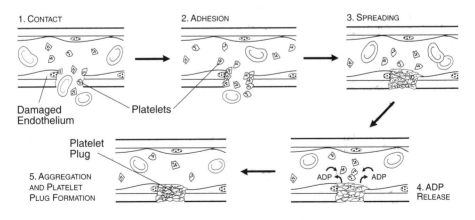

FIGURE 11.2 Steps in Platelet Plug Formation
The formation of a platelet plug is essential for the formation of a fibrin clot. A platelet plug is temporary until a stable fibrin clot is formed.

adhesion

(2) The second step involves adhesion. Platelets are attracted to the site of injury where they adhere to the damaged endothelial surface.

spreading

(3) The third step is called spreading. Platelets spread out along the damaged surface, changing their shape in this process.

ADP release

(4) The fourth step involves adenosine diphosphate (ADP) release. Adenosine diphosphate is a molecule that platelets release, thereby stimulating platelet aggregation in the damaged area.

aggregation

(5) The fifth and final step involves aggregation. Platelets aggregate at the site of injury forming a platelet plug.

Platelet Function in Fibrin Clot Formation

PF-3

Development of the platelet plug is only a temporary means to arrest blood flow. A platelet plug is sometimes called a white thrombus. As the platelet plug is forming, platelets release platelet factor 3 (PF-3). PF-3 binds certain clotting factors leading to fibrin clot formation over the platelet plug. Once the fibrin clot has formed, fibroblasts (connective tissue cells) trapped in the platelet plug and endothelial cells help repair the damaged endothelium. A molecule released by platelet granules, called platelet-derived growth factor, stimulates smooth muscle cells in the vessel wall to advance vessel healing.

fibroblasts
endothelial cells

platelet-derived
growth factor

Prostaglandins that Regulate ADP Release in Platelet Aggregation

thromboxane and
prostacyclin

Prostaglandins are molecules that regulate the amount of ADP released by platelets. The most important prostaglandins are thromboxane A_2 (TXA$_2$) and prostacyclin (PGI$_2$). These molecules work antagonistically to increase or decrease ADP release.

TXA$_2$ increases
ADP release

TXA$_2$ is synthesized by the platelet membrane. It increases ADP release to ensure that an adequate amount of platelets appears at the site of injury and

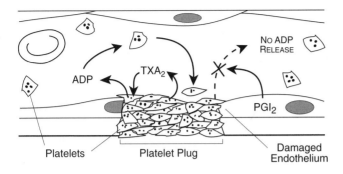

FIGURE 11.3 **Prostaglandins that Control Platelet Plug Formation**

When endothelial tissue is damaged, platelets release ADP. This chemical promotes the aggregation of platelets. The prostaglandin TXA_2 in platelet membranes increases the release of ADP. The prostaglandin PGI_2 is produced by endothelial cells and decreases the release of ADP. Together the prostaglandins maintain platelet aggregation at the site of injury.

forms a platelet plug. If there is an inadequate number of platelets, or platelet quality is poor, no plug forms.

Prostacyclin is synthesized by the endothelial cells lining blood vessels. It inhibits ADP release, therefore, PGI_2 prevents platelets from aggregating past the site of endothelial damage where they can block blood flow through the vessel.

PGI_2 inhibits ADP release

Role of Aspirin

Aspirin interferes with normal platelet aggregation. Doctors often prescribe aspirin for patients, as they say, "to help thin the blood." Aspirin does not thin the blood, however, but it does help to reduce the formation of blood clots. Because aspirin blocks the action of TXA_2, it prevents ADP release and platelet aggregation. The ability to form a platelet plug or a stable fibrin clot is diminished. The theory behind aspirin therapy is to prevent patients from forming clots that lead either to a cerebral vascular accident (CVA; stroke) or to a heart attack (coronary artery

aspirin blocks action of TXA_2 and prevents ADP release and platelet aggregation

thrombosis). Aspirin is not recommended as a pain reliever anytime the potential for bleeding exists, for example, following surgery or labor and delivery.

Platelet Aggregation on Foreign Surfaces

All foreign surfaces can initiate platelet aggregation and inappropriate clot formation. A foreign surface is any substance to which blood is not normally exposed, such as catheters, needles, immune complexes, and plastic containers. When blood comes into contact with a foreign surface, platelets aggregate and attach to the surface. When platelets aggregate, they release molecules (such as ADP, PF-3, and vWF) and clot formation is initiated.

Platelet Disorders

quantitative
qualitative

Platelet disorders are congenital or acquired abnormalities that prevent platelets from performing their intended function of forming a stable, functioning platelet plug and ultimately a fibrin clot. The disorders can be (1) quantitative, referring to platelet numbers and/or (2) qualitative, referring to platelet quality. Quantitative disorders are diagnosed by platelet count while qualitative disorders are assessed by the bleeding time.

Thrombocytosis

increased
platelet count
↓
platelet aggregation
and/or bleeding

There are three types of thrombocytosis that cause an increase in the platelet count. They are: (1) transitory, (2) reactive, and (3) primary, also called essential thrombocythemia. Increased platelet numbers may cause platelet aggregation and/or the tendency to bleed.

platelets released from
sequestration sites

Transitory Thrombocytosis   This form of thrombocytosis occurs, for example, following exercise, physical stress, and following the administration of epinephrine. It is believed that an increase of platelet numbers, in the range of 450 to 600 x 10^9/L, occurs because platelets are released from sequestration sites, such as the lungs, spleen, and other yet unidentified sites. They are circulating platelets; in other words, transitory thrombocytosis cannot be attributed to increased platelet production within the bone marrow. After the initiating event platelet numbers return to normal.

Reactive Thrombocytosis When the platelet numbers range from 600 to 800 x 10^9/L, reactive thrombocytosis is indicated. It is the result of increased platelet production in the bone marrow. Certain disease states, such as inflammatory disorders, iron deficiency anemia, trauma, lymphomas, other malignancies, hemolytic anemias, and certain chemotherapeutic agents are associated with reactive thrombocytosis.

increased platelet production in bone marrow

Primary Thrombocythemia This condition is a myeloproliferative disorder of stem cells indicated by a large increase in platelet numbers. Platelet numbers may be as high as 1,000 x 10^9/L. Defective stem cells cause myeloproliferation of megakaryocytes. Primary thrombocythemia is treated by radiation therapy or cytotoxic drug therapy to destroy some of the platelets. Platelet numbers can also be reduced by plateletpheresis. Increased platelets can make an individual more susceptible either to abnormal thrombus formation within blood vessels or to increased bleeding episodes. Thrombocythemia usually indicates that platelet quality is defective. Therefore, bleeding is the more common finding.

myeloproliferative disorder

Thrombocytopenia

A low platelet count indicates thrombocytopenia. Bleeding is likely to occur when platelet numbers are low because there are not enough platelets available to form a plug over the damaged endothelium. Thrombocytopenia is diagnosed when the count falls below 100 x 10^9/L. This disorder most commonly causes increased bleeding, but usually bleeding is not a problem until the platelet count falls below 50 x 10^9/L. When platelet numbers are dangerously low (20 x 10^9/L), brain and gastrointestinal hemorrhage can be major causes of mortality. A classic sign of decreased platelets is easy bruising of the skin.

low platelet count

Causes   A low platelet count can be due to decreased or ineffective production in bone marrow, shortened survival due to either increased consumption or increased destruction of platelets, sequestration in the spleen or liver, and finally, dilution of platelets in the circulation following massive transfusion. Causes of thrombocytopenia include the following:

thrombasthenia

- Thrombasthenia is a congenital stem cell disorder that prevents platelets from aggregating because they cannot release chemicals.

storage pool disease

- Storage pool disease is an congenital disorder that causes platelets to be larger than normal and prevents platelets from aggregating.

surgery and medical conditions

- Platelet destruction occurs following some types of surgery or is due to medical conditions.

treatment and transfusion reactions

- Platelet destruction can occur from radiation, chemotherapy, and transfusion reactions.

diseases

- Platelet destruction can occur from certain diseases, such as bone tumor, other cancers, chronic infections, and leukemia.

alloimmunization

- Alloimmunization (alloantibody formation) to platelet antigens following platelet transfusions causes platelet destruction.

hypersplenism

- Hypersplenism (premature removal of platelets) can lead to platelet destruction.

DIC

- Platelet destruction occurs in disseminated intravascular coagulation (DIC), a disorder in which platelets are consumed in a clotting event (see Ch. 12, Coagulation).

alcoholism

- Alcoholism can destroy platelets.

Platelet Quality

ability or inability to form stable platelet plug

Platelet quality refers to the ability or inability of platelets to form a stable platelet plug. When platelet quality is affected, platelets do not function properly and are unable to form a stable platelet plug, therefore, bleeding occurs. Aside from thrombocytosis or thrombocytopenia, there are many diseases and conditions that affect the platelets' ability to form a platelet plug. For example, certain drugs can affect the quality of platelets. Withholding these drugs can help restore platelet quality.

Drugs that affect platelet function include:

- Aspirin and ibuprofen, which depress platelet function (They should not be given to individuals likely to bleed.)
- Exogenous heparin (derived from animal products), which causes platelets to clump together even though it is an anticoagulant
- Protamine, which is used to reverse the effects of heparin
- Dextran, which is used as a volume expander following blood loss (see Ch. 17, Component Therapy)
- Some antibiotics, such as penicillin
- Some anesthetics, such as halothane

Conditions and diseases that affect platelet quality include:

- Bernard-Soulier Syndrome (congenital)
- Glanzmann's Disease (congenital)
- Transfusion reactions
- Splenomegaly
- Autoimmune disorders
- Multiple myeloma
- Cirrhosis
- Uremia
- Storage of platelets at cool temperatures, which causes them to clump and become dysfunctional
- Fibrin split products (FSPs), small pieces of fibrin released into circulation once a clot is dissolved, which prevent platelet plug formation if their concentrations are high (see Ch. 12, Coagulation)

Diagnostic Tests for Platelet Disorders

Bleeding time and platelet count are two diagnostic blood tests that help determine whether a patient has

platelet count
bleeding time

a platelet disorder. By comparing these two tests, a physician can diagnose whether the disorder is due to an inadequate number of platelets (platelet count) or due to poor platelet quality (bleeding time; see Blood Tests).

Treatment for Platelet Disorders

Depending on the cause of the disorder, a platelet transfusion can sometimes reverse inadequate platelet numbers by adding good quality donor platelets to the circulation. There are certain situations in which platelet transfusion may not alleviate bleeding, for example, if platelets are destroyed by immune reactions.

▪ QUESTIONS ▪

1. What is another name for platelets?

2. Platelets are enucleated formed elements. True or False?

3. Describe the vital role of platelets in hemostasis.

4. At some point in their life span, platelets change from a flattened to a spherical shape. When does this happen?

5. Explain sequestration.

6. Compare thrombocytosis and thrombocytopenia.

7. Define vascular integrity.

8. Identify the four steps in the hemostatic process.

9. Normal, intact vascular endothelium does not support platelet adhesion or fibrin clot formation. Describe the functioning of damaged endothelium.

10. A platelet plug is a temporary phenomenon. What five steps are involved in its formation? When is it replaced?

11. What is another name for a platelet plug?

12. What are the molecules that regulate the amount of ADP release by the platelets called? Name two.

13. Does aspirin really "thin the blood"? Explain your answer.

14. What happens when blood comes into contact with a foreign surface such as catheter tubing?

15. Describe the three types of thrombocytosis and their causes.

16. What happens in thrombocytopenia that may be life-threatening?

17. List at least five causes of thrombocytopenia.

18. Identify three drugs that affect platelet function.

19. What are the two major diagnostic tests for platelet disorders?

CHAPTER **12**

Coagulation

Introduction

Coagulation is the process whereby soluble plasma proteins become activated in response to vascular injury and form a blood clot that arrests blood flow. Fibrin is the end product of coagulation and forms a net, or meshwork, over a platelet plug stabilizing it and anchoring it in place. Fibrin formation following vessel damage is a natural response to endothelial damage and occurs by a chain reaction called the coagulation cascade. Following vessel repair, clot dissolution must occur so that blood flow through the vessel returns.

Vascular spasm and platelet plug formation make up primary hemostasis while coagulation is responsible for secondary hemostasis. Both primary and secondary hemostasis are essential for generating a stable fibrin clot. In addition to preventing further blood loss, secondary hemostasis assists in repairing the endothelial lining.

primary hemostasis
secondary hemostasis

Deficiencies of coagulation factors lead to hemostatic disorders that cause bleeding. Disorders of hemostasis can also cause thrombus (blood clot) formation within the vasculature, which leads to tissue necrosis.

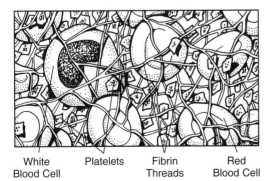

White   Platelets   Fibrin   Red
Blood Cell   Threads   Blood Cell

FIGURE 12.1 Fibrin Clot

This schematic representation depicts fibrin threads trapping blood elements within the fibrin clot.

Pathways of Coagulation

intrinsic and
extrinsic pathways

The coagulation cascade involves two pathways: the intrinsic and the extrinsic. The traditional theory of coagulation states that either pathway can initiate coagulation. The activating event determines which pathway is activated: damaged tissue activates the extrinsic, whereas a foreign (nonendothelial) surface activates the intrinsic. Current evidence indicates that only the extrinsic pathway initiates in vivo (inside the body) clot formation, whereas the intrinsic pathway is essential for adding fibrin to the developing blood clot.

The term extrinsic is used to indicate that tissue factor, which activates the extrinsic pathway, is not normally found in the blood; it comes from sources outside the blood. The term intrinsic is used to indicate that all components necessary for coagulation are found within the blood.

Knowledge of the intrinsic and extrinsic pathways and how they are activated is attained from (1) studying individuals with clotting factor deficiencies and (2) in vitro experiments (outside the body). However, what happens in vivo is not necessarily the same as that which happens in vitro and, therefore, theories about in vivo coagulation can only be assumed.

Coagulation Components

coagulation factors
TF (TT)
PF-3
Ca^{++}

The chemical components required to form a stable fibrin clot include: coagulation factors, also called coagulation proteins; tissue factor (TF), also called tissue thromboplastin (TT); platelet factor 3 (PF-3), also called platelet membrane phospholipid; and calcium ions (Ca^{++}).

circulate in the
inactive form

Coagulation factors are glycoproteins, with each factor having a molecular weight greater than 40,000 daltons (unit of mass). The majority of coagulation factors are synthesized by hepatocytes within the liver. When released from the liver, clotting factors circulate in their inactive form. If they circulated in their active form, clot formation would occur throughout the vasculature.

The coagulation proteins are referred to by Roman numerals assigned in the order in which the factors were discovered and not in the order in which they react in the coagulation cascade. The exceptions are factor III, which is typically referred to as tissue factor, and factor IV, which is referred to as calcium. A Roman numeral followed by "a" (for example, Va) indicates that the factor has been cleaved (split) and, therefore, is activated and ready to activate the next factor in the sequence.

Coagulation proteins are grouped according to their function in coagulation. Factors XII, XI, IX, VII, and II are serine protease cleavage enzymes: they split other factors. Factors V, VIII, and tissue factor are referred to as cofactors or helper factors: their presence is required for a reaction to occur. Factors II, VII, IX, and X are called vitamin K-dependent factors because they require vitamin K for their synthesis.

coagulation proteins:

serine protease
cleavage enzymes
cofactors

vitamin K-
dependent factors

Accessory Elements of Coagulation

Tissue Factor   Tissue factor is a complex molecule released from the membranes of damaged cells. It contains both a protein and phospholipid component, each of which is essential for initiating the coagulation cascade via the extrinsic pathway. Tissue factor is found in the cell membranes of blood cells, skin, bowel, heart and lungs, among others. It has a molecular weight of 44,000 daltons.

Platelet Factor 3   Platelet factor 3 (PF-3) is a phospholipid released by aggregated platelets. This molecule is essential for coagulation factors to bind to the platelet membrane. Platelet factor 3 is not usually present in plasma except when released by the membranes of aggregated platelets.

Calcium   Calcium (Ca^{++}) is a positive ion, or cation, found in plasma. It has many important functions within the body, and one of them is to assist in fibrin clot formation. Calcium is needed in coagulation to form a chemical bridge between a coagulation factor and PF-3. Its concentration is 8.5 to 10.5 mg/dL.

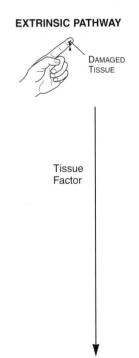

EXTRINSIC PATHWAY

DAMAGED
TISSUE

Tissue
Factor

Coagulation Factors and Their Functions

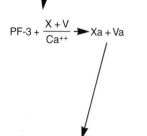

VIIa ◄──── VII + Ca++

IX + VIII ➤ IXa + VIIIa

PF-3 + $\dfrac{X + V}{Ca^{++}}$ ➤ Xa + Va

Factor VII/Proconvertin   Factor VII has a plasma concentration of 0.05 mg/dL and a molecular weight of 48,000 daltons. It is a vitamin K-dependent factor produced in the liver. Factor VII is the first vitamin K-dependent factor affected if a vitamin K deficiency occurs. Factor VII is a stable factor; that is, it is not easily degraded. It reacts with tissue factors and Ca++ to form VIIa in order to initiate coagulation.

Factor IX/Christmas Factor   Factor IX is a vitamin K-dependent factor with a molecular weight of 55,000 daltons. It has a plasma concentration of 0.3 mg/dL. Factor IXa, along with factor VIIIa, converts factors X and V to Xa and Va. Factor IX is deficient in plasma of individuals with hemophilia B or Christmas disease.

Factor VIII/Antihemophilic Factor   Factor VIII has a molecular weight of 330,000 daltons and a plasma concentration of 0.01 mg/dL. The function of factor VIII is to speed up the conversion of factor X to factor Xa by factor IXa. This reaction requires Ca++ and PF-3. Factor VIII is deficient in individuals with classic hemophilia, also called hemophilia A.

Von Willebrand Factor   Von Willebrand factor (vWF) is synthesized by vascular endothelium and platelets. It has a plasma concentration of 1 mg/dL and a molecular weight of 250,000 daltons. Von Willebrand factor functions as a carrier molecule for factor VIII. It also plays an essential role in primary hemostasis by allowing platelets to adhere to damaged endothelium. Individuals with von Willebrand's disease have either a deficiency of or low levels of vWF and, therefore, have a bleeding disorder.

Factor X/Stuart Factor   Factor X is another vitamin K-dependent factor. Its plasma concentration is 1 mg/dL and its molecular weight is 59,000 daltons. Along with factor Va, factor Xa cleaves factor II (prothrombin) to its active form factor IIa (thrombin).

Factor V/Proaccelerin   Factor V has a molecular weight of 330,000 daltons. It is produced in the liver and has a plasma concentration of 1 mg/dL. Although factor V is not a serine protease, it functions as a cofactor, or helper factor, in coagulation. Factor Va assists factor Xa in cleaving prothrombin. Proaccelerin is a labile factor, that is, easily degraded. It is deficient in certain stored blood components, such as Whole Blood, but is retained in fresh frozen plasma.

Factor II/Prothrombin   Prothrombin is a vitamin K–dependent coagulation factor synthesized in the liver. It has a plasma concentration of 10 mg/dL and a molecular weight of 70,000 daltons. When prothrombin is cleaved by factors Xa and Va it forms thrombin (factor IIa). Thrombin production requires PF-3 and Ca^{++} as well. In addition to cleaving fibrinogen, thrombin activates factor XIII and protein C.

Factor I/Fibrinogen   The inactive form, or precursor, of fibrin is fibrinogen. It is a soluble plasma protein with a molecular weight of 340,000 daltons. Factor I is produced in the liver and has a plasma concentration of 200 to 400 mg/dL. The plasma level of fibrinogen is determined by its production in the liver. Fibrinogen is cleaved (split) by the enzyme thrombin to produce fibrin, the tough, insoluble threads that form the net over the platelet plug.

Factor XIII/Fibrin Stabilizing Factor   Factor XIII has a molecular weight of 320,000 daltons and a plasma concentration of 1 to 2 mg/dL. This factor is converted to XIIIa by the enzymatic action of thrombin. Factor XIIIa stabilizes the platelet plug by crosslinking the fibrin threads with one another. A deficiency of factor XIII leads to increased bleeding, poor wound healing, and an increased incidence of abortion.

Contact Activation Factors

The following factors are called contact activation factors because they become activated when blood comes into contact with foreign surfaces. "Foreign" refers to nonendothelial substances not normally present in the blood. Contact activation factors are not involved in in vivo (inside the body) coagulation.

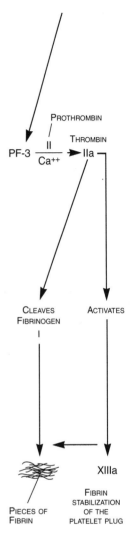

Factor XI/Plasma Thromboplastin Antecedent (PTA)
Factor XI is a serine protease enzyme with a molecular
weight of 160,000 daltons and a plasma concentration
of 0.5 mg/dL. It has a very limited function in in
vivo coagulation. In the traditional description of the
intrinsic pathway, factor XI activates factors IX and VIII.

Factor XII/Hageman Factor   Factor XII is a serine
protease with a molecular weight of 80,000 daltons and
a plasma concentration of 3 mg/dL. Factor XII has no
function in in vivo coagulation; it is activated only
when blood contacts foreign surfaces.

The Extrinsic Pathway

Traditional Theory   The extrinsic pathway, or tissue
factor pathway, is activated by the release of tissue
factor from damaged tissue into the bloodstream. Along
with Ca^{++}, tissue factor binds factor VII converting it
to factor VIIa. Factor VIIa in turn activates factors X
and V. Factors Xa and Va then split prothrombin into
thrombin. Factors X and V are the starting point of
the final common pathway, where the intrinsic and
extrinsic pathways share the same chemical reactions.

Current Theory   All in vivo coagulation is activated
by the release of tissue factor into the bloodstream.
The most recent evidence indicates that factor VIIa
activates factors IX and VIII rather than activating
factors X and V as held in the traditional theory.
Factors IXa and VIIIa in turn activate factors X and V.

The Intrinsic Pathway

Traditional Theory   The intrinsic pathway is initiated
through the contact of clotting factor XII with surfaces
not normally present in blood, such as plastic catheters,
blood collection bags, and molecules, such as collagen.
Factor XIIa activates factor XI to XIa. Factor XIa
activates factors IX and VIII. Factors IXa and VIIIa
then activate factors X and V. Factors Xa and Va
convert prothrombin to thrombin.

The intrinsic pathway, or contact activation pathway, is
activated when blood comes into contact with any

INTRINSIC PATHWAY

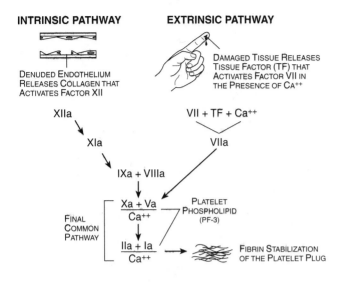

DENUDED ENDOTHELIUM
RELEASES COLLAGEN THAT
ACTIVATES FACTOR XII

EXTRINSIC PATHWAY

DAMAGED TISSUE RELEASES
TISSUE FACTOR (TF) THAT
ACTIVATES FACTOR VII IN
THE PRESENCE OF Ca^{++}

XIIa

XIa

VII + TF + Ca^{++}

VIIa

IXa + VIIIa

FINAL
COMMON
PATHWAY

$\dfrac{Xa + Va}{Ca^{++}}$

PLATELET
PHOSPHOLIPID
(PF-3)

$\dfrac{IIa + Ia}{Ca^{++}}$

FIBRIN STABILIZATION
OF THE PLATELET PLUG

FIGURE 12.2 **Traditional Coagulation Cascade**

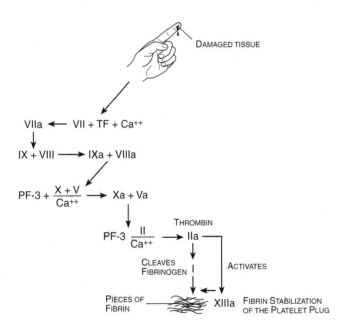

DAMAGED TISSUE

VIIa ⟵ VII + TF + Ca^{++}

IX + VIII ⟶ IXa + VIIIa

PF-3 + $\dfrac{X + V}{Ca^{++}}$ ⟶ Xa + Va

PF-3 $\dfrac{II}{Ca^{++}}$ ⟶ IIa

THROMBIN

CLEAVES
FIBRINOGEN   I

ACTIVATES

PIECES OF
FIBRIN

XIIIa

FIBRIN STABILIZATION
OF THE PLATELET PLUG

FIGURE 12.3 **Current Theory of In Vivo Coagulation**

foreign surface, such as glass or plastic, among numerous other substances not normally found in blood.

Current Theory   Present research indicates that factor XII has no function in the initiation of in vivo coagulation. Also, activation of factors IX and VIII is believed to occur by factor VIIa rather than factor XIa.

Monitoring the Coagulation Pathways

PT

aPTT

PTT

The prothrombin time (PT) is the coagulation test that monitors the extrinsic pathway. The activated partial thromboplastin time (aPTT) and the partial thromboplastin time (PTT) are the coagulation tests that monitor the intrinsic pathway (see Blood Tests).

The Final Common Pathway

Traditional Theory   In the traditional theory of coagulation the final common pathway is so named because the intrinsic and extrinsic pathways converge and share the same reactions leading to fibrin formation. Through activation by the extrinsic pathway, factors X and V is activated by factor VIIa. Through the intrinsic pathway, factors X and V is activated by factors IXa and VIIIa. Factors Xa and Va along with PF-3 and Ca^{++} cleaves prothrombin (factor II) into thrombin. Factor IIa (thrombin) with Ca^{++} and PF-3 split factor I (fibrinogen) into smaller units of fibrin called fibrin monomers. Fibrin monomers attach themselves to the platelet plug. Through the activation of factor XIII the fibrin threads are crosslinked, creating a meshwork over it and anchoring it place.

fibrin monomers

Current Theory   The activation of factors X and V occurs by factors IXa and VIIIa and not by factor VIIa. Fibrin monomers create a meshwork over the platelet plug. This is referred to as the soft clot. The soft clot is stabilized by factor XIIIa forming the hard clot.

soft clot

Clot Retraction

Clot retraction is the contraction, or firming up, of the platelet plug forming the hard clot. The shortening of protein fibers and microtubules in the platelet membrane is responsible. Clot retraction aids in vessel repair because during retraction the wound edges of the damaged vessel come closer together. As the vessel heals, the fibrin clot is slowly broken down (lysed) by plasmin, allowing blood flow to resume through the vessel. Vascular integrity is restored when endothelial damage is repaired and blood flow resumes.

Clot Lysis and Vascular Repair

Clot lysis, also called fibrinolysis, is the dissolution (breakdown) of the fibrin clot in a vessel. Fibrinolysis is nature's way of restoring blood flow through a blood vessel that has been injured and repaired itself. A clot must dissolve slowly or bleeding will resume if dissolution progresses before adequate healing takes place.

fibrinolysis

Although coagulation and fibrinolysis are two separate cascades, each assists in the repair of vascular injury. Coagulation controls the formation of fibrin, and fibrinolysis controls the breakdown of fibrin. Both processes work together to restore endothelium and the return of blood flow.

Plasminogen and Plasmin

Clot lysis is regulated by the protein plasmin. This protein is a serine protease that breaks the fibrin clot into small pieces called fibrin split products (FSPs) or fibrin degradation products (FDPs). Plasmin circulates in its inactive form called plasminogen, which is produced in the liver. Plasminogen has a molecular weight of 90,000 daltons and a plasma concentration of 20 to 40 mg/dL.

tissue cells
↓
tissue plasminogen
activators
(tPA, urokinase)
↓
plasminogen
↓
plasmin
↓
clot lysis
↓
FSPs

The cleavage of plasminogen by tissue plasminogen activators produces plasmin. Tissue plasminogen activators are molecules released by tissue cells and include tissue plasminogen activator (tPA) and urokinase. Streptokinase is a plasminogen activator produced by the bacteria beta-hemolytic streptococci. Urokinase and streptokinase have little function in in vivo clot lysis, but are used therapeutically to break down inappropriate clot formation within the vasculature, for example, following a myocardial infarction.

plasma inhibitors:
PAI-1 inactivates tPA
and urokinase

a_2-PI prevents
plasminogen from
binding to fibrin

Plasmin production is regulated by plasma inhibitors, which maintain low levels of plasmin within the blood. Plasma inhibitors include plasminogen activator inhibitor (PAI-1) and alpha$_2$-plasmin inhibitor (a_2-PI). PAI-1 is released into the blood by endothelial cells where it inactivates tPA and urokinase. Alpha$_2$-plasmin inhibitor is a fast-acting inhibitor that blocks the binding of plasminogen to fibrin.

Natural Anticoagulants

AT-III, proteins C and S

Within plasma are natural anticoagulants, such as antithrombin III (AT-III) and proteins C and S. These molecules help prevent thrombosis (inappropriate clot formation) within the vasculature. Most natural anticoagulants inactivate thrombin formation by destroying any thrombin that forms. They also neutralize other activated clotting factors, such as Va, VIIIa, and Xa. Neutralization helps maintain fibrin formation at the site of vascular damage and prevent its occurrence elsewhere.

Vitamin K and Coumadin™

Vitamin K is a fat-soluble vitamin essential for blood coagulation. Its presence is necessary for the liver to synthesize factors II, VII, IX, and X, as well as proteins C and S. Vitamin K is found in green leafy vegetables, vegetable oils, and tomatoes.

warfarin

Coumadin™ is a synthetic anticoagulant that blocks the action of vitamin K by inhibiting a step in the synthesis of vitamin K-dependent clotting proteins. Coumadin's chemical name is warfarin. Coumadin is used for treating patients susceptible to developing blood clots. Individuals with mechanical heart valves and those susceptible to strokes are treated with Coumadin. Because Coumadin is not a fast-acting anticoagulant, it must be administered for a few days before clotting factor levels are low enough to prevent blood clotting.

Fibrin Split Products

When a fibrin clot dissolves, small pieces of fibrin, called fibrin split products (FSPs), are released into circulation. They must be removed from the blood, otherwise they become potent inhibitors of coagulation. Fibrin split products interfere with coagulation by preventing fibrin threads from crosslinking. They also inhibit platelet function by preventing platelets from adhering to damaged endothelium.

The concentration of FSPs in blood depends on the rate of clot breakdown and on the removal of FSPs by the reticuloendothelial system (RES) of the liver. High concentrations of FSPs in blood occur (1) when excessive clotting causes excess FSP formation and (2) when the liver is unable to clear FSPs from blood due to liver disease or liver failure.

Hemostatic Disorders

Hemostatic disorders are congenital or acquired defects that cause either (1) hemorrhage or (2) thrombosis within the vasculature. Hemorrhage manifests itself by bleeding. Hemorrhagic disorders include abnormalities in the vascular system, platelets, or coagulation factor deficiencies. Thrombotic disorders, called thrombophilia, manifest themselves through inappropriate clot formation within a blood vessel. Thrombus formation interferes with blood flow leading to tissue necrosis.

hemorrhagic

thrombotic/ thrombophilia

Congenital hemostatic disorders are caused by defective genes. They usually affect a single gene, afflict a person throughout life, and are relatively rare in the population.

congenital

acquired

Acquired hemostatic disorders are caused by conditions extraneous to the blood itself, such as drugs and kidney and liver disease. They usually exhibit a sudden onset and are more common than congenital disorders. For example, many clotting disorders are caused by liver disease because the liver synthesizes most coagulation proteins.

Hemorrhagic Disorders

Hemorrhagic disorders can be caused by any of the following congenital or acquired defects. Some examples are given.

Vascular disorders

- Hereditary telangiectasia (see below)
- Senile purpura (see below)
- Purpura of infection
- Penoch-Schonlein syndrome (blood vessel abnormality)
- Connective tissue disorders

Platelet disorders

- Thrombocytopenia
- Disorders of platelet function
- Aspirin therapy
- Uremia
- Heparin therapy
- Increased destruction of platelets
- Splenomegaly
- Von Willebrand's disease
- Autoimmune disorders

Coagulation factor disorders

- Hemophilia A or B
- Vitamin K deficiency
- Factor VII deficiency
- Antibodies to factor VIII
- Liver disease
- Coumadin™ therapy

Miscellaneous disorders

- Complications due to massive transfusions
- Renal disease
- Liver disease
- Disseminated intravascular coagulation
- Multiple myeloma

Vascular Disorders   Vascular defects can occur within the vessel wall or within the supporting tissue surrounding the vessel. Easy bruising and spontaneous bleeding from small blood vessels characterize vascular defects. Vascular defects appear mainly as ecchymoses (bruising; black and blue spots) or petechiae (pinpoint-size purple spots), both of which are indicators of bleeding into the skin. Bleeding associated with vascular defects can also occur from mucous membranes of the intestines, mouth, and nasopharynx.

ecchymoses
petechiae

An example of a genetic disorder is hereditary hemorrhagic telangiectasia, a defect that causes microvascular swelling most commonly in the blood vessels of the skin, mucous membranes, and internal organs. There are numerous acquired vascular defects, such as senile purpura (bleeding into the skin in the elderly), and purpura associated with infectious organisms, scurvy (a vitamin deficiency), and connective tissue disorders.

Platelet Disorders   For platelet disorders, see Chapter 9, Platelets and Hemostasis.

Coagulation Factor Disorders   Coagulation factor deficiencies are responsible for bleeding disorders, such as hemophilia A and B and von Willebrand's disease (vWD), a condition resulting from a deficiency of von Willebrand factor (vWF). Von Willebrand's disease affects both platelet aggregation and clot formation. This disease is a defect within the coagulation system that promotes increased bleeding. Platelet aggregation does not occur and there are decreased levels of factor VIII in the blood. Von Willebrand's disease can be due to either congenital or acquired defects.

vWD:
vWF deficiency

hemophilia A:
factor VIII deficiency
inhibitors against
factor VIII

Hemophilia A is a congenital hemostatic disorder that causes bleeding because the body cannot form a fibrin clot. It is due to a deficiency of coagulation factor VIII or the presence of inhibitors against factor VIII. It is predominantly found in males. Males receive a defective X chromosome from their mother.

hemophilia B:
factor IX deficiency
inhibitors against
factor IX

Hemophilia B, also called Christmas disease, is a disorder due to a deficiency of factor IX or the presence of inhibitors against it. Both instances cause increased bleeding. A deficiency of other factors, such as VII, X, XI, and I, also causes coagulation disorders.

Treatments for Hemorrhagic Disorders

Hemorrhagic disorders are treated according to the defect or deficiency. Many times vascular defects are not treatable. Preventive measures need to be taken. Platelet defects, for example, can be treated with platelet transfusions. Coagulation deficiencies are treated with clotting factor concentrates, fresh frozen plasma, or cryoprecipitate. Mild cases of von Willebrand's disease can be treated with the drug vasopressin (desmopressin acetate; DDAVP). More serious forms of vWD are treated with certain factor VIII concentrates, fresh frozen plasma, or cryoprecipitate, although the latter two are rarely used.

Tests for Bleeding Disorders

PT
aPTT

Bleeding time, platelet count, prothrombin time (PT), activated partial thromboplastin time (aPTT), and factor assays are tests used to diagnosis bleeding disorders (see Blood Tests for a list of tests that detect these disorders).

Thrombophilia

Thrombophilia refers to thrombotic disorders due to thrombosis within arteries and veins. Thrombus formation within arteries and veins differ as to cause. Arterial thrombi develop because platelets adhere to atheroma (plaque) built up along the arterial wall. The platelet-atheroma complex can break free and release tissue factor, thereby stimulating clot formation.

When clot formation occurs in arteries, organ failure results. Blood flow can not occur unless the clot is removed or dissolved.

Inappropriate clot formation within arteries is responsible for conditions such as myocardial infarction (MI; heart attack), cerebral vascular accident (CVA; stroke), and pulmonary embolus (PE). Arterial thrombus formation causes tissue necrosis because blood flow distal to the thrombus is decreased or lacking.

The most common cause of venous thrombi is due to a deficiency of proteins C and S. Venous thrombi can also develop due to decreased or slowed blood flow through the vessel, which is called venous stasis. Venous stasis can occur after long periods of immobility. Clot formation within veins usually does not lead to tissue necrosis. An example of venous occlusion is deep vein thrombosis (DVT). DVT can occur, for example, from prolonged sitting in one position on an airplane flight.

venous thrombi: proteins C and S deficiency

venous stasis

DVT

The following conditions carry an increased risk of developing inappropriate clot formation:

- Prolonged and postoperative immobility
- Fibrinolytic defects
- Pregnancy
- Atherosclerosis
- Cancer
- Cardiac disease
- DIC
- Liver disease
- AT-III deficiency

Treatments for Thrombotic Disorders

Physicians treat thrombotic disorders by using thrombolytic drugs (primary approach), such as streptokinase, urokinase, and tissue plasminogen activator (tPA) to dissolve the clot. Removing the clot surgically is called thrombophlebectomy. Like hemorrhagic disorders, thrombotic disorders have the potential to be fatal.

thrombolytic drugs

thrombophlebectomy

Disseminated Intravascular Coagulation

triggering event
↓
abnormal bleeding
and clot formation

Disseminated intravascular coagulation (DIC) is a pathologic condition caused by a triggering event that leads to abnormal bleeding and clot formation and clot lysis within the body. The major manifestation of DIC is excessive bleeding.

All critically ill individuals should be evaluated for the presence of DIC. The more critically ill the individual the more likely DIC is to occur and also the more severe the DIC is. Ill newborns have increased chances of developing DIC because their body systems are immature and sometimes incapable of responding to DIC. Pregnant women at full term are susceptible to DIC because they have increased coagulation proteins, that is, they are hypercoaguable.

Causes and Complications

In children, DIC is most often caused by burns, infections, and trauma. Adults usually develop DIC in association with malignancies and infections.

Complications associated with DIC include: tissue necrosis, organ dysfunction, and hemorrhage. Thrombus formation in the microvasculature of the lungs, brain, and kidneys has very serious consequences because it prevents blood flow leading to tissue necrosis. Hemorrhage always has serious effects because loss of blood is incompatible with life.

Triggering Events

coagulation and
clot lysis

Many medical conditions, diseases, and disorders, known as triggering events, can initiate DIC. Triggering events initiate both coagulation and clot lysis in a diffuse, uncontrolled manner within the capillaries. Triggering events cause the release of phospholipids or phospholipidlike substances into the bloodstream that activate coagulation. The release of these substances occurs when there are large areas of endothelial damage, platelet aggregation, and tissue destruction, such as crush injuries and burns.

Triggering events of DIC include: (1) many obstetrical complications, such as amniotic fluid embolus and retained placenta, among others; (2) malignancies, such as leukemias and certain solid organ tumors; (3) infectious organisms, such as viruses and gram-negative bacteria; (4) widespread tissue damage that occurs with burns and crush injuries; (5) vascular tumors and vascular defects; (6) immunologic disorders, such as allergic and anaphylactic reactions as well as formation of immune complexes; (7) toxins released by certain bacteria or the release of cytokines in response to infection; (8) pieces of particulate matter, such as hemolyzed red cells (stroma); and (9) some snake and spider venoms.

Signs

The most obvious sign of DIC is the excessive bleeding, which usually manifests itself as bleeding into the skin and mucous membranes (bruising). Continued bleeding from either traumatic or surgical wounds is another sign of DIC. Bleeding occurs as a result of decreased levels of platelets and coagulation proteins, especially factors II, V, and fibrinogen. The increased amounts of FSPs generated during clot lysis accentuate bleeding.

The excessive bleeding associated with DIC is caused by several factors that include: (1) consumption of coagulation proteins, (2) consumption of platelets, and (3) increased levels of circulating FSPs. Consumption of coagulation proteins and platelets promote bleeding because there are insufficient levels of them to promote clot formation. Fibrin split products interfere with platelet aggregation and stabilization of the platelet plug.

consumption of coagulation proteins and platelets and increased FSPs
↓
excessive bleeding

Diagnosis

Lab tests used in diagnosing DIC include: peripheral blood smear, the prothrombin time (PT), activated partial thromboplastin time (aPTT), platelet count (PC), fibrinogen level, and the D Dimer assay.

peripheral blood smear, PT, aPTT, PC, fibrinogen level, D Dimer assay

Lab results can vary depending on the specific cause of DIC. For example, lab results from hypoxic individuals can show a normal platelet count and fibrinogen level, a slightly decreased PT, and increased levels of FSPs. Bacterial and viral infections can present quite different results, such as a low platelet count, increased levels of FSPs, decreased amounts of fibrinogen, a slightly increased PT, and a normal aPTT.

Management

The management of DIC is controversial because there are no set treatment modalities; physicians cannot agree about how it should be treated. However, there is agreement that identifying, treating, and resolving the triggering event is the first and most important step. Blood components used in treating DIC are determined from the lab results and the clinical picture of the individual.

To restore hemostasis in DIC, cryoprecipitate, Platelets, and fresh frozen plasma are administered to replenish depleted clotting factors and platelets. If shock is evident, fresh frozen plasma is administered to (1) maintain blood volume, (2) increase clotting factors, and (3) for the osmotic effect of the plasma proteins. Drugs used in DIC therapy include: (1) heparin, which although it is used occasionally is controversial because it potentiates bleeding; (2) specific factor replacements, such as protein C and antithrombin III; and (3) antifibrinolytics, the use of which is also controversial.

▪ QUESTIONS ▪

1. What initiates the coagulation process?

2. Describe the role of fibrin in the coagulation process.

3. Both primary and secondary hemostasis are essential for generating a stable fibrin clot. Describe the difference between these two processes.

4. Coagulation involves two pathways: the intrinsic and the extrinsic. What do these two terms represent?

5. List the four chemical components required to form a stable fibrin clot.

6. Coagulation factors are synthesized in the liver. True or False?

7. Coagulation proteins are referred to by Roman numbers. How are factors III and IV excepted?

8. Calcium has an important role in the coagulation process. Describe this role.

9. What coagulation factor is deficient in classic hemophilia?

10. If Mr. Jackson has a deficiency in vWF, what disease does he have?

11. Describe coagulation factor I.

12. Factor XIII is also known as fibrin stabilizing factor. What serious conditions can a deficiency of this factor cause?

13. Explain the function of factor XII in in vivo coagulation.

14. List the three laboratory tests that monitor the coagulation pathways.

15. Describe the process of clot retraction.

16. A clot must dissolve slowly or bleeding will resume if dissolution progresses before adequate healing takes place. How do coagulation and fibrinolysis allow this to happen?

17. How do plasmin and plasminogen contribute to the coagulation process?

18. Describe tissue plasminogen activators and how they are used therapeutically.

19. Identify three natural anticoagulants and their actions.

20. Vitamin K is a fat-soluble vitamin essential for blood coagulation. Where can an individual find it?

21. Where can an individual obtain Coumadin™, and what is its relationship to vitamin K?

22. What happens after a fibrin clot dissolves?

23. Why must FSPs be removed from circulation?

24. Contrast hemorrhagic disorders with thrombotic disorders.

25. Why are many clotting disorders caused by liver disease?

26. Identify the major symptoms of vascular disorders.

27. How does hemorrhagic telangiectasia occur? and what are its symptoms?

28. Describe von Willebrand's disease.

29. Describe the main difference between hemophilia A and hemophilia B.

30. List three serious conditions caused by inappropriate clot formation.

31. Explain venous stasis and give an example of its occurrence.

32. Name the two chief events in disseminated intravascular coagulation (DIC).

33. Identify two causes of DIC.

34. List at least five triggering events for DIC.

35. What causes the excessive bleeding associated with DIC?

36. The management of DIC is controversial. What blood components may be used?

CHAPTER **13**

ABO and Rh Blood Group Systems

Introduction

Red cells express a number of antigens on their membranes. These antigens can provoke an immune response when transfused into a recipient. Groups of related antigens define a blood group system. ABO, Rh, Kidd, Kell, Duffy, and Lewis are examples of several blood group systems. The ABO blood group system is the most important in transfusion medicine because differences between ABO groups cause immediate immune reactions. This system was discovered at the beginning of the twentieth century by Karl Landsteiner, an Austrian researcher.

red cell membrane
antigens
↓
immune response

Antigens in the Rh system were discovered by Weiner, Levine, and other scientists around 1940. They include the Cc, Ee, and D antigens. The most prominent Rh antigen is referred to as D. In transfusion medicine, ABO blood groups and D antigen are always expressed together, as A+, O-, or AB+, for example. A positive sign (+) indicates the presence of D antigen on the red cell membrane, and a negative sign (-) denotes its absence. Positive and negative signs refer specifically to the D antigen of the Rh system. A commonly used example of Rh incompatibility occurs between a D- mother and a D+ fetus. Hemolytic disease of the newborn (HDN) may result from this incompatibility (see p. 215).

D antigen

ABO Blood Group System

A and B Antigens

Blood groups of the ABO system are classified by the presence or absence of two distinct antigens—

A group: A antigen
B group: B antigen
AB group:
A and B antigens
O group: neither
A nor B antigens

the A and the B. These antigens are oligosaccharides (complex carbohydrates) found on the red cell membranes. Red blood cells with the A antigen are called group A; those with the B antigen, group B; those with both A and B antigens, group AB; and those with neither antigen present, group O.

Antigens are inherited from one's parents. In actuality the A and B genes do not produce antigens directly, but code for enzymes that add sugar (oligosaccharide) molecules on the red cell membrane. The A and B antigens develop early on in fetal development.

Isoagglutinins

preformed antibodies in:
- A and O groups: anti-B antibodies
- B and O groups: anti-A antibodies
- O group: anti-A and anti-B antibodies

isoagglutinins/antibodies of ABO blood group

isoimmune

Normally the body does not produce antibody unless it is exposed to antigen. Landsteiner made the significant discovery that humans have preformed antibodies in their plasma against ABO antigens they do not have. Landsteiner found that group A and O individuals have anti-B antibodies, group B and O have anti-A antibodies, group AB have no antibodies, and group O have both antibodies. Antibodies of the ABO blood group are referred to as isoagglutinins because they cause agglutination of red cells. The anti-A and anti-B antibodies do not develop in fetal life but during the first months of life. The prefix "iso" means the same, and the term isoimmune refers to immunization against the blood of a member of the same species.

ABO Compatibility

ABO-incompatible blood
↓
AHTR

Landsteiner's discoveries are significant in blood transfusion therapy. Donor and recipient blood must be compatible, that is, both individuals usually must have the same blood group. A transfusion of ABO-incompatible blood causes an acute (immediate) hemolytic transfusion reaction (AHTR) in a recipient. Before medical personnel administer a transfusion of allogeneic (donor) blood, they must be certain that the donor's blood group is compatible with the recipient's. Administration of the wrong blood group is usually due to clerical error and occurs very rarely.

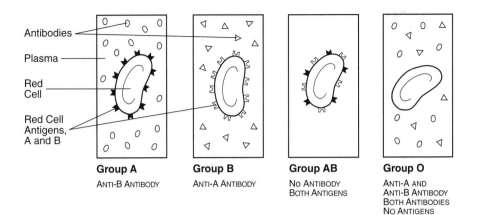

	Group A	**Group B**	**Group AB**	**Group O**
Antibodies	Anti-B Antibody	Anti-A Antibody	No Antibody Both Antigens	Anti-A and Anti-B Antibody Both Antibodies No Antigens

Plasma

Red Cell

Red Cell Antigens, A and B

FIGURE 13.1 ABO Blood Groups

This schematic representation shows ABO blood groups and the different antibodies associated with each group. Individuals have preformed antibodies directed against the ABO antigens that they do not have. If an individual receives a transfusion of incompatible blood, an acute (instant) hemolytic transfusion reaction occurs. For example, if group B blood is transfused into a group A individual, the anti-B antibodies circulating in the plasma of group A blood will attack the antigens on the group B red cells which activates complement and causes hemolysis.

- Group A can receive group A or O Packed Red Cells.   A: A or O
- Group B can receive group B or O Packed Red Cells.   B: B or O
- Group AB can receive group A, B, AB, or O Packed   AB: A, B, AB, or O
  Red Cells.
- Group O can receive *only* group O Packed Red Cells.   O: O only

Packed refers to blood that has had the plasma removed. The red cells are concentrated.

In the early days of blood transfusion, group O blood was considered the universal donor because there are no antigens on its red cell membranes and it could be administered to people of any ABO group. Group AB blood was considered the universal recipient. Lacking antibodies in its plasma, group AB could receive red cells from donors of any ABO group. Today, identical blood groups are preferentially used, but group O–Packed Red Cells can be given in an emergency when an individual's specific blood group is not available.

FIGURE 13.2 Compatible Blood Groups

This chart indicates which donor blood groups can be transfused into which recipient. Compatible blood groups are indicated by "C" and incompatible blood groups by "I."

RECIPIENT BLOOD GROUP

DONOR BLOOD GROUP (PACKED RED CELLS ONLY)	O	A	B	AB
O	C	C	C	C
A	I	C	I	C
B	I	I	C	C
AB	I	I	I	C

ABO Incompatibility in Transfusion

An acute hemolytic transfusion reaction occurs immediately after an ABO-incompatible transfusion. Preformed antibodies in a recipient's plasma attach themselves to donor red cell antigens and stimulate complement activation. Complement attaches to the antigen-antibody complex and causes red cell lysis. An AHTR leads to intravascular hemolysis, that is, cells are lysed within the vasculature, which is an event that can trigger coagulation leading to clot formation in the microvasculature of the lungs and kidneys (see Ch. 15, Transfusion Complications). Red cell destruction causes anemia. The remnants of destroyed red cells, called stroma, or ghosts, are removed from circulation by the reticuloendothelial system (RES) of the spleen, also referred to as the mononuclear phagocytic system (MPS).

complement and antigen-antibody complex
↓
red cell lysis

Symptoms of an Acute Hemolytic Transfusion Reaction

Symptoms of an AHTR can include: shock, chills, fever, chest pain, dyspnea (shortness of breath), back pain, and disseminated intravascular coagulation (DIC). Death also can result.

The first indications that the wrong blood group has been used for an anesthetized patient is excessive bleeding from the microvasculature (DIC). Other signs include: hypotension (low blood pressure), hemoglobinuria (red urine), and hemoglobinemia (decreased hemoglobin levels). These may not always be evident due to the effects of anesthesia.

ABO in Solid Organ Transplantation

The A and B antigens are expressed on the endothelial lining of blood vessels. Therefore, ABO compatibility between donor and recipient is required for the success of solid organ transplantation, such as kidney, liver, lung, and heart. Any ABO mismatch leads to hyper-acute graft rejection (see Ch. 9, The Immune System). Recipient anti-A and anti-B antibodies react with donor antigen causing endothelial damage within the transplanted organ. This reaction leads to thrombus formation and ultimately graft failure. Thrombi prevent blood flow through the transplanted organ.

Rh Blood Group System

Rh antigens are protein molecules found on red cell membranes. Approximately 85% of the population has the most prominent, the D antigen, while 15% does not.

The D Antigen in Transfusion

The presence of the D antigen always poses a risk to a transfusion recipient who does not have it because he or she will produce antibody against the D antigen. A D- individual produces anti-D antibody only after being exposed, or alloimmunized, to D antigen following transfusion, transplant, or pregnancy. Anti-D antibody is of the IgG type and persists in the individual for many years. Because anti-D is the IgG isotype that does not bind complement, anti-D antibody usually is not implicated in intravascular hemolysis but is hemolyzed extravascularly in the spleen.

RhIG:
anti-D antibodies

Rh immune globulin (RhIG), which is a concentrated form of anti-D antibodies, is available to prevent a transfusion reaction. However, the assumption is that most male transfusion recipients do not require RhIG. Females of childbearing potential are given RhIG following transfusion of an Rh+ blood product. RhIG is administered primarily to prevent hemolytic disease of the newborn (HDN; see below).

Rh Compatibility

A transfusion recipient should receive Rh-compatible blood. D+ blood is preferentially given to a D+ individual. D- blood can be given to either a D- or a D+ individual but is usually saved for D- individuals.

first transfusion of
D+ blood sensitizes
D- person to form
anti-D antibody

second transfusion of
D+ blood in D- person
↓
antigen-antibody response
↓
red cell hemolysis
↓
anemia

If D+ blood is transfused into a D- individual, there are usually few complications with the first incompatible transfusion. With the first exposure, an individual becomes immunized (sensitized) to the D antigen. Because it takes time for the antibody titer (level) to reach an amount sufficient enough to cause hemolysis, there is no immediate reaction. When a D- individual receives D+ blood a second time, however, anti-D antibody formed during the first exposure has reached a titer high enough to cause a severe antigen-antibody reaction (immune response). The antigen-antibody reaction causes the recipient's red cells to hemolyze, resulting in anemia.

Rh Hemolytic Disease of the Newborn

Causes

isoimmune hemolytic
anemia

Hemolytic disease of the newborn (HDN) is a form of isoimmune hemolytic anemia that results from an antigen-antibody response between incompatible fetal antigen and maternal antibody of the IgG type. Many red cell antibodies can cause HDN, including anti-A, anti-B, anti-C, anti-D, anti-Duffy, anti-Kell, anti-Kidd, and others. When HDN is caused by these antigens, the disease is less severe than when it is caused by anti-D. When the fetus inherits a red cell antigen from the

1. and 2. On exposure to fetal red cells, a D– mother develops anti-D antibody to the D+ antigen of the fetus

3. Administration of RhIG prevents maternal antibodies from binding to fetal antigens

4. If RhIG is not given, preformed maternal antibodies will attack the red cells of the subsequent D+ fetus causing HDN

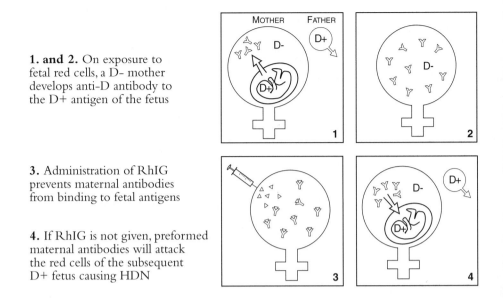

FIGURE 13.3 A D– Mother with a D+ Fetus

father that the mother does not have and she is exposed to fetal blood cells, her immune system is stimulated to make antibody against the foreign antigen. Fetal red cells can enter maternal circulation during an induced abortion, amniocentesis, ectopic pregnancy, spontaneous abortion (miscarriage), cesarean section, or vaginal delivery.

HDN due to anti-D has been the most important historically. Hemolytic disease of the newborn caused by the D antigen is very serious. The first D+ fetus usually does not experience harm because the mother's antibody titer is too low to cause hemolysis. However, antibodies produced by the mother at the time of sensitization (the first D+ fetus) can cross the placenta and attack the red cells of subsequent D+ fetuses. The anti-D IgG antibody crosses the placenta and attacks fetal red cells bearing the D antigen. Once maternal antibodies destroy fetal red cells, the fetus becomes anemic and produces large numbers of immature red cells called erythroblasts. At one time, HDN was called erythroblastosis fetalis.

erythroblasts

Symptoms of HDN

The fetus with HDN can experience mild to severe symptoms of anemia. Mild forms of HDN can go undetected or present with symptoms of mild jaundice or hepatomegaly (enlarged liver due to extramedullary hematopoiesis). Severe forms of HDN compromise the fetus's health with the following: anemia, heart disease, hypoxia, poor liver function, severe jaundice, DIC, kernicterus (high bilirubin levels in the brain leading to mental retardation), and hydrops fetalis (generalized edema of the body). Hydrops fetalis is the term used to describe the most serious form of HDN.

hydrops fetalis

Hemolytic disease of the newborn begins during fetal life and can progress into the early neonatal period (first months of infancy.) The level of hemolysis is greatest at birth because the fetus has been continuously exposed to maternal antibodies. Hemolysis diminishes following birth because the number of maternal antibodies in the newborn declines over time.

Therapies for HDN

Severe forms of HDN can be treated with an intrauterine transfusion or, if necessary, an exchange transfusion. A female with anti-D antibody and a D+ fetus can also undergo plasmapheresis (withdrawal of plasma) to lessen the amount of anti-D in their plasma. This is rarely performed, however.

Intrauterine Transfusion

This procedure is performed after a careful clinical assessment. It is rarely done prior to 20 weeks gestation. Once the decision is made to perform the transfusion, a fetal transfusion must be administered about every 2 weeks until birth to maintain the red cell count. An intrauterine transfusion differs from a regular blood transfusion in that blood is injected into the abdominal cavity of the fetus. The physician uses ultrasound to view the fetus during the procedure. Transfused red cells administered through the fetus's abdominal cavity are absorbed by the lymphatic channels in the fetal peritoneum (abdomen). Intrauterine transfusion can also be administered intravenously directly through the umbilical vein.

Blood used in fetal transfusion should meet the following criteria:

- Blood preferably should be less than 5 days old to provide the longest survival time of transfused red cells in fetal circulation.

- The percentage of red cells (Hct) should be at least 0.80 (80%) or greater to minimize the possibility of fluid overload in the fetus.

- Blood should be group O, Rh-.

- Blood products transfused should be irradiated in order to destroy donor lymphocytes, thereby preventing transfusion associated graft-versus-host disease (TAGVHD) in the fetus. Steps should be taken to reduce the likelihood of the transmission of cytomegalovirus (CMV). Frozen deglycerolized red cells are recommended by some physicians because these cells have normal levels of 2,3-DPG and contain no anticoagulant or plasma.

less than 5 days old

Hct: 0.80+

O, Rh-

irradiated blood products

Exchange Transfusion

This is a technique used to transfuse a neonate (newborn) with HDN. In this instance, all fetal blood is replaced with that of a donor. The technique usually is reserved for severe cases of HDN. A total blood exchange lessens the amount of bilirubin and circulating antibodies in fetal blood. Exchange transfusion of neonates is more common than intrauterine transfusion of the fetus.

Rh Immune Globulin

Use of Rh immune globulin (RhIG) has greatly reduced the incidence of D alloimmunization and

HDN. Rh immune globulin is a concentrated form of anti-D antibody. It should be administered to a D- mother within 72 hours following sensitization by the D+ antigen to prevent her from forming antibodies against the D antigen. Rh immune globulin binds to D antigen and thus blocks the formation of anti-D antibody. However, RhIG does not prevent a reaction if anti-D antibody has already formed, nor does it prevent other forms of HDN caused by other antibodies, such as anti-A or anti-B.

RhIG binds D antigens to block formation of anti-D antibodies

Rh immune globulin has all but eliminated the incidence of hemolytic disease of the newborn (HDN) due to anti-D and Rh alloimunization. One of several commercial drug preparations of RhIG is called RhoGAM™.

Indications for the use of RhIG include:

- A D- individual who receives a transfusion of D+ blood or blood product
- A D- woman during the 28th week of pregnancy
- A D- woman following delivery if the fetus is D+
- A D- woman who has an abortion, ectopic pregnancy, or amniocentesis when fetal Rh status is unknown
- A D- woman of childbearing potential who has received a transfusion of D+ red cells

ABO Hemolytic Disease of the Newborn

ABO HDN

Group A and B mothers produce the IgM type of anti-A and anti-B antibodies, whereas group O mothers produce IgG type of anti-A and anti-B. IgG antibody can cross the placenta, thus a group A or B fetus carried by group O mothers can experience what is known as ABO HDN. This form of HDN is less severe than Rh HDN and often requires no treatment. Newborns with moderate jaundice are treated with phototherapy (ultraviolet light) to assist in breaking down the bilirubin so that it can be removed from the body.

■ QUESTIONS ■

1. Why is the ABO blood group system important in transfusion medicine?

2. What is the most prominent antigen in the Rh system?

3. How are blood groups identified in the ABO system?

4. Identify the blood group associated with the presence of each of the following red cell antigens: (a) A and B antigens, (b) A antigen, (c) B antigen.

5. How is blood group O different from other blood groups in the ABO system?

6. Explain the presence of isoagglutinins in the ABO system.

7. Explain ABO compatibility.

8. What are Packed Red Cells?

9. What can happen in an ABO-incompatible transfusion?

10. List seven symptoms of AHTR.

11. Why is ABO compatibility necessary in organ transplant procedures?

12. Explain the Rh blood group system.

13. Why does the Rh antigen (D+) present the risk of transfusion reaction following an initial transfusion?

14. What causes hemolytic disease of the newborn (HDN)?

15. Identify six circumstances whereby fetal red cells can enter maternal circulation.

16. List symptoms identified with both mild and severe forms of HDN.

17. When does HDN become apparent?

18. How is HDN treated?

19. What blood group is used for an intrauterine transfusion?

20. What is RhoGAM™ and how is it used?

21. Contrast ABO HDN with Rh HDN.

CHAPTER **14**

Blood Transfusion

Introduction

Blood transfusions are used to treat a variety of surgical and medical conditions. Also called transfusion therapy, blood transfusion involves the infusion of allogeneic (someone else's) blood, autologous (one's own) blood, or any blood component or its substitute. A blood transfusion is given (1) to replace blood lost during trauma or surgery, (2) to treat anemia, hemophilia, and internal bleeding, and (3) to replace a specific component destroyed by disease or chemotherapy.

Before the discovery of blood groups in the early part of this century, blood transfusion was hazardous and successful only by chance. Over time, the risks associated with transfusions—disease transmission and transfusion reactions—have been greatly reduced. Transfusions save many lives.

All testing and storage of blood in the United States are carried out according to standards established by the American Association of Blood Banks (AABB) and the Food and Drug Administration (FDA). The AABB and FDA also establish all transfusion policies within the United States.

AABB
FDA

Prior to and during a transfusion, it is necessary to follow specific procedures. Whole Blood from a donor or patient is collected in a blood bag that contains an anticoagulant-preservative. Whole Blood is usually separated into its components: Packed Red Cells, Platelets, and Plasma. Usually components are separated immediately following collection. Blood components are stored in blood banks and available for transfusion.

Whole Blood:
Packed Red Cells
Platelets
Plasma   **223**

Prior to transfusion, Whole Blood and its components are tested for transmissible viral and bacterial diseases (see Ch. 16). Once a donor's and recipient's ABO and Rh groups are determined, cross matching between donor and recipient is carried out (see Ch. 13). Blood or its components are always transfused through a blood filter. During infusion, a patient must be closely monitored for the signs and symptoms of a transfusion reaction (see Ch. 15).

Blood Collection

donation

Collection of blood or blood components used for transfusions is called donation. Eligible adults who meet AABB donation requirements can donate 450 mL +/- 45 mL of whole blood (approximately 1 pint) once every 8 weeks, the time it takes for red cells to replace their numbers.

450 mL +/- 10%

The amount of whole blood collected in a typical donation is a unit that contains 450 mL +/- 10%. To prevent anemia or volume-associated problems, a donation should not exceed 1/10 of the donor's total blood volume.

Donor Screening

Prior to donation, a donor undergoes extensive medical questioning and basic physical screening that includes: temperature, pulse, blood pressure, hematocrit (Hct) level or hemoglobin (Hgb) concentration. Persons with certain conditions and diseases are precluded from donating, either permanently or temporarily.

As long as a donor meets all other criteria and wishes to donate, blood is usually withdrawn from veins in the antecubital fossa at the bend of the elbow. A tourniquet is tightened around the upper arm to make the veins bulge and the insertion of the needle easier. A needle with a large bore is connected to a plastic bag containing an anticoagulant-preservative solution added to maintain red cell viability and prevent clotting. Blood should enter the blood bag at an even rate, with collection taking no longer than 10 minutes. These collection criteria are necessary to avoid hemolysis and clot formation within the unit.

Donor Deferral

Donors are temporarily deferred for the following reasons:

temporary deferral

- Low Hct or Hgb
- Pregnancy
- Recent injection of immunoglobulins (antibodies)
- Blood transfusions or tissue transplants received within a year
- Recent immunizations against measles, mumps, and certain other communicable diseases
- Drug therapy, such as nonrecombinant growth hormones, antibiotics, anticoagulants, and aspirin in the case of platelet donors
- Tatoos obtained within a year
- Sexual contact with an individual in a permanent deferral category
- Individuals who have had malaria in the past must be asymptomatic for 3 years before they can donate blood

Permanent preclusions for blood donation include: a history of hepatitis, heart disease, HIV infection, homosexual activity, and I.V. drug use.

permanent deferral

Testing of Donated Blood

Serum is tested for the bacterium that causes syphilis. All blood components are tested for the following antibodies and antigens that indicate the presence of transmissible diseases:

antigens and antibodies
transmissible diseases

- HBsAg (hepatitis B surface antigen)
- Anti-HBc (antibody to hepatitis B core antigen)
- Anti-HCV (antibody to hepatitis C virus)
- Anti-HTLV I/II (antibody to human T cell lymphotropic virus type I and II)

- Anti-HIV 1/2 (antibody to human immunodeficiency virus types 1 and 2)
- HIV-1-Ag (HIV antigen). It is believed that this test will show a positive result before the anti-HIV 1/2.
- Alanine aminotransferase (ALT; a liver enzyme). This test is no longer required by AABB, but is still performed by some centers to assess liver function.

If all tests of donor blood are negative, the blood component(s) can be used for transfusion.

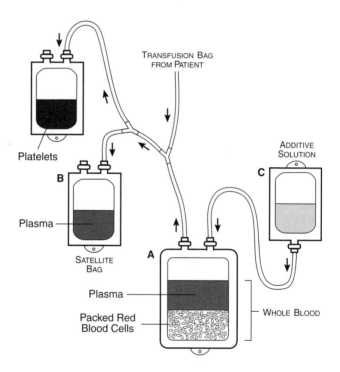

FIGURE 14.1 A Typical Blood Donation Set-up

Once whole blood is collected from the donor (bag A), plasma and platelets are separated by centrifugation and run into a satellite bag. These components are centrifuged again to isolate the platelets. Remaining Packed Red Cells are mixed with an additive solution to increase their storage shelf life up to 42 days.

Citrate Anticoagulants-preservatives for Whole Blood Collection

CPD, CP2D, and CPDA-1 are collectively known as citrate anticoagulants-preservatives. They are commercially prepared solutions placed in blood collection bags and used only for collection and storage of Whole Blood and blood components that will be transfused. CPD, CP2D, and CPDA-1 are used (1) to preserve Whole Blood, Packed Red Cells, Platelets, and Plasma and (2) to prevent collected blood from clotting, which can happen within minutes of collection.

CPD
CP2D
CPDA-1

Whole Blood
Packed Red Cells
Platelets
Plasma

Functions of Anticoagulant-preservative Components

CPD, CP2D, and CPDA-1 contain citrate, phosphate, and dextrose. Citrate is the anticoagulant. The other additives are preservatives that aid in maintaining and extending the storage life of red cells. CP2D contains twice the amount of dextrose as the other solutions, and CPDA-1 contains adenine (A).

The components of the anticoagulant-preservative solutions have specific functions:

- Citrate prevents clotting by binding calcium ions (Ca^{++}) present in plasma and necessary for coagulation.

C: citrate anticoagulant

- Phosphate helps control pH and also maintain high levels of adenosine triphosphate (ATP) in the blood.

P: phosphate

- Dextrose, also known as glucose, is a simple sugar that helps to maintain the viability of red cells.

D: dextrose

- Adenine in CPDA-1 aids red cells in maintaining high levels of ATP.

A: adenine

Blood Storage

Whole Blood and blood components are stored in blood banks that carefully maintain and organize units to ensure their safety for transfusion; they are available as patients need them. For example, Platelets are ready for patients actively bleeding due to thrombocytopenia or abnormal platelets, and plasma derivatives are ready for patients with coagulation disorders. All blood and blood components are labeled by ABO and Rh blood group: A+, B-, AB+, and so on. Blood banks are operated by hospitals, the American Red Cross, and other regional facilities.

Shelf Life and Storage Temperature

Each blood component is stored for the appropriate length of time at a temperature that maintains its viability. Whole Blood and Packed Red Cells are refrigerated at 1 to 6C, a temperature range that slows down metabolic activity and inhibits the growth of bacteria. When collected in CPD or CP2D these components can be refrigerated for 21 days (shelf life). If collected in CPDA-1, their shelf life is 35 days. Platelets and Plasma require different storage temperatures and have different shelf lives. Platelets are maintained at 20 to 24C and slowly rocked to prevent clumping. They can be stored for 5 days. Plasma is usually frozen at -18C or lower. It can be stored for 1 year.

Whole Blood, Packed Red Cells: 1 to 6C

CPD or CP2D: 21 days
CPDA-1: 35 days

Platelets: 20 to 24C
5 days
Plasma: -18C or lower
1 year

Additive Systems for Packed Red Cell Storage and Preservation

additive system/ additive solution

An additive system, also known as additive solution, is the generic name used for commercially prepared chemical solutions that contain adenine, dextrose, saline, and mannitol (see Ch. 17, Component Therapy). Currently there are three solutions, AS-1, AS-3, and AS-5, approved by the FDA.

After plasma and platelets are removed by centrifugation from a unit of Whole Blood, Packed Red Cells remain in the collection bag and the additive system is added. Additive systems are added only to Packed Red Cells and extend their storage shelf life to 42 days. The components in additive systems aid in reducing red cell damage incurred during storage. They increase the storage shelf life of Packed Red Cells by allowing

Packed Red Cells: 42 days

these cells to carry on their metabolic processes. About 100 mL of an additive system is added to each unit of Packed Red Cells within 72 hours after blood is collected.

Storage Lesions in Banked Blood

Blood is a living tissue and must have a favorable environment to maintain viability and carry out cellular metabolism. Stored blood is subject to many chemical changes, and the longer it is stored, the less viable its elements become. Over time, all stored units of blood suffer damage, a condition called storage lesion.

damage/storage lesion

Examples of Storage Lesions Blood elements have different survival times. For example, after 24 hours, Whole Blood and Packed Red Cells have few viable platelets and granulocytes. Lymphocytes survive for many days. The levels of clotting factors V and VIII also decline. Due to their short shelf life, these clotting factors are called labile factors. The remaining clotting factors maintain their levels of activity during storage and therefore are called stable factors. Other examples of storage lesions include: decreased pH, low levels of 2,3-DPG and ATP, and, increased potassium (K^+) in the plasma.

labile factors

stable factors

Certain storage lesions are reversible, such as the levels of 2,3-DPG and ATP. They return to normal after donated cells have circulated within the recipient for a period of time. Other storage lesions are not reversible and do not return to normal, such as the labile clotting factors and red cells that have been hemolyzed.

reversible storage lesions

Blood Grouping and Cross Matching for Transfusions

Blood grouping and cross matching must be done before a recipient receives allogeneic blood. Identification of donor and recipient by ABO and Rh blood groups is called blood grouping. Determining that there is compatibility between a donor and a recipient is known as cross matching.

blood grouping

cross matching

Blood Group Identification

forward grouping:
A and B antigens
on red cells

reverse grouping:
antibodies in serum

The specific blood group of an individual is identified by two grouping tests: (1) forward, or front, which utilizes red cells, and (2) reverse, or back, which utilizes serum. Forward grouping determines the presence or absence of A and B antigens on red cell membranes. The testing laboratory uses reagent anti-A and anti-B antibodies to determine whether the A and/or B antigen is on the red cell membrane. A reagent is a strong concentration of antibodies commercially prepared. Reverse grouping determines the antibodies present in serum when they are mixed with reagent red cells known to have the A and B antigens. The anti-A and anti-B isoagglutinins in the serum are naturally occurring, unlike other red cell antibodies such as Kidd and Kell. Forward and reverse grouping test results must agree with one another in order for the blood group to be determined. For example, group A blood is determined in the following way:

reagent

FORWARD GROUPING TEST

Unknown red cells are mixed with reagents anti-A and anti-B. Hemolysis or agglutination with anti-A indicates that the red cells have A antigen. These cells are mixed with anti-B to detect group B. A negative reaction with anti-B indicates the A antigen only.

REVERSE GROUPING TEST

Unknown serum is mixed with reagent A and B red cells. Hemolysis or agglutination with reagent B cells indicates that the serum contains anti-B antibody. Anti-B antibodies are found in persons with group A blood.

D antigen determination:
red cells and reagent
anti-D antibody

The presence of the D antigen is determined by mixing red cells with reagent anti-D antibody. If the red cells contain the D antigen, they will agglutinate when mixed with the anti-D reagent.

Cross Matching

agglutination or
hemolysis:
incompatibility

In cross matching, donor red cells and recipient serum are mixed. Agglutination or hemolysis indicates that the recipient has antibodies against donor red cell antigens. A positive reaction indicates incompatibility between this donor and recipient. A smooth cell suspension, in which there is no agglutination or hemolysis, indicates that both blood groups are compatible.

smooth cell suspension: compatibility

Blood Filtering

All blood products should be transfused through a filter before being administered to a patient. Filters trap undesirable debris that form in blood during collection and over time in storage. They filter out particulate matter such as cell fragments and blood clots. Filters are designed to allow all red cells and platelets to pass through. They are placed in the I.V. line between the blood bag and the individual. Plasma derivatives, such as albumin, do not need to be filtered.

Filters

Filters are available in many sizes and shapes. Standard blood filters have a pore size of about 150 to 270µ. Microaggregate filters have a much smaller pore size (20 to 40µ). These filters trap microaggregate particles such as pieces of fibrin, fragments of red cells (called stroma or ghosts), platelets, and white cells.

microaggregate filters

Leukocyte-depletion Filters

Leukocyte-adsorption filters, also called leukocyte-depletion filters, are used to remove white cells from blood and blood components because these cells may cause transfusion reactions. Small amounts of white cells, which carry human leukocyte antigen (HLA) molecules on their membranes, are found in units of Packed Red Cells, Whole Blood, and Platelets. Individuals who have received multiple transfusions become alloimmunized to HLA. Therefore white cells are removed before an individual is transfused with Packed Red Cells, Whole Blood, or Platelets to prevent a transfusion reaction. Leukocyte removal from a unit of Whole Blood or Packed Red Cells is usually done with adsorption filters at the bedside as the individual is receiving the blood transfusion. It is preferable to

leukocyte adsorption

removal of HLA molecules

remove white cells before blood is stored because cytokines and biological response modifiers (BRMs) released by white cells during storage are responsible for febrile and other nonhemolytic transfusion reactions.

Leukocyte-adsorption filtration is the most efficient and preferred method of removing white cells from Whole Blood, Packed Red Cells, and Platelets. Leukocyte-adsorption filters are made of wool, acetate, cotton, cellulose, or chemically treated polyester fibers. They remove greater than 99% of the white cells yet retain almost all the red cells and platelets in the unit. The filters are also used to prevent or lessen an individual's chance of contracting cytomegalovirus (CMV).

The Blood Transfusion

Preliminary Cautions

bacterial contamination

When the decision is made to transfuse a patient, the blood bank is notified. Before releasing a unit of blood, blood bank personnel must examine it for various signs that indicate bacterial contamination: blood clots; air bubbles; or dark coloration, which indicates hemolysis. If any of these signs of contamination are present, that particular unit of blood should not be used.

identification numbers: patient and blood bag

After a blood unit arrives from the blood bank, it must be checked by medical personnel to be sure that the patient identification number on the blood bag matches the identification number on the patient. This step ensures that a patient receives the correct unit for which he or she was grouped and cross matched.

Transfusion

Individuals are infused with blood through a needle or catheter placed in a vein. All air in the tubing line must be expelled before the tubing is connected to the needle or catheter. This can be achieved if the person administering the blood opens the roller clamp on the I.V. line and allows the blood or blood product to fill the

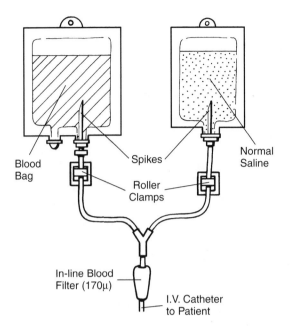

FIGURE 14.2 A Typical Blood Transfusion Set-up

The tubing set consists of spikes that go into the blood and NS bags, the roller clamps, the in-line blood filter, and the tubing that goes from the blood bag to the I.V. needle within the patient.

tubing until the blood flows from the end of the tubing. Once air is removed from the tubing, the end of it is attached to the needle or catheter. Each tubing set comes with a 170μ filter in place. A Y set allows for a unit of blood and a bag of saline, albumin, or compatible plasma to be infused at the same time if needed. Drugs are never added to any unit of blood or blood component. During transfusion, a patient's vital signs (pulse, blood pressure, temperature) are taken at regular intervals for any possible sign of a transfusion reaction.

170μ filter
Y set

no drugs
vital signs

Compatible Solutions for Transfusion

To decrease the viscosity of transfused blood cells, 0.9% normal saline (NS), ABO-compatible plasma, or 5% human albumin can be administered through the I.V. line. The addition of these solutions allows blood to flow more freely.

0.9% NS
ABO-compatible plasma
5% human albumin

Normal saline (0.9%) is the only crystalloid solution that can be used in conjunction with blood or blood components administered intravenously (see Ch. 17,

Component Therapy). This solution does not damage red cells like other crystalloid I.V. solutions do. A dextrose solution causes hemolysis. Lactated Ringer's contains 3 mEq/L of Ca^{++} and increases Ca^{++} levels in the blood. This solution can override the effect of the citrate anticoagulant and increase the risk of blood clots.

Blood Warmers

Blood warmers are devices used to warm blood as Whole Blood or blood components are being administered. Infusions of cold blood can cause cardiac arrhythmias and possibly death in some individuals. Patients requiring large volumes of blood and premature infants should be infused with blood that has been warmed. The temperature of the blood

37C

warmer should be maintained at about 37C to prevent hemolysis of red cells. At temperatures greater than 42C, hemolysis occurs and increased levels of K^+ (potassium ions) are likely.

warm water bath
countercurrent system

Blood warmers are a warm water bath or a countercurrent system. A warm water bath warms the blood as it flows through the I.V. tubing placed in the water bath. Blood warming systems are similar in that blood is warmed before entering a recipient.

▪ QUESTIONS ▪

1. What are the three main reasons for a blood transfusion?

2. In transfusion therapy Whole Blood is separated into what components?

3. How much blood can an eligible adult donate and how often?

4. What is the procedure for a blood donation?

5. There are a number of temporary reasons for deferring a blood donation, e.g., pregnancy or drug therapy. What are the permanent ones?

6. Besides syphilis, for what other diseases are donated blood products tested?

7. What are the four major components of anticoagulants-preservatives? and what role does each play in the safe storage of blood products?

8. What blood product is used for thrombocytopenia? for coagulation disorders?

9. What is the maximum storage time for Packed Red Cells and how is this achieved?

10. Over time all stored units of blood suffer damage, a condition called storage lesion. Identify which storage lesions are reversible and which are not.

11. What is blood grouping?

12. Determining that there is compatibility between a donor and a recipient is known as cross matching. True or False?

13. The specific blood group of an individual is identified by two grouping tests. How do these two tests differ? How are they used together?

14. What does agglutination indicate in the cross matching process?

15. What is the purpose of leukocyte-depletion filters? When are they used?

16. How can an individual's chance for contracting cytomegalovirus (CMV) be lessened?

17. What is done to assure the safety of blood products and decrease the possibility of transfusion reactions?

18. What compatible solution is used during a blood transfusion? Why?

19. In certain instances individuals must receive warm blood. Identify these individuals.

CHAPTER 15

Adverse Events in Transfusion

Introduction

Transfusion of allogeneic blood components is a safe and effective way to treat individuals with hemorrhage, disease, and hematologic defects. However, transfusion of allogeneic or autologous blood and components into the body always has the potential for causing an adverse event. Adverse events are transfusion complications and reactions that occur within the body during or following the infusion of blood or blood components. The term transfusion reaction is used when the adverse event is due to an immune response. In this book the term complication refers to nonimmune adverse events, such as circulatory overload. Although all adverse events are potentially life-threatening, their severity can vary from mild, non-life-threatening reactions to serious, possibly fatal ones.

transfusion reaction: an immune response

The following concepts are associated with adverse events in transfusion:

- Acute adverse events occur during or shortly after the infusion of a blood component.

  acute

- Delayed adverse events occur later at a time following the infusion, usually after 24 hours.

  delayed

- Transfusion reactions can be localized to the site at which the antigen entered the body. Rashes and welts are local reactions.

  local

- Transfusion reactions can be systemic. Reactions occurring throughout the body are usually more serious than local reactions. Hypotension (decreased blood pressure) and shock are systemic reactions.

  systemic

- Adverse events can be hemolytic and life-threatening. Hemolysis result in the destruction of infused red cells.

  hemolytic

nonhemolytic

- Nonhemolytic adverse events do not involve hemolysis of red cells but oftentimes have serious effects. Anaphylactoid reactions are examples.

immune

- An immune response in the recipient to some element in the transfused blood component is the cause of many transfusion reactions. Antigens that can be problematic in a blood transfusion include: the A and B antigens, HLA, and platelet-specific antigens among others. Plasma proteins can also generate an immune reaction when infused into another individual.

nonimmune

- Nonimmune transfusion complications are those not caused by an immune response to foreign antigen, for example, circulatory overload.

Adverse Events Involving an Immune Response

hemolytic
allergic
anaphylactic
febrile nonhemolytic
TRALI
PTP

Adverse events caused by antigen that binds antibody include: hemolytic, allergic, anaphylactic, febrile nonhemolytic transfusion-related acute lung injury, transfusion-associated graft-versus-host disease, and post-transfusion purpura. Females who have had multiple pregnancies develop antibodies to fetal antigens that they do not carry, which can present problems for them if a subsequent blood transfusion is required.

Hemolytic Transfusion Reactions

red cell hemolysis and removal of red cells

immune-mediated HTR:
recipient antibodies and donor antigens

A hemolytic transfusion reaction (HTR) is characterized by red cell hemolysis or an increased rate of removal of red cells from the circulation due to incompatibility between donor and recipient. Immune-related HTRs are caused when antibodies in the plasma of the transfusion recipient react with antigens on the donor's red cells. These reactions happen immediately after the transfusion. Antibodies to antigens in the ABO, Rh, Kidd, Duffy, and Kell systems may be responsible for an HTR.

acute or delayed

Hemolytic transfusion reactions (HTRs) are described as either acute or delayed. They are also classified according to the location where red cells are destroyed, that is, whether hemolysis occurs intravascularly (within the vascular system) or extravascularly (outside the vascular system, such as in the spleen). Acute HTRs usually are associated with intravascular hemolysis, whereas delayed HTRs are associated with extravascular hemolysis, although there are exceptions.

intravascular hemolysis
extravascular hemolysis

Acute Hemolytic Transfusion Reactions

One of the most severe and life-threatening immune reactions is the acute hemolytic transfusion reaction (AHTR). Acute HTRs are rare, however, because an occurrence is usually due to clerical error. In an AHTR, antigens on donor red cells react with recipient antibodies leading to complement activation and the intravascular destruction of red cells. Complement proteins bind to the antigen-antibody complex and lyse the red cell membrane via the membrane attack complex (MAC).

intravascular
hemolysis:
↓
complement activation
↓
red cell lysis

Causes   An AHTR is almost always caused by the transfusion of ABO-incompatible blood, and can be precipitated by small amounts of transfused blood, as little as 10 to 20 mL. An AHTR is life-threatening and should prompt immediate action.

ABO-incompatible
blood

Acute HTRs can also be caused by blood components that contain plasma, such as platelet concentrates and fresh frozen plasma. In this situation, donor plasma contains antibodies directed against recipient antigens, which when combined with complement causes hemolysis. Another instance, although rare, in which a recipient can have an AHTR is when he or she is receiving red cells from one donor and a plasma-containing component from another donor. The donor red cells are incompatible with plasma antibodies from the other donor and when mixed in the recipient leads to hemolysis. The degree of hemolysis is usually much less than that seen with red cell transfusions.

plasma-containing
components

Symptoms   The following are signs and symptoms of an AHTR: fever, chills, pain at the needle site, nausea, chest and back pain, hypotension (decreased blood pressure), shock, vomiting, flushed skin, shortness of breath, hemoglobinuria (pink or red urine), thrombocytopenia (low platelet numbers), an increased level of lactate dehydrogenase (LDH is an enzyme released by damaged tissue), increased amounts of bilirubin (a breakdown product of hemoglobin), little or no urine production, and generalized bleeding due to disseminated intravascular coagulation (DIC).

In an anesthetized individual, signs that can accompany an AHTR are DIC, hypotension, and hemoglobinuria.

renal failure

The most difficult complication to manage in an AHTR is renal failure. This complication involves the following: intravascular hemolysis, DIC, complement activation, cytokine release, hypotension, renal vasoconstriction, and formation of intravascular thrombi (clots). When renal shutdown occurs, the individual is slowly poisoned because the kidneys

uremia

cannot remove impurities from the blood and uremia develops. Dialysis is required to cleanse the blood if the kidneys no longer function and is conducted 3 to 4 times a week until kidney function returns to normal.

Treatments   The treatment for an AHTR consists of stopping the transfusion immediately, controlling DIC, maintaining blood pressure with drugs, providing cardiac support, and maintaining renal function with I.V. fluids and diuretics.

Delayed Hemolytic Transfusion Reactions

primary immunization: within 2 weeks

There are two types of delayed hemolytic transfusion reactions. One is caused by primary immunization, when an individual is first exposed to an antigen. This type of reaction occurs within 2 weeks following a transfusion. Antibody titers (levels) increase and cause extravascular hemolysis of any donor red cells still in circulation. Primary immunization rarely causes any problems in an individual other than a drop in Hct and Hgb levels.

The other type of delayed hemolytic transfusion reaction occurs in individuals who have been previously sensitized and is usually nonlife-threatening.

These individuals have an anamnestic (secondary) response to the sensitizing antigen. The response occurs within 3 to 7 days from the time of transfusion. Delayed reactions can also occur up to 6 weeks. The most noticeable effects are fever, drop in Hct and Hgb levels, possibly mild jaundice of the skin, and hemoglobinuria. The antigens most frequently responsible for this reaction are in the Kidd and Kell systems.

anamnastic response: within 3 to 7 days

Allergic Transfusion Reactions

Causes

Allergic transfusion reactions are common and usually nonlife-threatening. Proteins in donor plasma are thought to be the causative factor of allergic reactions in recipients. The causative factor is referred to as an allergen. A recipient reacts to the allergen by releasing histamine from mast cells and basophils during or following the transfusion. Histamine release is responsible for the signs and symptoms of the reaction.

donor plasma proteins

allergen
histamine release

Symptoms

Signs of an allergic reaction usually are hives (welts) and itching. An allergic reaction is called urticarial, from urticaria, meaning welts. Although an allergic reaction is usually mild, it can become more serious and lead to wheezing and stridor (abnormal breathing sounds).

utricarial reaction

Treatments

As soon as an allergic reaction becomes evident, the transfusion should be stopped. If the reaction remains localized, with hives or itching being the only symptoms, the transfusion can be restarted, provided antihistamines have been administered and are effective in relieving the local symptoms. Antihistamines, such as diphenhydramine (Benadryl™), are agents that block the action of histamine. If the reaction progresses and hives become more widespread over a major portion of a patient's body, the transfusion should not be restarted. Allergic reactions usually need no further treatment.

antihistamines

Allergic reactions to blood components can be prevented in individuals known to have them by pretransfusion administration of antihistamines.

Anaphylactic Transfusion Reactions

Causes

anaphylaxis: an immune–mediated reaction

Anaphylaxis is a serious, life-threatening, immune-mediated reaction in response to an allergen (bee sting, etc.). Anaphylaxis occurs after hypersensitive individuals, those who have developed IgE antibody (sensitivity) following primary immunization, are reexposed to the sensitizing allergen. The anaphylactic reaction is referred to as a type I hypersensitivity reaction. Anaphylactic reactions resulting from blood transfusions are rare, although they can occur in certain individuals. Anaphylactic transfusion reactions are almost always fatal unless immediate medical therapy is initiated. Only small amounts of an allergen are necessary to initiate an anaphylactic reaction (see Ch. 9, The Immune System).

type I hypersensitivity reaction

Features

IgE production

The major features of anaphylaxis include: the production of IgE, the release of histamine, and involvement of several organ systems, such as the skin, lungs, heart, and the gastrointestinal system. Fever is not usually associated with this reaction.

Anaphylactoid Reactions

Causes

no IgE production

The anaphylactoid reaction differs from the anaphylactic reaction. This reaction is not mediated by the action of IgE antibody but by anaphylatoxins, IgG antibody complexes, and cytokines released by activated macrophages.

anaphylatoxins, IgG antibody complexes, cytokines

Anaphylactoid reactions following a transfusion can

occur in a recipient after only a few mL of the component have been transfused. Antigen–IgG antibody complexes form and activate the classical complement pathway. Complement proteins C3, C4, and C5 are cleaved and in the process generate anaphylatoxins C3a, C4a, and C5a. When anaphylatoxins are released into the circulation they cause basophil and mast cell degranulation, which is the release of histamine and other chemicals.

Substances that cause anaphylactoid reactions include: nonsteroidal anti–inflammatory drugs, such as aspirin and ibuprofen; certain narcotics, such as morphine; blood products, such as plasma proteins; muscle relaxants, such as curare; and exercise. All of the above can cause the cleavage of complement components C3, C4, and C5 and the generation of anaphylatoxins.

antigen–IgG
antibody complex
↓
classical complement
pathway
↓
anaphylatoxins:
C3a, C4a, C5a
↓
histamine release

Symptoms

Symptoms of an anaphylactoid reaction are similar to those of an anaphylactic reaction although milder. Initial symptoms of anaphylactic and anaphylactoid reactions include: coughing, bronchospasm (closing of the bronchus), laryngeal edema (swelling of larynx), flushing of the skin, hypotension, rapid heart rate (tachycardia), nausea, abdominal cramping, bloated abdomen, vomiting, diarrhea, shock, loss of consciousness, and the impending feeling of doom. Temperature is not usually elevated and is one of the diagnostic indicators separating anaphylactic reactions from acute hemolytic transfusion reactions.

Treatments

If either an anaphylactic or anaphylactoid reaction occurs, the transfusion should be stopped immediately. An I.V. of 0.9% normal saline should be kept open, and such drugs as epinephrine (adrenaline) readily available for quick administration as well as endotracheal intubation equipment in the event that a patient develops severe laryngeal edema.

Vasovagal Response

Either an anaphylactic or anaphylactoid reaction can be confused with a vasovagal response, which is a reaction caused by stress or pain. Vasovagal responses are manifested by decreased heart rate and blood pressure, and possibly loss of consciousness, among others. If an individual is incorrectly diagnosed and treated for a vasovagal response rather than for a anaphylactoid reaction, the outcome can be fatal.

Other Causes of Anaphylactic and Anaphylactoid Reactions

There are many other causes of anaphylactic and anaphylactoid reactions. They include: the direct infusion of allergens, such as the drugs aspirin, penicillin, and heparin; foods, such as eggs, shellfish, and peanuts; chemicals, such as ethylene oxide, which are used in the sterilization of the blood bags and transfusion equipment; infusion of blood component containing IgE antibody; and blood components containing high levels of complement-derived anaphylatoxins.

IgA Deficiency Certain individuals are at greater risk for anaphylactic and anaphylactoid transfusion reactions, most notably people who are IgA-deficient and have anti-IgA antibody. This antibody may have developed in response to a previous exposure (transfusion) or may have arisen spontaneously.

A transfusion of IgA-deficient blood products is recommended for an IgA-deficient individual—but only if the individual has experienced a previous anaphylactic reaction. IgA-deficient blood products may be obtained from IgA-deficient donors. Another method for obtaining IgA-depleted blood includes washing units of plasma-containing cellular components. An individual with anti-IgA antibody can donate units of autologous blood and plasma that are kept frozen for use later.

Febrile Nonhemolytic Transfusion Reactions

Along with allergic reactions, febrile nonhemolytic transfusion reactions (FNHTRs) are the most common transfusion reactions. Traditionally an FNHTR has been defined as an increase in body temperature of 1C or higher following a blood transfusion.

1C increase in body temperature

Causes

Recipients can develop FNHTRs following the infusion of Red Cells, Granulocytes, Platelets, and peripheral blood progenitor cells (PBPCs). FNHTRs occur most often in individuals who have been sensitized to numerous leukocyte alloantigens following transfusions or in females who have had multiple pregnancies.

sensitization to leukocyte alloantigens

Current research indicates that the cause of FNHTRs is more complex than just antibody directed against leukocyte antigens. There are several mechanisms involved in FNHTRs, and not all reactions are associated with fever, released cytokines, or antigen-antibody complexes. It is clear that the length of component storage time and leukocyte numbers in the component play a role in FNHTRs. Most reactions occur toward the end of the transfusion or shortly thereafter. This indicates that the cause of FNHTRs is somehow dose-dependent, that is, the more of the component the recipient receives the greater the chance an FNHTR will occur.

storage time
leukocyte numbers

dose-dependent cause

Symptoms

The symptoms of FNHTRs include: fever (not always), chills, rigors, general feeling of malaise, and sometimes headache, nausea, and vomiting.

Packed Red Cells as Causes

Febrile NHTRs following the infusion of Packed Red Cells are caused by antibodies in the recipient that react to antigens on the leukocyte membrane (MHC/HLA and others). Therefore the likelihood of

BRMs

an FNHTR is dependent on the number of leukocytes in the unit of Packed Red Cells. FNHTRs are also caused by chemically active molecules called biological response modifiers (BRMs). Cytokines, complement proteins, and lipids are examples of BRMs that accumulate during storage. BRMs are dependent on the number of leukocytes in the unit.

leukocyte-reduction

It is known that if Packed Red Cell units are leukocyte-reduced to less than 5 x 10^8 leukocytes per unit, the incidence of FNHTRs is greatly reduced. Leukocyte-reduction is usually performed post-storage, before the Red Cells are infused into the recipient. Leukocytes can be removed by either centrifugation or filtration. Present filters on the market can leukocyte-reduce Packed Red Cells and Whole Blood to less than 5 x 10^6 leukocytes per unit.

antipyretics

Treatments Individuals who develop FNHTRs caused by red cell infusions are initially given antipyretics, such as acetaminophen, once a more serious reaction has been ruled out. Antipyretics are drugs that reduce fever, such as aspirinlike drugs. Individuals who have had at least two FNHTRs are provided with leukocyte-reduced Packed Red Cells and Whole Blood.

Platelets as Causes

Platelet concentrates are more likely to cause FNHTRs than Packed Red Cells. The cause seems to be due to two different mechanisms, (1) BRMs that accumulate during platelet storage and (2) antigen-antibody complexes that form in the recipient.

BRMs
antigen-antibody
complexes

leukocyte-reduction

Treatments Platelet-related FNHTRs caused by antigen-antibody complexes can be decreased with the use of leukocyte-reduced (leukocyte-poor) platelet units. Leukocyte-reduction should be performed before the unit is stored. While this will not prevent FNHTRs caused by BRMs, it reduces their occurrence. However, there are filters available that adsorb BRMs and thus decrease the incidence of FNHTRs. The disadvantage of filtering platelet units is that it activates complement, which in itself can precipitate an FNHTR.

Plasmapheresis also decreases the chances of an FNHTR by removing most BMRs. Plasma removal requires that the platelet-rich-plasma be centrifuged to separate the platelets and plasma. The only disadvantage to plasma removal is that the platelets cannot be infused for at least 1 hour to allow the platelets to separate from one another.

plasmapheresis

Leukocyte-reduced blood components should be used to prevent an FNHTR in sensitized individuals. Prevention can also be accomplished by the use of antipyretics before the transfusion is initiated. Acetaminophen is the antipyretic of choice. Aspirin should not be administered to donors or recipients of platelet transfusions because aspirin destroys platelet function.

acetaminophen

Transfusion–related Acute Lung Injury

Transfusion-related acute lung injury (TRALI) is a rare transfusion reaction. Individuals who develop TRALI do so within 1 to 6 hours following the administration of a plasma-containing blood product. TRALI most often occurs in the very young and the elderly and most have no prior history of a transfusion reaction.

within 1 to 6 hours

Symptoms

The obvious sign is acute pulmonary edema with no evidence of myocardial damage or volume overload. An individual experiences severe respiratory distress due to the release of fluid from the vascular system into the lung tissue. Blockage in the pulmonary vasculature forces fluid from the plasma into the interstitial spaces of the lungs and results in pulmonary edema. Other symptoms associated with TRALI are: fever, cyanosis, tachycardia (rapid heart rate), hypotension, and hypoxemia (low partial pressure of oxygen in the blood).

acute pulmonary edema

Causes

The blood components associated with TRALI include: Packed Red Cells; Whole Blood; granulocytes prepared by apheresis; platelet concentrates and Platelets collected by apheresis; and cryoprecipitate.

TRALI: possibly immune-mediated by donor antibodies or cytokines released by activated macrophages

The cause of TRALI is not entirely clear; it is assumed that TRALI is immune-mediated and that the antibodies are donor rather than recipient in origin. Antigen–antibody complexes within the recipient activate complement proteins that cause damage to the endothelial lining of the pulmonary microvasculature, thereby causing pulmonary edema. Cytokines released by activated macrophages in the recipient are also involved with TRALI.

The following agents induce pulmonary vascular damage:

- Agglutinins, which are antibodies that agglutinate antigens
- HLA antibodies in donor plasma that activate complement proteins within the recipient
- White cells that aggregate and settle in the small vessels of the pulmonary vasculature and cause endothelial cell damage

Diagnosis

There is no specific diagnostic test for TRALI. The diagnosis is made through an exclusion process by ruling out other possibilities for pulmonary edema and respiratory distress. Most patients recover without any ill effects within 2 to 4 days if respiratory support is provided.

Treatments

The treatment for TRALI usually consists of steroid administration to curb the immune response and mechanical ventilation and oxygen therapy for respiratory support.

Transfusion-associated Graft-versus-host Disease

Causes

Transfusion-associated graft-versus-host disease (TAGVHD) is a rare but serious immunologic reaction that occurs (1) in immunoincompetent individuals, (2) in individuals receiving a blood transfusion from a blood relative, and (3) in recipients who share an HLA haplotype with the donor. TAGVHD usually occurs within 8 to 10 days following a transfusion of a donor blood component that contains viable T lymphocytes.

TAGVHD: immune-mediated reaction within 8 to 10 days

Immunocompetent individuals receiving a blood transfusion can develop TAGVHD if they are transfused with blood products from a blood relative, such as a mother, father, or siblings or, in some cases, an unrelated donor. In the above situations the donor and recipient share an HLA haplotype. The donor T lymphocytes recognize the unshared HLA of the recipient as foreign and mount an immune response against recipient bone marrow, skin, and GI tract.

Symptoms

The most serious symptoms of TAGVHD are bone marrow aplasia and pancytopenia, resulting in a decrease in the number of all blood cells. Aplasia occurs when donor cytotoxic T lymphocytes attack and destroy the recipient's bone marrow. Once the marrow is destroyed, blood cell production cannot take place and pancytopenia ensues.

pancytopenia
aplasia

Other symptoms of TAGVHD include the following: watery diarrhea, liver function abnormalities, nausea, vomiting, and skin rash. The mortality rate from TAGVHD is as high as 90% due to infections and hemorrhage resulting from granulocytopenia and thrombocytopenia (decreased granulocytes and platelets).

Treatment

There is no known treatment for TAGVHD. Death usually follows within 3 to 4 weeks following the transfusion.

Prevention

TAGVHD can be prevented in susceptible individuals if donor blood components are irradiated prior to infusion. Irradiation destroys the T lymphocytes within the unit. The dose of irradiation that destroys most lymphocytes in the blood product is 2500 cGy (25 Gy = 1 rad). This amount of radiation does not destroy other cellular components in the unit. Blood components that have viable lymphocytes are Whole Blood, Packed Red Cells, and Platelets.

Candidates for irradiated blood products are donor-recipient relatives, patients who have received or are about to receive an autologous or allogeneic bone marrow transplant, neonates undergoing an exchange transfusion, fetuses having intrauterine transfusions, leukemia patients receiving high-dose chemotherapy, and individuals with lymphomas or severe combined immunodeficiency syndrome (SCIDS).

Post-transfusion Purpura

Causes

PTP:
anamnastic response
within 7 to 10 days

Post-transfusion purpura (PTP) is a transfusion reaction that occurs approximately 7 to 10 days following a transfusion of cellular components. This reaction is a classic example of an anamnestic response. It is most common in females who have become sensitized to platelet-specific alloantigens through pregnancy. PTP can also occur following blood transfusions in recipients who have received multiple transfusions.

Symptoms

Post-transfusion purpura is responsible for severe

thrombocytopenia. Antiplatelet antibodies within recipient plasma are directed against platelet-specific antigens on donor platelets. An immune response reduces the recipient's platelet numbers. Thrombocytopenia poses a risk of hemorrhage.

thrombocytopenia

Treatments

Most individuals with PTP are treated with corticosteroids, which lessen the immune response. The prognosis for recovery is usually good, and most recipients improve within several weeks. The course of thrombocytopenia can be slowed by plasmapheresis, which removes antibodies that destroy donor platelets. Another therapy is the use of intravenous gammaglobulin (IVGG).

corticosteroids

IVGG

Nonimmune Adverse Events

Although the following transfusion complications cause problems for recipients, they are not prompted by an immune response to foreign antigens. Nonimmune transfusion complications include: acute nonimmune hemolytic reactions, circulatory overload, hemosiderosis, and infections associated with blood transfusions.

acute nonimmune hemolytic reactions, circulatory overload, hemosiderosis, infections

Acute Nonimmune Hemolytic Transfusion Reactions

Causes Acute nonimmune hemolytic transfusion reactions (ANHTRs) result when blood is hemolyzed in any of the following situations:

red cell hemolysis

- Infusion of blood that has been improperly warmed in a malfunctioning blood warmer, left out at room temperature, or frozen improperly

temperature

- Infusion of a hypotonic (lower ionic concentration) normal saline solution

NS concentration

- Infusion of blood through a small bore needle

small bore needle

- Infusion of contaminated blood containing bacterial endotoxins

bacterial endotoxins

Symptoms An ANHTR can possibly have a fatal outcome, but this is very rare. Signs and symptoms can include: possible chest and back pain, shortness of breath, and hemoglobinuria.

Circulatory Overload

Causes When a transfusion adds more fluid to the circulatory system than the system can accommodate, circulatory overload results. This condition occurs most frequently in neonates, the elderly, and normovolemic patients who have cardiac disease, renal failure, or anemia.

Symptoms These include: pulmonary edema, dyspnea, and possibly hypertension.

Treatments Treatment for circulatory overload usually involves one, two, or all of the following steps: administration of diuretics to remove excess fluid, assistance of pulmonary function with oxygen therapy, and removal of a portion of blood through phlebotomy (rarely needed).

diuretics

oxygen therapy

phlebotomy

Any individual considered likely to develop circulatory overload should be transfused slowly and monitored closely for signs of overload. Complications due to circulatory overload illustrate the importance of administering the appropriate component in a transfusion.

Hemosiderosis

Causes and Symptoms Hemosiderosis is the accumulation of excess iron in vital organs such as the liver and heart, which cause these organs to malfunction. The buildup of iron usually results from transfusions of Whole Blood or Packed Red Cells over many years. A unit of Whole Blood or Packed Red Cells contains large amounts of iron present in hemoglobin.

excess iron in vital organs

Treatments Use of the chelating agent known as desferrioxamine can prevent iron buildup. Desferrioxamine binds excess iron and removes it

desferrioxamine

from the body. Recipients who require frequent Packed Red Cell transfusions sometimes receive infusions of neocytes (young red cells). Younger cells have a longer circulating time, which reduces the number of transfusions required.

neocytes

CHART 1: Adverse Events in Transfusion

Hemolytic Transfusion Reactions

Acute HTR

Description: A serious life-threatening reaction caused by an antigen-antibody-complement response to ABO incompatibility.

Causes: Transfusion of ABO-incompatible blood, Packed Red Cells, or other red cell-containing components, in which antibodies and complement in the recipient plasma attach to transfused donor red cells leading to intravascular lysis of transfused red cells.

Symptoms: Intravascular hemolysis, shock, DIC, renal failure, and others.

Actions: Stop the transfusion immediately. Monitor the patient closely. Maintain renal blood flow and treat DIC if it occurs.

Delayed HTR

Primary Immunization

Description: The primary immunization type of a delayed HTR is usually a nonlife-threatening reaction. It occurs approximately within 2 weeks following a transfusion.

Causes: Newly elicited antibodies within the recipient plasma attack donor red cells.

Symptoms: The only indication are drops in the Hgb and Hct.

Actions: No treatment is usually required for this reaction.

Anamnestic (Secondary) Response

Description: This type of delayed HTR is usually nonlife-threatening. It occurs within 3 to 7 days following the transfusion.

Causes: The most common cause is due to antibodies in the recipient that are directed against red cell antigens, often in the Kidd and Kell systems.

Symptoms: The most likely indications are fever, drops in the Hgb and Hct, and possibly a mild jaundice. Occasionally, hemoglobinuria occurs.

Actions: There is usually no treatment required for this response, but if hemoglobinuria occurs the patient should be monitored closely.

(continued)

CHART 1: **Adverse Events in Transfusion**, *continued*

Nonhemolytic Transfusion Reactions
Allergic Reactions
Description: This reaction is usually nonlife-threatening. Allergic reactions are recognized by itching and hives (welts) formation.

Causes: Some recipients of allogeneic blood products react to donor plasma proteins. The recipient releases histamine.

Symptoms: Itching and hive formation (urticaria). More serious reactions may lead to stridor.

Actions: Stop the transfusion immediately and monitor the patient closely. Antihistamine is used for treatment of symptoms.

Anaphylactic Transfusion Reactions / Type I Hypersensitivity Reaction
Description: One of the most serious transfusion reactions. Anaphylaxis occurs in hypersensitive individuals following reexposure to the offending antigen. This reaction has the strong possibility of being fatal. True anaphylactic reactions require the presence of IgE.

Causes: Many situations, such as bee stings and food allergies, can cause an anaphylactic transfusion reaction, but rarely by the infusion of blood plasma and components. Also implicated are IgA deficiencies.

Symptoms: Coughing, bronchospasm, laryngeal edema, flushing, hypotension, tachycardia, nausea, bloated abdomen, vomiting, diarrhea, shock, sense of doom, involvement of several organ systems, and other symptoms. Fever is not usually associated with this reaction.

Actions: The transfusion should be stopped immediately and the I.V. kept open with normal saline (0.9% NS). Epinephrine should be readily available. The individual may need to be intubated if laryngeal edema is serious.

Anaphylactoid Transfusion Reaction
Description: This is reaction very similar to an anaphylactic transfusion reaction, but IgE is not produced in response to the sensitizing antigen. The reaction is mediated by anaphylatoxins, IgG antibody complexes, and cytokines. Histamine and other chemicals are released.

Causes: Nonsteroidal anti-inflammatory drugs, some narcotics, blood products, muscle relaxants, exercise are causes.

(continued)

CHART 1: **Adverse Events in Transfusion,** *continued*

Symptoms: Similar to those in an anaphylactoid reaction but milder.

Actions: The reaction is treated the same way as an anaphylactic reaction. Like the anaphylactic reaction it can be fatal.

Other Causes of Anaphylactic and Anaphylactoid Reactions

The following are responsible for anaphylactic and anaphylactoid reactions: preexisting antibodies to MHC, and other substances, such as albumin, aspirin, penicillin, food allergens, chemicals introduced in making blood bags, blood components containing IgE, antibodies to penicillin, blood components with high levels of complement-derived anaphylatoxins, among others.

Febrile Nonhemolytic Transfusion Reactions (FNHTRs)

Description: Along with allergic reactions, FNHTRs are the most common transfusion reactions. They occur most often in individuals who have received multiple transfusions or have had multiple pregnancies.

Causes: Recipient antibodies react against antigens on donor platelets, granulocytes, and lymphocytes, and PBPCs. FNHTRs may also be caused by cytokines that accumulate in the component during storage.

Symptoms: Possible temperature increase of 1C, chills, and general feeling of malaise. An FNHTR usually does not progress to a more serious reaction.

Actions: Treat the fever with antipyretics. Leukocyte-depleted blood components to decrease the likelihood of an FNHTR. Plasmapheresis also removes BRMs.

Transfusion-Related Acute Lung Injury (TRALI)

Description: A rare reaction characterized by the presence of pulmonary edema not caused by cardiac problems or volume overload. Occurs most often in the very young and elderly.

Causes: TRALI occurs within 1 to 6 hours in individuals following administration of a plasma-containing blood product. The exact cause is not clear, although it is possibly immune-mediated.

(continued)

CHART 1: **Adverse Events in Transfusion,** *continued*

Symptoms: The classic sign is pulmonary edema and respiratory distress. Other symptoms are fever, cyanosis, tachycardia, hypotension, and hypovolemia.

Actions: Stop the transfusion and administer steroids, oxygen therapy, and ventilation.

Transfusion–Associated GVHD (TAGVHD)

Description: The most serious form of GVHD. It typically occurs within 8 to 10 days of an immunoincompetent individual or immediate blood relative or haplotype identical blood donor receiving a blood transfusion.

Causes: Donor T cells attack recipient bone marrow, skin, and gastrointestinal tract.

Symptoms: Bone marrow aplasia, pancytopenia, diarrhea, nausea, vomiting, skin rash, and liver function abnormalities

Actions: There is no real treatment for TAGVHD; therefore, prevention is key. In susceptible individuals, blood transfusion products containing viable lymphocytes should be irradiated.

Post–Transfusion Purpura

Description: Post-transfusion purpura (PTP) occurs approximately 7 to 10 days following a blood transfusion in sensitized individuals (previously transfused or having had multiple pregnancies). It is marked by a severe drop in platelet numbers. PTP usually is nonlife-threatening.

Causes: Antiplatelet antibodies that develop in the recipient following a previous blood transfusion or pregnancy. Subsequent transfusion with a blood product that contains platelet antigens can cause thrombocytopenia.

Symptoms: Marked thrombocytopenia

Actions: Corticosteroids are used to reduce platelet destruction. Plasma exchange can reduce the amount of antibodies. Intravenous gammaglobulin (IVGG) may be useful.

Nonimmune Transfusion Complications

Acute Nonimmune

Causes: Infusion of blood via small bore needle, blood kept at room temperature, contaminated blood, and hypotonic NS can cause this complication.   *(continued)*

CHART 1: **Adverse Events in Transfusion,** *continued*

Symptoms: Possible chest and back pain, dyspnea, hemoglobinuria

Actions: Stop the transfusion immediately and monitor the patient, making sure it is not a more serious reaction.

Circulatory Overload

Description: A transfusion complication marked by congestive heart failure with subsequent pulmonary edema following the rapid infusion of a blood component. This complication is most likely to occur in the elderly or very young and usually is not life-threatening, but it has the possibility to create serious problems for the recipient.

Causes: The circulation contains more volume than it can accommodate. Circulatory overload occurs most often in normovolemic individuals with cardiac disease, renal failure, and anemia, and in neonates and the elderly.

Symptoms: Pulmonary edema, dyspnea, and possibly increased hypertension

Actions: Stop the transfusion. Diuretics may be required to decrease the amount of fluid. Rarely is the removal of excess volume (blood) by phlebotomy necessary.

Hemosiderosis

Description: This usually is not an immediate threat to life, but if left untreated may become a chronic problem.

Causes: Chronic transfusions of Whole Blood or Packed Red Cells. These products contain Hgb, which consists of iron. Iron buildup in vital organs can lead to organ failure.

Symptoms: Liver function abnormalities and dysrhythmias

Actions: The use of desferrioxamine, a chelating agent, is used to bind excess iron. The use of neocytes or Packed Red Cells in transfusion therapy reduces the number of transfusions necessary.

Bacterial Contamination

Infectious Complications: See Chapter 14, Transfusion and Disease Transmission

CHART 2: Steps to Follow When Symptoms of an Adverse Event Occur

- Stop the transfusion immediately
- Maintain I.V. of 0.9% normal saline to maintain venous access for drug administration
- Report incident to physician and blood bank
- Check blood bag tags with patient identification band
- Treat symptoms appropriately
- Send unused portion of blood in blood bag and the administration set to the blood bank
- Collect and send blood and urine samples to the lab
- Document the transfusion reaction and treatment thoroughly

CHART 3: Symptoms of Adverse Events in the Unconscious or Anesthetized Patient

Symptoms:
- Weak or absent pulse
- Decrease in blood pressure
- Small amount of urine: possibly none produced
- Fever
- Increase or decrease in the heart rate
- Increase in amount of bleeding during surgery
- Visible signs of Hgb in the urine (hemoglobinuria)

Actions:

Stop the transfusion immediately and monitor the patient closely
Initiate treatment

■ **QUESTIONS** ■

1. Contrast transfusion reaction with transfusion complication.

2. Define acute versus delayed and local versus systemic adverse events.

3. List six types of immune response caused by transfusion therapy.

4. What occurs when the antibodies in the plasma of the transfusion recipient react with the antigens on the donor's red cells?

5. How is the phenomenon described above classified?

6. What is the most common cause of an AHTR?

7. What is the most difficult adverse event to manage in an AHTR? Why?

8. What is the first step taken by a health care worker during a transfusion reaction?

9. Compare and contrast the two types of delayed hemolytic transfusion reactions.

10. Describe the signs and symptoms of an allergic transfusion reaction.

11. What is the immediate treatment for an allergic transfusion reaction?

12. What type of allergic reaction is sometimes fatal? and what causes it?

13. Identify five causes of anaphylactoid reactions.

14. How are anaphylactic or anaphylactoid trans fusion reactions treated?

15. Define a vasovagal response.

16. What population is at greatest risk for an anaphylactic or anaphylactoid reaction?

17. How is a febrile nonhemolytic transfusion reaction (FNHTR) defined?

18. What population is most susceptible to incurring an FNHTR?

19. Febrile nonhemolytic transfusion reactions are caused by biological response modifiers (BMRs). What are they?

20. There are two categories of cause for FNHTR. What are they? and how is each treated? Explain your answer.

21. Transfusion-related acute lung injury (TRALI) occurs within 24 to 72 hours of the transfusion. True or False?

22. What symptoms are associated with TRALI?

23. List three agents that can induce pulmonary vascular damage.

24. How is TRALI usually treated?

25. In what populations does transfusion-associated graft-versus-host disease (TAGVHD) occur?

26. Why is TAGVHD most often fatal?

27. How can TAGVHD be prevented?

28. What condition would a diagnostician suspect in an individual who has had many platelet transfusions and is showing signs of bleeding?

29. How is this condition treated?

30. Identify four transfusion complications not prompted by an immune response.

31. List four potential causes of an acute nonimmune hemolytic transfusion reaction.

32. Ms. Hayes, a 74-year-old woman, has a long history of cardiac problems. Immediately after her blood transfusion for anemia she had difficulty breathing while getting off the table and into her coat, her lungs were congested on auscultation (by stethoscope, and her blood pressure was 178/92. From what condition was she most likely suffering?

33. How is hemosiderosis, the accumulation of too much iron in certain vital organs, treated?

CHAPTER **16**

Transfusion and Disease Transmission

Introduction

During the 1980s, fear of contracting AIDS forced the public and medical community to question the safety of allogeneic blood and blood products. Three developments have greatly reduced the incidence of disease transmission via blood transfusions: (1) newly developed blood tests, which are 99% accurate; (2) more stringent donor standards; and (3) ability of donors to exclude themselves anonymously. Nevertheless, diseases transmitted through transfusions remain a threat to recipients.

Hepatitis and AIDS are two viral diseases of major concern to most transfusion recipients and health care professionals. These viruses are discussed in this chapter along with other viruses and bacteria that can contaminate blood.

Blood Testing

All blood donations must be screened for certain transmissible bacterial and viral diseases. Tests for these diseases detect antigenic markers or antibodies against them. Testing of blood and blood components is required by the American Association of Blood Banks (AABB) and the Food and Drug Administration (FDA). These organizations set definitive standards for all blood banking and transfusion policies in the United States.

antigenic markers
antibodies

AABB, FDA

The following assays test serum for infectious agents in blood:

HBsAg
(1) The hepatitis B surface antigen (HBsAg) assay detects antigenic particles.

anti-HBc
(2) Anti-HBc assay detects antibody to hepatitis B core antigen.

anti-HCV
(3) Anti-HCV assay detects antibody against hepatitis C.

anti-HIV 1/2
(4) Anti-HIV 1/2 assay detects antibody produced in response to HIV. Human immunodeficiency viruses 1 and 2 (HIV 1/2) lead to AIDS.

HIV-1-Ag
(5) HIV-1 antigen (HIV-1-Ag) is a test that detects the presence of HIV directly. It is believed that a positive result may provide an indication of HIV infection before antibody can be detected in the blood. AABB and FDA standards require all blood and blood components be negative for the HIV-1 antigen.

anti-HTLV-I/II
(6) Anti-HTLV-I/II assay detects antibody to the human T cell lymphotropic virus type I/II, which is a viral precursor to a rare type of leukemia, a specific type of cancer known as lymphoma, and a paralytic disease that affects the nervous system. HTLV-I is predominantly found in individuals of Japanese and Caribbean ancestry. HTLV-II is predominantly found in Native Americans and I.V. drug users. The only disease associated with HTLV-II is HTLV-associated myelopathy (HAM).

syphilis antibody to a lipid antigen
(7) Serologic test for syphilis (STS) detects antibody in the serum to a lipid antigen.

Other Transfusion-transmissible Diseases

malaria

babesiosis

Malaria, babesiosis, cytomegalovirus (CMV), and Epstein-Barr Virus (EBV) are other transfusion-transmissible diseases. Babesiosis is the most common parasitic disease associated with transfusions. It is sometimes fatal and caused by a protozoan parasite that attacks red cells. It is transmitted by the bite of a deer tick and occurs mostly in the northeastern United States. The parasite has the ability to survive in blood stored at 4C. Cytomegalovirus is a problem only for immunoincompetent individuals and newborns weighing 1250 g (approximately 3 lb) or less. This disease is discussed later in this chapter. Epstein-Barr virus rarely precipitates disease in immunocompetent recipients.

cytomegalovirus

Epstein-Barr virus

Donation Deferral

If a donor's blood tests positive for any of the diseases highlighted in this section, the blood is discarded and the donor is deferred from donation. Individuals who have been in an area in which malaria is endemic are not permitted to donate blood for one year.

Seronegative donor blood means that the tested serum does not contain antibody and/or antigen against infectious organisms. Seropositive donor blood means that the serum does contain antibody and/or antigen to infectious agents.

seronegative

seropositive

Hepatitis

Hepatitis is the inflammation of liver cells. There are five, possibly seven, viruses in the *Hepadnaviridae* family. These viruses include: (1) hepatitis A (HAV); (2) hepatitis B (HBV); (3) hepatitis C (HCV), formerly referred to as non-A non-B; (4) hepatitis D (HDV), previously called delta; and (5) hepatitis E (HEV). Hepatitis F and G are new viruses whose identities are being established. The hepatitis viruses are very hardy and cannot be destroyed even if donor blood is frozen or washed.

inflammation of liver cells

HAV

HBV, HCV

HDV

HEV

Hepatitis A and E viruses are usually not transmitted by blood but by contaminated food or water and unsanitary conditions. Transfusion-related hepatitis most often is caused by the B and C viruses. Hepatitis D can infect a person already infected with hepatitis B or a past history of hepatitis B infection. Most hepatitis cases run a course of infection to recovery. Anyone

transfusion-related hepatitis: B and C

who has had hepatitis after his or her 11th birthday is deferred permanently from donating blood.

Signs and Symptoms

The signs and symptoms of hepatitis include: jaundice, fatigue, weight loss, and loss of appetite, among others.

Hepatitis B

HBV

Hepatitis B (HBV) is the most serious form of hepatitis and was previously referred to as serum hepatitis. It is so infectious that as little as 1 pg (picogram) can cause an infection in a recipient. A picogram is equivalent to 0.000000000001 g or 1×10^{-12} g. Individuals infected with HBV usually experience liver damage, and 10% become chronically infected. Chronic HBV carriers can transmit HBV and have an increased risk of developing liver cancer later in life, which is also true for chronic hepatitis C carriers. Seemingly healthy individuals can be carriers and transmitters of HBV.

incubation:
6 to 8 weeks

Hepatitis B is transmitted through blood, body secretions, and vaginal secretions and semen during sexual contact. There are approximately 300,000 new cases in the United States each year. The incubation period is from 6 to 8 weeks.

Blood Tests

surface antigen HBsAg

anti-HBc

Blood tests for HBV reveal the presence of the surface antigen HBsAg, formerly known as the Australia antigen. HBsAg ("s" indicates surface) is the first indicator to appear in the blood of an individual infected with hepatitis B. All persons exposed to hepatitis B form antibody, called anti-HBc, to core antigen. A positive test result on a blood unit warrants that it be discarded.

Hepatitis B Vaccine

The hepatitis B vaccine provides protection against HBV. Vaccination is strongly recommended for health care workers and other persons in routine contact with blood and body fluids. The HBV vaccine is also recommended for newborns. The vaccine stimulates an individual's immune system to produce antibody against HBV. If exposed to the virus, the individual mounts an immune response before the virus can do damage.

The HBV vaccine is given at three separate intervals. Following the initial injection, the second one is given at 1 month and the third at 6 months. A booster shot may be needed at a later time if an individual has a low antibody titer (low levels of antibody to HBV). The HBV vaccination schedule for an infant is somewhat different from the adult's.

Hepatitis B Immune Globulin

Any unvaccinated health care worker accidentally exposed to blood or body fluids of an HBV-infected individual should receive hepatitis B immune globulin (HBIG). HBIG is derived from the plasma of individuals who have developed antibody against HBV. It should be administered as soon as possible or within 7 days from the time of exposure. Health care workers can contract HBV if they puncture themselves with a contaminated needle or get infected blood in open cuts or on any mucosal surface, such as those within the mouth and nose. Babies born of infected HBV mothers should receive HBIG at the time of birth. Those who require HBIG can receive the initial dose of hepatitis B vaccine at the same time.

HBIG

Hepatitis C

Hepatitis C is responsible for 90 to 95% of all transfusion-related hepatitis. This virus has the strong likelihood of causing chronic disease that progresses to cirrhosis. The majority of HCV-positive individuals are asymptomatic and become chronic carriers. Hepatitis C is apt to be a milder infection than hepatitis B. The incubation period is anywhere from 2 to 26 weeks. There are approximately 150,000 to 170,000 new cases in the United States each year.

incubation:
2 to 6 weeks

FIGURE 16.1 The Structure of HIV

This schematic representation shows the basic physical characteristics of HIV. Although it is not a hardy virus, HIV can mutate and form new strains.

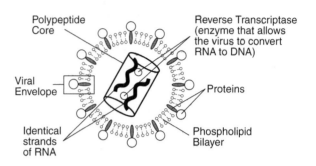

HIV and AIDS

HIV-1
HIV-2

Two strains of virus can transmit AIDS: HIV-1 and HIV-2. HIV-2 is found mostly in West Africa and rarely seen in the United States. It is somewhat different from HIV-1 in that it has a longer incubation time and less chance of progressing to AIDS. Transmission of HIV-2 seems to be less efficient than transmission of HIV-1.

retrovirus

HIV belongs to the family of viruses called *Retroviridae*. HIV is a retrovirus, called a lentivirus, that causes chronic infections. It attacks CD4+ T lymphocytes (see Ch. 6 for functions of CD4+ T cells) and other CD4+-bearing cells, such as macrophages. Most viruses, including HIV, are so small that a billion can fit on the head of a pin.

Transmission

HIV is transmitted by many routes that include: contaminated needles, sperm and vaginal secretions, menstrual blood, breast milk, blood transfusion, or other body fluids passed directly from infected individuals to recipients. Although risk of HIV transmission through transfusion is small because donor blood is tested, contaminated blood will transmit the virus to a recipient.

Blood Tests for HIV

ELISA The enzyme-linked immunosorbent assay (ELISA) is a test that screens serum for antibody to

HIV. When the ELISA is positive for HIV, the serum sample in question is further tested by the Western blot, a more specific confirmatory test. A positive Western blot for HIV indicates that an individual is seroconverted and has detectable antibody to HIV in the blood. Seroconversion refers to the presence of antigen or antibody to HIV in the blood.

Western blot

seroconversion

These tests for antibody to HIV are not foolproof. Although they measure antibodies produced in response to HIV infection, they do not determine the presence of the virus itself. Production of antibody in response to an infection is not immediate because the body takes time to build up an antibody titer (level) that registers a positive test result. The time between the day an infected individual becomes infectious and the appearance of antibody to HIV in the bloodstream is approximately 22 days, which is called the window period, or lag period. An individual recently infected by HIV may not have sufficient antibody titers to test positive. In this case, the ELISA will be negative and donor blood can transmit the virus. An individual who wants to confirm HIV negativity after testing negative to HIV should be retested in 6 months.

antibody titer

window, or lag, period:
22 days

HIV-1-Antigen Test   As of March 1996, the FDA requires that all blood be tested for the presence of the virus itself. The test is called the HIV-1-Antigen Test.

Reproduction of HIV and Development of AIDS

Like all viruses, retroviruses need the genetic material of a cell to reproduce more of themselves. They are equipped with a special enzyme called reverse transcriptase. All retroviruses have RNA (ribonucleic acid) as their genetic material, whereas most organisms, including humans, have DNA (deoxyribonucleic acid). After they gain entry into the host cell, retroviruses use the reverse transcriptase enzyme to convert their RNA into viral DNA. They insert this newly formed viral DNA into the host's DNA. At this point, viral DNA controls the host cell, which is converted into an HIV factory and used to produce more viruses. Newly made

RNA

reverse transcriptase
enzyme

viral DNA

viruses assemble within the host cell. When ready for release, they migrate to the cell membrane and burst through the cell membrane in a process called budding. They are then free to infect other cells.

budding

Immunosuppression

Persons with AIDS lack major components of the immune system: CD4+ T lymphocytes and macrophages. The body cannot conquer any disease without these immune cells because CD4+ T lymphocytes and macrophages are essential to the lines of communication

CD4+ T lymphocytes
macrophages

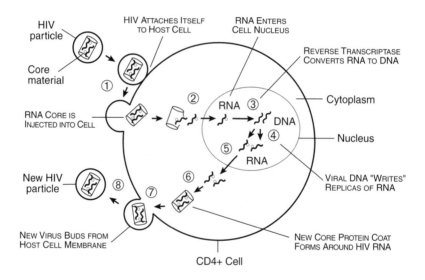

FIGURE 16.2 **HIV Infecting a CD4+ T Cell**
1. The virus attaches to the CD4 cell surface marker (molecule) and releases its core material into the cell. 2. The viral core is disrupted and releases its contents (RNA and enzyme reverse transcriptase). 3. In reverse transcription, viral RNA is converted into DNA. 4. The viral DNA is inserted into the host cell's DNA. At this point the virus takes control of the cell. 5. New viral RNA is made from the host cell's chemicals. 6. New core protein forms a coat around the new viral RNA. 7. The core material moves to the cell membrane. 8. In a process called budding, HIV is released from the host cell. The newly released viruses are free to attack other CD4+ T cells and macrophages.

in the immune response. When HIV invades CD4+ T cells and macrophages, HIV replicates itself and destroys these T cells and macrophages, which can no longer alert other cells—phagocytes, cytotoxic T cells, B cells—to mount an immune response. Because HIV destroys CD4+ cells, the following cannot take place: antigen recognition, conversion of T cells to become cytotoxic cells, and antibody production. As the number of CD4+ T cells declines, infections become more prevalent and also more difficult to treat.

Clinical Definition

The Centers for Disease Control and Prevention (CDC) uses certain standards to indicate that an individual has progressed from being HIV-positive to having AIDS. The number of CD4+ T lymphocytes (greater than 200/μL) *along* with the presence of any of the numerous opportunistic infections associated with HIV is considered diagnostic of AIDS. However, in the absence of severe opportunistic infections AIDS is defined as a CD4+ T cell count of 200/μL or less. A normal blood T cell count is between 800 and 1500 CD4+ T cells/μL.

CDC standard for AIDS: number of CD4+ T lymphocytes

opportunistic infections

Along with decreased numbers of CD4+ T cells, AIDS is clinically defined by the presence of any numerous disease states, such as Kaposi's sarcoma, *Pneumocysitis carinii* pneumonia, toxoplasmosis, and candidiasis, among many others.

Symptoms

An HIV-positive individual can be symptom-free from infection for a while, but over the course of time, the person usually develops minor to severe bacterial, viral, fungal, and protozoan infections. Severity of these infections depends on the number of CD4+ T lymphocytes available to provide immunity. The average time from HIV infection to development of AIDS is approximately 7 years from seroconversion.

HIV→AIDS: 7 years

Classic symptoms of AIDS include: fever, night sweats, fatigue, and infections and tumors such as

Kaposi's sarcoma, a form of cancer characterized by a purplish skin lesion; *Pneumocystis carinii* pneumonia, caused by a ubiquitous protozoan microorganism; thrush, a fungal infection; and lymphadenopathy (enlarged lymph nodes). Diseases associated with AIDS arise because an individual cannot generate an immune response.

Infections associated with AIDS are typically opportunistic infections, so called because they appear in individuals with severely weakened immune systems but not in those with healthy immune systems. Individuals can live with HIV and AIDS for years, but ultimately most succumb to the ravages of the disease.

Treatments

AZT

At the present time, there is no cure for AIDS. Some drugs, such as azidothymidine (AZT), can prolong the onset of AIDS, but these drugs are potent and have many side effects. Treatment can cause chronic problems such as anemia, liver damage, thrombo-cytopenia, neutropenia, and many other blood disorders. Drugs on the market and in clinical trials attempt to make the course of AIDS manageable.

protease inhibitors

At the present time drugs known as protease inhibitors show promise in decreasing the amount of virus in the blood.

Human T Cell Lymphotropic Viruses

HTLV I/II

Human T cell lymphotropic viruses (HTLV-I/II) are a group of retroviruses known to cause disease in blood transfusion recipients who receive infected lymphocytes. Plasma does not transmit HTLV-I/II. Like other retroviruses, HTLV-I/II can lie dormant in cells for years. For this reason, they are said to have a

long latency period

long latency period between the time of infection and the actual signs of disease.

Transmission   Both HTLV-I/II have been found in seronegative individuals who have been transfused with blood from a seropositive donor.

Tests   Tests have been developed that detect antibody to HTLV-I/II. The incidence of positive donors is small, approximately 2 in 10,000 donors. Any unit of blood that tests positive for HTLV-I is discarded. The donor should be notified and permanently deferred from donating.

HTLV-I

HTLV-I appears in some individuals with adult T cell leukemia and lymphoma. It has also been identified as the causative agent of a neurologic condition called tropical spastic paraparesis, which is now called HTLV-associated myelopathy (HAM). HAM attacks and damages the individual's spinal cord. HTLV-I is seen most frequently in Japan, the Caribbean, and other areas.

HAM

HTLV-II

HTLV-II has not been proved to cause any specific disease. The virus has been found in Native Americans and I.V. drug users and in individuals who have HAM.

Syphilis

Transfusion-associated syphilis is a rare occurrence in the Western hemisphere, whereas in earlier times it was a serious health problem. The decrease in transfusion-associated syphilis is mainly due to the storage of blood at 1 to 6C and the universal use of penicillin for the treatment of syphilis.

Transmission

Syphilis is a venereal disease caused by the bacterium *Treponema pallidum*. It is called a venereal disease because it is most often contracted through sexual intercourse. The organism enters the body through the mucous membranes of the genitourinary tract or through any other contact site. *Treponema pallidum* is also transmitted by contact with contaminated material, blood transfusion, and from mother to fetus. The incubation period following a contaminated blood

incubation period: 4 to 5 weeks

transfusion is approximately 4 to 5 weeks, although it can be as long as 10 weeks.

Symptoms

Syphilis causes lesions (sores) to appear on most organs and tissues, especially the skin. The disease can remain undetected for many years.

Stages

There are three stages associated with syphilis:

primary

(1) *Primary stage* Initially lesions called chancres appear on the skin of the penis and vulva about 2 weeks following exposure to the organism. Lymph nodes may swell at this time.

secondary

(2) *Secondary stage* Approximately 6 weeks after the appearance of the primary lesions other lesions appear on the skin and mucous membranes. Fever, headache, rashes, and generalized malaise may or may not occur.

tertiary

(3) *Tertiary stage* When syphilis reaches this stage it affects the blood vessels, heart, and nervous system. Affects on the nervous system include a form of paralysis and different types of psychoses occur.

Blood Donation

There are several tests available for detecting syphilis in the blood (see Blood Tests). Plasma products do not transmit syphilis, but plasma collected from a unit of positive blood should not be used for transfusion.

Treatment

penicillin

Penicillin is the drug of choice. However, if the patient is unable to take penicillin, other drugs are available that are effective against the organism.

Cytomegalovirus

CMV: herpes virus

Cytomegalovirus (CMV) is a member of the herpes family of viruses. Unlike retroviruses, herpes viruses have DNA as their genetic material. CMV has the ability to infect many different types of cells, such as white cells, kidney, liver, lung, and epithelial cells. Various organs can harbor CMV. Within the blood, it is believed that CMV infects white cells, specifically the CD4+ mononuclear cell subsets (T cells and macrophages). The virus can survive indefinitely and become reactivated in individuals whose immune systems are suppressed or compromised.

Transmission

The transmission of CMV can occur through contact with urine, blood, semen, vaginal secretions, airway secretions, and breast milk. Fetuses and newborns can be infected. Most adults contract CMV through sexual contact with an infected individual. Children usually acquire CMV through close contact, such as nursery schools and day care centers.

Approximately 30 to 60% of the adult population have been exposed to CMV. These percentages have been confirmed by the presence of antibody to CMV detected in donor blood. However, only a small percentage of adults are infective (less than 10%; 1 to 4% of blood donors).

CMV Infections

There are three types of CMV infections: primary infection, reactivated infection, and secondary infection. An individual with a primary infection contracts CMV for the first time. The virus can also remain latent in infected cells for many years and then become reactivated. A different strain of the virus is responsible for secondary infection.

A variety of antibodies is produced in response to exposure to CMV. The first is IgM, which is followed by IgG, and IgA. The body sheds the virus in saliva, sperm, cervical secretions, urine, and breast milk.

Evidence of CMV exposure is indicated by (1) seroconversion, denoting antibody in serum, (2) viral shedding in all body secretions, (3) elevated

DNA

white cells

primary infection

reactivated infection
secondary infection

IgM, IgG, IgA

body temperature, and (4) increased lymphocyte production.

Symptoms

mild mononucleosis-like syndrome

The symptoms of CMV vary. Within healthy adults, symptoms may include those of a mild mononucleosis-like syndrome. Primary infection is usually not serious in individuals with a competent immune system. In a person with a reactivated infection, the clinical course is usually milder than it is in a primary infection.

immunoincompetent individuals

graft rejection
superinfection

CMV

The most serious effects of CMV are seen in immunoincompetent individuals who can develop pneumonitis, retinitis, gastritis, and other inflammatory conditions. In immunocompromised individuals, a CMV infection can cause rejection of an allogeneic graft and superinfection, (a combination of infectious agents that attack the body simultaneously). Immunosuppressed or immunincompetent individuals also can experience a latent infection in which CMV is reactivated. In transplant recipients with compromised immune systems, superinfection contributes significant morbidity and mortality.

Tests

Enzyme immunoassay, immunofluorescence, and hemagglutination are among the tests used to detect CMV in blood and body tissues, for example, for individuals receiving bone marrow and organ transplants. These tests determine the presence of antibody to the virus.

Treatments

gancyclovir

IgG

IVIG

There are treatments available for CMV infection in immunoincompetent or immunosuppressed individuals. The drug of choice is gancyclovir, which has shown the most promise in infected newborns and in bone marrow and organ transplant recipients. Immunoglobulin G (IgG) prepared from individuals with high CMV antibody titers can also be administered. Intravenous IgG (IVIG) has shown promise as an effective means of treating CMV.

CMV-Safe Components

Immunoincompetent individuals and premature infants are susceptible to CMV infection following a blood transfusion or a tissue or organ transplant. For this reason, they should receive CMV-safe blood cell components. "Safe" means that the blood product, organ, or bone marrow is obtained from a seronegative donor, that is, a person who has no antibody to CMV.

seronegative blood

Transfusion or transplant candidates susceptible to CMV who should receive seronegative blood include:

- Newborns weighing less than 1250 g (approximately 3 lb) who are seronegative
- Pregnant females who are seronegative and require an intravenous or intrauterine transfusion
- Seronegative individuals who are to receive a bone marrow or organ transplant from a seronegative donor
- Recipients of autologous bone marrow who are seronegative
- Seronegative individuals with AIDS

Alternatives to Safe Components

There are alternatives to safe blood components for seronegative recipients. Frozen red cells that have been deglycerolized (washed of the cryoprotective agent glycerol) can be given. Use of leukocyte-depletion blood filters is considered a way to decrease the chances of CMV infection, although this method is still controversial.

Bacterial Contamination of Blood

Bacterial contamination of a donor unit of red cells is a rare occurrence, while bacterial contamination of platelet products is more common. With platelet contamination, bacteria tend to be ordinary gram-positive organisms, such as cocci and diptheroids. Contamination of red cells is caused by cold-growing, gram-negative bacteria. Donor blood can also contain

platelet contamination: gram-positive bacteria red cell contamination: cold-growing, gram-negative bacteria

endotoxins

endotoxins produced by these organisms. (Gram-negative bacteria that contaminate red cells grow at low temperatures.) Gram stains are a way of classifying bacteria. If an organism takes a gram stain, it is positive, and if it does not, it is negative.

Transmission

venipuncture site
bacteremia

It is believed that most bacterial contamination of blood comes from the donor via either of two ways: improper cleansing of the venipuncture site or from an undiagnosed bacteremia, such as might occur following dental extraction, sigmoidoscopy, or barium enema. Autologous donors may contaminate a unit of predonated blood through bacteremia associated with an indwelling I.V. or urinary tract catheter.

Transfusion of blood or blood components contaminated with bacteria has very serious consequences with fatal complications about 25% of the time. Red cells infected with organisms such as *Escherichia coli* (*E. coli*), *Yersinia*, and *Pseudomonas*, among others, produce endotoxins that cause septic reactions.

Signs and Symptoms

A recipient's reaction to bacterially contaminated blood are elevated temperature, bright red flushing of the face, abdominal cramping, a feeling of warmth, vomiting, diarrhea, and possibly shock. If disseminated intravascular coagulation (DIC) occurs, it should be treated immediately. Bacterial endotoxins that contaminate red cells can cause severe hemolysis and shock.

Treatment

antibiotics

Treatment for bacterial infection usually consists of antibiotics to reduce infection.

Transfusion Precautions

Packed Red Cells Prior to transfusion, a unit of Packed Red Cells should be examined for signs of bacterial contamination. These include: blood clots, large gas bubble in the unit, and dark appearance of plasma due to extensive destruction of red cells. To help prevent bacterial contamination special care should be taken to prepare the venipuncture site of a donor prior to collection. The skin should be prepped according to standards established by the AABB and FDA.

Another means of preventing bacterial contamination of Packed Red Cells is to make sure that a unit is infused within 4 hours from the time that the transfusion was initiated. Packed Red Cells for transfusion should not be kept at room temperature (25C) any longer than necessary.

Platelets   Platelet transfusions are associated with bacterial contamination as well. The reactions are less severe and mortality caused by contaminated platelets is much less than with red cells. Symptoms can appear during the transfusion or in the 2 weeks following infusion. Platelet transfusions are associated with both gram-positive and gram-negative organisms.

gram-positive, gram-negative organisms

▪ QUESTIONS ▪

1. Since the 1980s there have been three major developments in transfusion therapy that have greatly reduced the incidence of disease transmission via blood transfusions. What are they?

2. Identify the two diseases of most concern to transfusion recipients and health care professionals. What kind of disease are they?

3. The National Institutes of Health (NIH) and the Food and Drug Administration (FDA) set the standards for blood banking and transfusion policies in the U.S. True or False?

4. Besides the two diseases mentioned in Question 2, there are five other transfusion-transmissible diseases. List them.

5. Ms. Carter-Jones' blood has tested seropositive. Can she donate blood?

6. Hepatitis is a constant subject of study in the medical profession. Currently seven hepatitis viruses have been identified in the *Hepadnaviridae* family. What are they?

7. Hepatitis has many signs and symptoms. What are the four best known ones?

8. What is the most serious form of hepatitis and how is it transmitted?

9. A seemingly healthy individual can be a chronic carrier and transmitter of HBV. True or False?

10. How can an individual be protected against contracting HBV, and what individuals especially require protection?

11. Why is HBV vaccine recommended for newborns?

12. What can be done for an unvaccinated health care worker accidentally exposed to the virus?

13. Contrast and compare hepatitis C with hepatitis B.

14. How is HIV transmitted?

15. Name three tests available for determining HIV status.

16. Briefly, how does HIV affect the immune system?

17. How is the progression from being HIV-positive to having AIDS defined?

18. List four diseases associated with the clinical definition of AIDS.

19. Describe the classic symptoms of AIDS.

20. How is AIDS treated?

21. Human T cell lymphotropic viruses have a long latency period. What does this mean?

22. What is HAM?

23. Transfusion-associated syphilis is a rare occurrence in the Western hemisphere today. How is it transmitted?

24. Describe the course of a syphilitic infection.

25. How prevalent is the cytomegalovirus (CMV)? and what does it have in common with other herpes viruses?

26. How is CMV detected?

27. Who is at greatest risk for contracting CMV?

28. Who should receive CMV-safe blood products?

29. How does bacterial contamination of blood occur?

30. What are the signs and symptoms of bacterially contaminated blood?

31. What are the three main precautions against the bacterial contamination of blood?

CHAPTER 17

Component Therapy

Introduction

In the early days of transfusion medicine, Whole Blood was given to individuals who needed blood for any reason. Today, Whole Blood is rarely administered to individuals because there is no clear advantage to it. Component therapy has radically changed the way all blood and blood products are used.

Blood components are Packed Red Cells, Platelets, and Plasma that have been processed from Whole Blood. With component therapy, individual blood products are used to treat many conditions and diseases. For example, Packed Red Cells can be transfused to treat anemia, Platelets to treat thrombocytopenia, and Plasma to treat coagulation defects.

blood components:
Whole Blood
Packed Red Cells
Platelets
Plasma

Blood products are used only when no other therapeutic measures are available to meet the medical needs of a patient. The component of choice is the one that best treats the patient's existing medical condition. Use of the appropriate component is essential to avoid complications. Nevertheless, allogeneic blood components pose the possibility of causing adverse reactions in recipients and transmitting viral and bacterial diseases via transfusion.

For many clinical conditions, Whole Blood or blood components are not required. Volume expanders and hematopoietic growth factors can be used therapeutically instead. Crystalloid or colloid solutions are volume expanders that can be given to maintain blood volume. The decision to administer blood components or volume expanders depends on many factors related to a patient's health status.

Whole Blood

volume:
450 mL

A unit of Whole Blood is composed of red cells, white cells, platelets, and plasma. It has a volume of 450 mL (+/- 45 mL). Units that contain between 300 and 404 mL are labeled "Low Volume" and other components cannot be prepared from them. A unit of Whole Blood also has 63 mL of a citrate anticoagulant-preservative (CPD, CP2D, or CPDA-1) added (see Ch. 14, Blood Transfusion).

In most instances, Whole Blood is processed into its components (Packed Red Cells, Platelets, and Plasma) soon after collection, allowing many individuals to benefit from one unit of blood. Blood banks prepare these components. Pharmaceutical companies use outdated plasma to make purified concentrations of plasma proteins. Plasma proteins include: coagulation factor concentrates, albumin, plasma protein fraction, and immune serum globulins.

Hematocrit

0.36 to 0.44

The hematocrit (Hct) of Whole Blood is typically between 0.36 and 0.44 (36 and 44%).

Uses

for treatment of
massive blood loss

Although Whole Blood is rarely used in transfusion therapy, it may be justified for a patient who has suffered massive blood loss, usually greater than 25% of total blood volume. In a unit of stored Whole Blood, there are no viable granulocytes and decreased levels of clotting factors V and VIII and platelets. Lymphocytes may still be viable, however. An infusion of Whole Blood improves an individual's ability to transport oxygen, as indicated by the increased Hct, and increases the circulating blood volume (plasma). A unit of Whole Blood raises an adult's Hct by about 0.03 (3%) and Hgb concentration by about 1 g/dL.

Cautions

Transfusion of Whole Blood when Whole Blood is not needed is wasteful and medically unsound.

Whole Blood can cause circulatory overload in a normovolemic (normal circulating blood volume) individual. Circulatory overload can induce serious complications, such as congestive heart failure or pulmonary edema. Usually, a blood component can more effectively treat a problem than Whole Blood can. Packed Red Cells, for example, are given to anemic patients to increase their Hct.

circulatory overload

Leukocyte-reduced Blood Components

Whole Blood, Packed Red Cells, and Platelets are components that have white cells removed if the recipient so requires. When white cells are removed from a component it is called leukocyte-reduction and the component is referred to as leukocyte-reduced. For certain transfusion recipients white cells are removed to prevent (1) disease transmission, such as CMV; (2) FNHTRs; and (3) alloimmunization to human leukocyte (HLA) antigens, also known as major histocompatibility complex (MHC) molecules. It is best to remove white cells before storage because cytokines and other biological response modifiers (BMRs) released by white cells during storage accumulate in the unit and can cause FNHTRs in recipients.

for prevention of disease transmission, FNHTRs, and alloimmunization to HLA

Packed Red Cells

Uses and Preparation

Packed Red Cells are given to individuals who lose blood during surgery or trauma, or who are anemic and need to improve the oxygen-carrying capacity of their blood to meet tissue demands.

for treatment of blood loss and anemia

Packed Red Cells are prepared from a unit of Whole Blood. The term packed refers to the concentration of red cells that remains after most of the plasma has been removed. Removal of plasma increases the

packed: concentration of red cells after removal of plasma

concentration of red cells and, therefore, the unit's Hct. Between 200 and 250 mL of plasma is removed and frozen creating fresh frozen plasma (FFP).

Cautions

Packed Red Cells should not be transfused pre-operatively to expand blood volume. They should not be used to improve wound healing.

Compatibility

ABO and Rh

Recipients should receive Packed Red Cells that are ABO and Rh compatible with theirs. In some emergency situations, when a specific blood group is not available, O negative cells are administered.

Shelf Life

Packed Red Cells collected in CPD or CP2D have a shelf life of 21 days and a Hct of 0.70 to 0.80. Those collected in CPDA-1 have a shelf life of 35 days and a Hct of 0.70 to 0.80. Packed Red Cells are stored at temperatures between 1 to 6C. The shelf life of Packed Red Cells can be extended to 42 days with 100 mL of additive solution, but the Hct will be lower. Those stored in additive solutions have a Hct of 0.55 to 0.60. Additive solutions are used *only* for Packed Red Cells and cannot be added to any other blood component.

Frozen Red Cells

for rare blood types

Uses   Frozen red cells are prepared for individuals with rare blood types who may have problems finding a donor. Freezing is also used for storing units of autologous blood.

Preparation and Storage   Frozen red cells are mixed with a cryoprotective agent, usually glycerol, and stored frozen at - 65C or lower. They can be stored frozen for up to 10 years. Blood bags made of the plastic agent called polyolefin seem to cause less hemolysis during storage and are used routinely for frozen blood. Polyvinyl chloride bags seem to cause hemolysis of red cells when placed in frozen storage. The thawing of frozen red cells is accomplished by placing the unit in a 37C waterbath or blood warmer. Thawing should take between 25 and 40 minutes and no longer.

Before the unit can be transfused it must be washed with a series of saline solutions to remove glycerol. Washing of frozen cells is called deglycerolization. Once deglycerolized, the cells can be used immediately or stored at 1 to 6C for up to 14 days. If deglycerolized in an open system (exposed to room air), they can be stored at 1 to 6C for a period of 24 hours.

washing of frozen cells/ deglycerolization

Platelets

Uses

Platelets are transfused into individuals whose numbers are low and cannot form a platelet plug. They are used to treat individuals whose bleeding is due to thrombocytopenia or functionally abnormal platelets. Platelet functions are affected by certain diseases and conditions such as drugs, liver disease, bypass surgery, and sepsis, among others.

for treatment of low numbers and bleeding

Platelets usually are not successful in arresting bleeding in certain situations because they are destroyed faster than they can be replaced. Excessive platelet destruction occurs in idiopathic thrombocytopenia (ITP), untreated DIC, septicemia (infection), and hypersplenism (increased removal of platelets).

Preparation

Platelets are collected for transfusion from units of Whole Blood or from individual donors by plateletpheresis. An individual who has taken aspirin within 3 days of donation should not be used as a platelet donor. Platelets can have some white cells within the unit and therefore may need to be leukocyte-depleted before storage or before transfusion into a recipient. FNHTRs are more common following transfusion of platelet concentrates than Packed Red Cells.

Because platelets are less dense (lighter) than other blood cells, they are obtained from Whole Blood by soft spin centrifugation that separates the red cells from platelet-rich-plasma. The platelet-rich-plasma is then centrifuged using hard spin centrifugation that separates the platelets from plasma.

Compatibility

Rh compatibility

Platelets should be Rh compatible with a recipient. Although ABO compatibility is preferable, it is not necessary because of the small number of red cells present in platelet concentrates. Rh-compatible Platelets prevent sensitization to donor D antigen. If only Platelets from a D+ donor are available for transfusion into a D- recipient, the recipient should receive Rh immune globulin (RhIG) to prevent Rh sensitization, particularly if the individual is a female of childbearing potential.

Storage and Shelf Life

To prevent clumping, Platelets are stored at 20 to 24C with gentle agitation. At colder temperatures, platelets clump and become functionless. Platelets have a shelf life of 5 days.

Complications

During or after a Platelet transfusion, it is not uncommon for recipients to have fever and chills. If a transfusion reaction does occur, the transfusion should be stopped immediately and the physician notified.

Pooled Platelets

Uses and Preparation

Platelets prepared from units of Whole Blood are often pooled for individuals needing many units. Pooled platelets must be transfused within 4 hours because they are prepared in an open system shortly before use. They are administered to individuals with very low platelet counts, for example, following heart and liver surgery. Use of pooled platelets, however, increases a patient's exposure to numerous donor antigens and transmissible diseases.

Plasma Components

Uses and Preparation

Collected blood plasma can be frozen or separated into various components: cryoprecipitate (Cryo), liquid plasma, coagulation factor concentrates (factors VIII and IX), albumin, plasma protein fraction, immune serum globulins, and antiprotease concentrates. Plasma components are used for many conditions, including bleeding disorders, liver disease, massive blood loss, and hemophilia.

for treatment of many conditions

Fresh Frozen Plasma

Uses and Preparation Fresh frozen plasma (FFP) is separated from whole blood within 8 hours following collection and quickly frozen. If FFP is treated in this manner, clotting factors V and VIII retain most of their effectiveness (clotting activity). FFP contains all clotting factors, including the labile factors V and VIII.

contains all clotting factors

This product is useful for treating individual clotting factor deficiencies as well as multiple factor deficiencies resulting from liver disease, vitamin K deficiency, deficiency of antithrombin III, deficiency of proteins C and S, dilutional coagulopathy following bypass surgery, and DIC, among others. FFP is the preferred replacement fluid for plasma exchange. (Dilutional coagulapathy refers to the washing out, or loss of, coagulation factors and platelets.)

Cautions FFP should not be used for volume expansion, as protein supplement for nutrition, or to improve wound healing.

Storage FFP can be stored up to 1 year at -18C or lower. The volume of a unit ranges from 200 to 250 mL. FFP is thawed in a water bath with a temperature range of 30 to 37C immediately prior to transfusion.

Liquid Plasma

Uses and Preparation Liquid plasma can be separated from a single donor unit of Whole Blood any time up to 5 days following the expiration date of the unit. This component is used to treat clotting factor deficiencies for which there is no specific concentrate available, such as factor XI and XII. Liquid plasma is rarely indicated for the treatment of patients requiring component therapy.

Pharmaceutical companies purchase liquid plasma and use it in the preparation of albumin and immune serum globulin.

Storage Liquid plasma collected in the above manner can be frozen and stored for 5 years and is called Plasma. If not frozen, it is stored at 1 to 6C with a shelf life of not more than 5 days past the expiration of the unit from which it was obtained. It is then referred to as liquid plasma.

Cryoprecipitate AHF

Uses Cryoprecipitate AHF (antihemophilic factor) is primarily used to treat congenital and acquired fibrinogen and factor XIII deficiencies, and, uncommonly, von Willebrand's disease, and occasionally hemophilia A. This product is often referred to as Cryo.

for treatment of fibrinogen and factor XIII deficiencies

Cryo

Preparation Cryo is a 20 to 50 mL concentrated solution of coagulation proteins. The proteins include: factor VIII, von Willebrand factor, fibrinogen, and factor XIII.

To prepare Cryo a unit of FFP is thawed at 1 to 6C. During the thawing process a white precipitate called cryoprecipitate forms within the FFP unit. The plasma is removed and Cryo remains in the bag. Cryo is resuspended in a small volume of plasma and refrozen.

Before Cryo is infused, it is thawed, between 30 and 37C. Transfusion of Cryo should occur within 6 hours after it has thawed. CPD, CPDA-1, and ACD are the preferred anticoagulant-preservatives for the collection of plasma used in the preparation of Cryo.

Pooled Cryo   Cryo may be pooled before freezing. Once pooled it should be quickly refrozen. The unit should be labeled as such with the number of units used in pooling indicated. If it has been removed from FFP, this fact must also be stated on the FFP label. It must be used within 4 hours after thawing.

Compatibility   Because Cryo contains minimal amounts of plasma, it does not need to be ABO compatible with the recipient's blood group. If pooled, Cryo should be ABO compatible with the recipient's blood group because donor antibodies are present in the Cryo. The first choice is ABO compatibility but this is not necessary especially in an emergency. If the volume of Cryo infused is large (due to pooling) in comparison to the recipient's blood volume, it should be ABO compatible; for example, for a neonate or child.

ABO compatibility

Fibrin Glue   Cryo is also used to create fibrin glue, which is applied topically to stop bleeding that cannot be controlled by other means. For example, it can be used surgically in an area where sutures cannot control bleeding. Fibrin glue is prepared by mixing Cryo and bovine (cow) thrombin. Although the mixture is applied topically to the bleeding area rather than injected, it can transmit disease if it was prepared from infected plasma.

Coagulation Factor Concentrates

Uses   Factor VIII concentrate, also called Antihemophilic Factor (AHF), is used to treat hemophilia A, which is a congenital disorder in which little if any factor VIII is produced. Factor IX concentrate is used to treat hemophilia B (Christmas disease), which is a congenital disorder affecting the production of factor IX. Because this concentrate contains factors II, VII, and X, it can also be used to treat other factor deficiencies.

AHF for hemophilia A

factor IX concentrate for hemohilia B, etc.

Preparation   Coagulation factor concentrates are lyophilized (powdered) concentrates processed from units of (1) pooled donor plasma, (2) cryoprecipitate, or (3) through recombinant DNA technology by pharmaceutical companies. At the present time, two recombinant factors, VIII and IX, are available for use. Coagulation factor concentrates undergo extensive processing so that if viruses, such as hepatitis or HIV, are present they will be inactivated.

Cautions An infusion of factor IX concentrates can cause thrombosis. Recently a factor IX concentrate has been produced containing minimal amounts of factors II, VII, and X. It therefore has decreased the chances of causing thrombosis.

Immune Serum Globulins

gammaglobulins

There are three types of immune serum globulins, also called gammaglobulins, that can be prepared from plasma.

IVIG

(1) Intravenous immune globulin (IVIG) is a solution of mostly IgG molecules and very small amounts of IgM and IgA. It is used to treat individuals with immune deficiency disorders, HIV infection, and autoimmune disorders, among others.

hyperimmune globulins

(2) Hyperimmune globulins provide passive immunity to individuals who have been exposed to diseases such as hepatitis B, tetanus, and chicken pox, among others. Rh immune globulin (RhIG) is an example of a hyperimmune globulin.

immune globulins for IM

(3) Immune globulins prepared for intramuscular administration (IM) are not specific and contain antibodies against a variety of infectious organisms, such as measles and hepatitis A, among others. If these immune globulins are administered I.V., decreased blood pressure and anaphylactic reactions can occur.

immunoglobulins

to provide already-formed anibodies

passive immunization

Uses and Preparation Immune serum globulins are concentrated solutions of antibodies (immunoglobins) prepared from plasma. Antibodies are removed from donor plasma and administered to the recipient to provide already-formed antibodies against the antigen. Immunity provided from sources outside the body is called passive immunization.

Complications Administration of IVIG can cause headache, vomiting, allergic reactions, and circulatory overload, among others.

Antiprotease Concentrates

Uses and Preparation Antiprotease concentrates are prepared from plasma; they are protein substances found in the plasma, such as antithrombin III (AT-III), alpha-1-antitrypsin, and C1-esterase inhibitor, that are used to treat various conditions. Individuals deficient in AT-III have the tendency to form clots within the vasculature. AT-III deficiency is due to either congenital or acquired defects.

for treatment of protein deficiencies

AT-III concentrate is referred to as Thrombate™. Liquid plasma and FFP are alternative sources for AT-III replacement. Alpha-1-antitrypsin is used in the treatment of alpha-1-antitrypsin deficiency, which causes respiratory problems. C1-esterase inhibitors are used to treat individuals with defects in the complement system that cause hereditary angioedema, which leads to urticaria and edema of the skin and mucous membranes.

AT-III/Thrombate™

alpha-1-antitrypsin

C1-esterase inhibitors

Protein C Concentrate

Individuals with defective production or deficiency of protein C have increased susceptibility to thrombotic episodes. Protein C concentrate is now available for infusion.

Vitamin K

Vitamin K is a fat-soluble vitamin necessary for complete synthesis of certain clotting proteins, including factors II, VII, IX, X, and proteins C and S. The body can only store vitamin K for about 2 weeks. There are several reasons for low levels of vitamin K—nutrition, antibiotic use, and malabsorption syndrome. The anticoagulant Coumadin™ inhibits the synthesis of vitamin K. The best therapy for vitamin K deficiency is treating the cause of the deficiency and intravenous infusion of vitamin K.

for treatment of low levels

Granulocytes

Uses and Preparation

rarely used for
transfusion

Granulocytes are usually prepared by leukapheresis and are rarely used in blood transfusion therapy. The indication for granulocytes is to treat (1) neutropenia, (2) patients with bacterial sepsis unresponsive to antibiotics, and (3) individuals with defective white cell production.

If granulocytes are collected, they are stored at 20 to 24C, but should be infused as soon as possible following collection and certainly within 24 hours. Granulocyte concentrations should not be leukocyte-reduced before infusion. Some physicians feel that the unit should be irradiated to prevent transfusion-associated graft-versus-host disease (TAGVHD).

Volume Expanders

Uses

to maintain adequate
blood volume

crystalloids, colloids

Volume expanders are solutions used to maintain adequate blood volume when blood loss occurs due to trauma or surgery. Crystalloids and colloids are the two types of volume expanders.

When either crystalloids or colloids are infused into the vascular space, they increase the circulating blood volume, which is critical for homeostasis. If blood volume is inadequate (hypovolemia), many organ systems, especially the heart, brain, and kidneys, do not function properly. Hypovolemia can present serious problems for an individual and possibly lead to death.

Although used differently in volume replacement therapy to treat blood loss, both crystalloids and colloids are administered I.V. A physician determines which type of fluid is optimal in a given situation.

Crystalloid Solutions

Crystalloid solutions include: normal saline, lactated

Ringer's, dextrose, and various combinations of these. Normal saline and lactated Ringer's are simple solutions made up of anions, Cl^- and HCO_3^-, cations, such as Na^+, Mg^{++}, and Ca^{++}. Dextrose is a liquid solution containing the simple sugar glucose.

lactated Ringer's

Uses

Crystalloids often are used to replace blood loss, provide fluid for dehydrated patients, and maintain direct access to the vascular system (via the I.V.) for emergency drug administration. Crystalloids expand blood volume but only for a short time. They tend to diffuse into the interstitial space (within 30 minutes) or are removed by the kidneys. They are usually used when rapid volume expansion is required. If possible, the cardiac status of an individual should be assessed before large volumes of a crystalloid are administered because their infusion can possibly cause congestive heart failure (CHF) and/or pulmonary edema.

rapid volume expansion

Normal Saline

Normal saline (NS) is a salt solution found in the body in its ionic form of sodium (Na^+) and chloride (Cl^-). It is prepared by pharmaceutical companies for use in fluid replacement. Normal saline is an ideal I.V. solution because it is easily removed by the kidneys. It is the only crystalloid solution that can be transfused along with blood or blood components. Normal saline (0.9%) is infused with Packed Red Cells and other components because it decreases blood viscosity and does not hemolyze red cells.

NS for fluid replacement

transfused with blood or components

Lactated Ringer's

The most widely used volume expander is lactated Ringer's (LR), which is similar to normal saline solution except that it contains added calcium (Ca^{++}) and magnesium (Mg^{++}) ions. It must not be infused in the same line as blood because Ca^{++} can induce blood clotting.

LR

must not be infused with blood

Dextrose

must not be infused
with blood

This is a simple sugar solution often administered I.V. to patients. It is never used with blood transfusions because it causes red cell hemolysis.

Colloids

Colloids include: albumin, plasma protein fraction, dextran, and Hespan™. Colloids resemble plasma.

Uses

for maintaining blood
volume and for
treatment of bleeding

Colloids are very useful in maintaining blood volume. They are used to treat certain individuals, including burn patients and patients in shock from bleeding. Because of their protein concentration, colloids are effective in maintaining osmotic pressure, although they can cause hypersensitivity in some individuals.

natural colloids:
albumin, PPF

synthetic colloids:
dextran, hetastarch

Natural and Synthetic Colloids   There are two types of colloid volume expanders: (1) natural colloids, which include albumin and plasma protein fraction (PPF) and (2) synthetic colloids, which are dextran and hydroxyethyl starch, also called hetastarch or Hespan™. Synthetic colloids are made up of long-chain polymers. Due to their molecular size and chemistry, both natural and synthetic colloids tend to remain within the vascular system longer than crystalloids and, therefore, do not diffuse readily into the interstitial space.

Albumin

for treatment of liver
disease and blood loss

Uses   Albumin is used mainly to treat individuals with liver disease or those who have lost large volumes of blood from burns, trauma, surgery, or plasma exchange. These conditions involve a protein deficiency due either to decreased protein synthesis by the liver or plasma loss. Albumin functions in the transport of molecules, such as bilirubin in the blood; therefore, albumin can be used in treating neonatal hyperbilirubinemia, which is an excessive amount of bilirubin in the bloodstream.

Preparation   Albumin is a naturally occurring blood protein that is the major protein in blood plasma. It is processed from disease-free blood plasma by pharmaceutical companies. Prepared albumin comes in 5% and 25% concentrations. The 5% concentration is similar to plasma. The 25% concentration has X5 the albumin concentration of plasma. During the preparation process, albumin is heated to 60C for 10 hours and therefore inactivates viruses.

Compatibility   ABO testing is not required before a transfusion.

Administration   Albumin can be administered in conjunction with blood components used in exchange or intrauterine transfusions for the treatment of hemolytic disease of the newborn (HDN). This is a disease in which the presence of Rh antibodies of a D- mother hemolyze the D+ red cells of her fetus or newborn. Albumin does not need to be administered through a blood filter because it does not contain clots or debris. This blood product only circulates within the vasculature for about 24 hours.

Complications   Individuals receiving albumin can experience nausea, vomiting, fever, and allergic reactions, possibly even an anaphylactoid reaction. Because albumin infusions increase intravascular volume, they can cause pulmonary edema and hemodilution.

Plasma Protein Fraction

Uses and Preparation   Like albumin, plasma protein fraction (PPF) is used to treat individuals with burns, massive bleeding, or liver failure. PPF is another protein component that can be separated from plasma. It can be used to expand volume. Less pure than albumin, it contains a higher percentage of other plasma proteins, such as globulins. PPF does not transmit disease via transfusion because it is pasteurized (heated to kill organisms) during preparation.

for treatment of liver disease and blood loss

to expand volume

Cautions   PPF is likely to cause hypotension (decreased blood pressure) when infused and, therefore, is used less often than albumin, the preferred colloid.

Dextran

Uses and Preparation   Several concentrations of dextran, which are differentiated by molecular weight, are prepared for therapeutic use. Because of its molecular size and shape, dextran stays within the vasculature for approximately 6 hours, much longer than crystalloids.

to increase blood volume

Dextran is one of two synthetic plasma volume expanders (the other being Hespan™) used to replace lost blood volume or hypovolemia. It is a solution consisting of polymerized glucose molecules (long chains of glucose).

Complications   Individuals receiving dextran can experience hypersensitivity reactions such as rash, dyspnea, decreased blood pressure, and nasal congestion. When used in large volumes, dextran can cause hemostatic disturbances, such as platelet inactivation, and reduction in levels of clotting proteins V, VIII, IX, and fibrinogen. It also can interfere with blood grouping and cross matching tests.

Cautions   Dextran should be used cautiously in individuals with heart failure, kidney failure, severe bleeding disorders, such as hemophilia, and liver disorders.

Hespan™

to expand blood volume

Uses   The synthetic colloid Hespan is used to expand blood volume following burns, surgery, and sepsis, among other conditions. It has about the same osmotic pressure as a 5% albumin solution. Hespan is also used in the collection of granulocytes by apheresis. Because it acts as a sedimenting agent for red cells, it decreases the number of red cells collected with the granulocytes.

Hespan is a 6% solution consisting of a long-chain polymer of amylopectin (starch). The molecular size and shape of Hespan restrict it to the vasculature, where it remains for approximately 24 hours.

Complications   Hespan has the potential to cause hypersensitivity reactions as well as fever, chills, rash, nausea, and vomiting. Like dextran, Hespan can interfere with hemostasis.

Cautions The amount infused should be closely monitored. It is usually not used for individuals with congestive heart failure or kidney disease.

Hematopoietic Growth Factors

Uses and Preparation

Hematopoietic growth factors stimulate the growth and differentiation of stem and progenitor cells into mature blood cells (see Ch. 1, The Concept of Blood). When hematopoietic growth factors were first produced through recombinant DNA (genetic) technology, they were regarded as potential sources for treating diseases in which blood cell production was decreased. Now some of these recombinant factors are marketed and used therapeutically to increase the numbers of red and white cells. Recombinant growth factors are used (1) after a bone marrow transplant to induce engraftment, (2) prior to hematopoietic progenitor cell apheresis to increase the number of progenitor cells in circulation, (3) following high-dose chemotherapy to increase the numbers of certain white cells, and (4) to increase red cells for some patients with anemia. Many growth factors, other than those on the market today, are under clinical investigation and may have a therapeutic role in the future. Despite some side effects, recombinant hematopoietic growth factors continue to show great promise in treating patients.

recombinant growth factors increase progenitor cells, red cells, white cells

Hematopoietic growth factors in use presently include: recombinant erythropoietin (rEPO) and two colony-stimulating factors, granulocyte colony-stimulating factor (G-CSF) and granulocyte-macrophage colony-stimulating factor (GM-CSF). Recently, a recombinant thrombopoietin (TPO) has become available for studies involving thrombocytopenic patients.

rEPO

G-CSF
GM-CSF
TPO

Recombinant Erythropoietin

Uses Recombinant technology has developed synthetic erythropoietin, which is proving to be a very effective therapeutic drug. As with the naturally

rEPO
red cells

occurring hormone, rEPO stimulates stem cells to make red cells. Following the initiation of rEPO therapy, it takes about 2 weeks before red cell production increases and 2 to 3 months before an individual's Hct reaches the desired level. Recombinant EPO can be administered either intravenously (I.V.) or subcutaneously (s.c.).

end-stage renal disease

to treat anemia
and malignancies
for perioperative surgery

Recombinant EPO is used for individuals with anemia due to end-stage renal disease. Before the discovery of rEPO, kidney patients were given Packed Red Cells to maintain a normal Hct. Recombinant EPO has almost eliminated the need for blood transfusions in these individuals. This growth factor is also being used to treat some forms of anemia in individuals with AIDS and certain malignancies and is licensed for perioperative (before surgery) use as well.

Complications Although individuals can experience headache and bone pain, rEPO causes few other side effects. Blood pressure can increase slightly following therapy, but this usually is due to the increased Hct.

Granulocyte Colony-Stimulating Factor and Granulocyte–Macrophage Colony-Stimulating Factor

Uses Recombinant granulocyte colony-stimulating factor (G-CSF) and granulocyte-macrophage colony-stimulating factor (GM-CSF) are used therapeutically in the following situations:

- After a bone marrow transplant to enhance engraftment of neutrophils and macrophages.
- After intensive chemotherapy to increase the number of neutrophils and macrophages.
- Prior to peripheral blood progenitor cell collection (PBPC) to increase the number of peripheral blood progenitor cells (see Ch. 18, Apheresis and Ch. 20, Bone Marrow Transplantation).

stimulates neutrophil
production

Recombinant G-CSF This protein has an important role in blood therapy because it stimulates stem cells to differentiate into neutrophils, which are the body's main defense against bacterial infections. Use of G-CSF improves the body's production of neutrophils thereby promoting the control of bacterial infections. In patients undergoing intensive chemotherapy and bone marrow transplant, bacterial infections are a major cause of mortality.

Recombinant G-CSF can be administered either I.V. or s.c. Recombinant G-CSF should be diluted with dextrose in water, not with saline.

The main adverse effect of G-CSF about which individuals most often complain is bone pain. Individuals receiving G-CSF can also experience anemia and thrombocytopenia. Leukocytosis can occur following therapy.

Recombinant GM-CSF This is a glycoprotein used to increase the number of granulocytes and macrophages in the following individuals: those undergoing bone marrow transplant, high-dose chemotherapy, or peripheral blood progenitor cell collection. The drug can be administered either I.V. or s.c.

increases granulocytes and macrophages

Side effects from GM-CSF include: diarrhea, rash, malaise, fever, chills, and headaches.

CHART 4: Blood Components

PRODUCT	WHOLE BLOOD	PACKED RBCS	PACKED RBCS	PLATELETS	GRANULOCYTES	FRESH FROZEN PLASMA (FFP)
AC/P	CPD, CP2D, CPDA-1	CPD, CP2D, CPDA-1	CPD-preferred additive system	CPD, CPDA-1	CPD, CPDA-1	CPD, CPDA-1
HCT OF PRODUCT	0.36–0.44	0.70–0.80	0.55–0.60	—	—	—
VOLUME OF UNIT	450 mL	250 mL	300–350 mL	50–70 mL	200–400 mL with platelets;100–200 mL in unit if no platelets in units	200–250 mL
DISEASE TRANSMISSION	Yes	Yes	Yes	Yes	Yes	Yes, not CMV
ABO/Rh COMPATIBILITY	ABO and Rh	ABO and Rh	ABO and Rh	Rh compatibility necessary; ABO compatibility preferred, not necessary	ABO and Rh	ABO
USES IN TREATMENT	Rarely used; may be used for massive blood loss	Red cell replacement; often used with crystalloids to increase Hct and volume	Red cell replacement; often used with crystalloids to increase Hct and volume	To increase platelet count or unresponsive to antibiotics	For individuals with low white cell count	To increase clotting factor levels; valuable in treating factor deficiencies when concentrates not available
INCIDENTALS	Rh- blood may be given to Rh+ individuals; presence of white cells and platelets may cause sensitization; should be filtered. Storage: 21 days in CPD or CP2D, 35 in CPDA-1	2 times the Hct of unit of whole blood; should be filtered. Storage: 21 days in CPD or CP2D, 35 in CPDA-1	Additive systems increase storage time to 42 days; should be filtered	Rh- patients may need Rh+ platelets and possibly Rh immune globulin. Multiple platelet transfusions may sensitize patients to HLA antigens, requiring HLA-matched platelets. Blood filter (170m). Storage: 20-24C Shelf life: 5 days	Not accepted by Food and Drug Administration (FDA). HLA complications possible with transfusions. Storage: 20- 24C. Shelf life: 24 hrs	Often used after bypass surgery. Storage: -18C Shelf life: 1 yr

Chart 4: Blood Components, *continued*

Product	Cryoprecipitate	Coagulation Factor Concentrate; Factor VIII	Factor IX	Colloid Solutions Albumin	Plasma Protein Fraction (PPF)	Immune Serum Globulins
AC/P	—	—	—	—	—	—
Hct of Product	—	—	—	—	—	—
Volume of Unit	25–50 mL	Amount of FVIII in mgs varies by manufacturer	Amount of FIX in mgs varies by manufacturer	—	5% protein solution	Varies by manufacturer
Disease Transmission	Yes	No; reduced risk	No; reduced risk	No	No	Yes, some, but not AIDS
ABO/Rh Compatibility	Preferred, but not necessary	Plasma compatible, but not necessary	Plasma compatible, but not necessary	No	No	—
Uses in Treatment	To increase levels of factors VIII, XIII, fibrinogen, and von Willebrand factor	For treatment of FVIII deficiency (Hemophilia A)	Hemophilia B (Christmas disease)	Volume expansion when crystalloids inadequate (shocks, burns, liver failure, hemorrhage); used in severe liver disease	Used for hemorrhagic and hypovolemic shock, burns, plasma replacement during plasmapheresis	Provides immune protection; used to treat patients with low levels of gamma globulin
Incidentals	Can be pooled; 0.9% normal saline may be needed to assist transfusion; used to prepare fibrin glue	Lyophilized plasma derivative; obtained by fractionation; allergic reactions reduced over Cyro	Also has factors II, VII, X; prepared from large pools of donor plasma; contains Vitamin-K dependent coagulation factors for treating warfarin overdose in certain patients	5% solution equivalent to plasma; 25% is 5 times the protein concentration of plasma	—	Concentrated solution of gamma-globulin; prepared from pools of random donors; prepared from donors with large amounts of antibody; extracted from patients exposed to certain viral and bacterial diseases

■ **QUESTIONS** ■

1. With component therapy, how is Whole Blood used?

2. What are volume expanders?

3. What is the volume of a unit of Whole Blood? What is its hematocrit?

4. Whole Blood is administered only when blood loss is significant, usually greater than 25% of the total blood volume. True or False?

5. List three conditions for which white cells are removed from blood components.

6. How is the blood component known as FFP created?

7. Which additive solution will give plasma the longest shelf life?

8. Packed Red Cells are collected in an anticoagulant-preservative. Name two.

9. What is deglycerolization, and when does it occur?

10. Ms. Brown has developed an ITP with signs of bleeding. Why is she not receiving platelets?

11. Why is ABO classification not as important in platelet transfusion?

12. What is meant by pooled platelets?

13. The use of pooled platelets presents problems. Describe one.

14. Identify five components that may be derived from plasma.

15. What two clotting factors remain viable in fresh frozen plasma?

16. For how long can FFP be stored?

17. What is liquid plasma specifically used for?

18. Define cryoprecipitate and explain how it is produced.

19. Give two uses for Cryo.

20. What is fibrin glue made of? and how is it used?

21. Identify two coagulation factor concentrates and the conditions for which they are indicated.

22. One of the coagulation factor concentrates has been known to cause thrombosis in the past. What has been done to remedy this situation?

23. What are immune serum globulins? They are also know by another name. What is it?

24. Identify the three main categories of immune serum globulins.

25. What are C1-esterase inhibitors? and what conditions do they help treat?

26. Why is vitamin K necessary for a healthy individual?

27. Granulocytes are rarely used in blood transfusion therapy. Describe three conditions for which they may be necessary.

28. Why is an adequate circulating blood volume important to maintaining life?

29. What crystalloid solution is commonly used with transfusion therapy? What are its advantageous characteristics?

30. What are the other two commonly used crystalloid solutions? and why can't they be used with blood transfusion products?

31. There are two types of colloid volume expanders. What are they? and what are they used for?

32. Describe three conditions for which albumin is used.

33. Why is plasma protein fraction (PPF), another colloid, used less often than albumin?

34. Compare and contrast the two synthetic colloid volume expanders.

35. Explain what hematopoietic growth factors are.

36. How long does it take for red cell production to increase and the Hct to reach the desired level in a individual who has received rEPO?

37. What groups of patients benefit particularly from rEPO?

CHAPTER 18

Apheresis

Introduction

Apheresis is the removal of whole blood from a donor/recipient for the purpose of isolating a specific component or components. The component or components collected may be used in a transfusion, or a diseased component is removed and discarded. Unused components are recombined and reinfused back into the donor/recipient. Apheresis is most frequently performed to collect plasma and platelets, respectively referred to as plasmapheresis and plateletpheresis. Occasionally, granulocytes are separated from whole blood by leukapheresis. Autologous and allogeneic peripheral blood stem/progenitor cells (PBSCs/PBPCs) are isolated from whole blood by cytapheresis and used alone or in conjunction with bone marrow stem cells for transplantation. Technically there is a difference between the terms stem cell and progenitor cell, but they often are used synonymously.

plasmapheresis
plateletpheresis
leukapheresis

cytapheresis

Therapeutic apheresis is the removal of a diseased or defective component from an individual's blood. Depending on the condition to be treated, the component may or may not be replaced. For example, diseased plasma can be removed and replaced with albumin, crystalloids, or fresh frozen plasma (FFP). Therapeutic apheresis is used to treat such conditions as Waldenström's macroglobulinemia, myasthenia gravis, hyperviscosity syndrome, thrombocythemia, and leukocytosis caused by some leukemias.

therapeutic apheresis

Apheresis donors must meet the same requirements for donation as donors of whole blood. All components collected by apheresis must be ABO and Rh grouped and screened for antibodies and transmissible diseases.

ABO and Rh
grouped and screened
for antibodies and
disease testing   **307**

Complications

Complications that can arise in a recipient during apheresis include: hemolysis due to the equipment, infectious disease transmission and bacterial infection due to the vascular catheter, allergic reactions due to administration of FFP, pulmonary complications from fluid overload, and, rarely the following: fatalities caused by anaphylactic reactions, hemorrhage, thrombosis of the vasculature, and perforation of the blood vessel. Citrate toxicity is another complication that can occur in the individual undergoing apheresis.

Citrate Toxicity

Citrate in ACD and CPD binds ionized calcium in the plasma. Calcium is an essential electrolyte for normal physiologic function. Large amounts of citrate can lead to citrate toxicity. High levels of citrate in the plasma can cause cardiac arrhythmias possibly leading to death. Citrate toxicity evolves from the amount of citrate returned to the donor/recipient in the apheresis procedure.

Symptoms The symptoms of citrate toxicity are numbness and tingling around the mouth and extremities and muscle cramps. At times, individuals can also experience chest pain, vomiting, nausea, chills, and fever.

Treatments Some physicians treat citrate toxicity by administering calcium gluconate or calcium chloride. Both agents replace the ionized calcium in the plasma. Other physicians feel citrate toxicity can be more effectively treated by decreasing the amount of citrate anticoagulant delivered to the donor. This is accomplished by decreasing the speed of the anticoagulant pump.

Apheresis Techniques

Apheresis can be performed with several different separation techniques, such as centrifugation, membrane filtration, and adsorption. Cellular components are separated by centrifugation only, whereas plasma and plasma components can be separated from whole blood by centrifugation, membrane filtration, and adsorption.

Centrifugation

An automated cell separator, also referred to as an apheresis machine, is used to collect plasma or cellular blood component(s) from a donor or patient. One needle for a single puncture site, two needles for double puncture sites, or an indwelling subclavian catheter is attached to tubing connected to a centrifuge bowl within the cell separator. Two mechanical pumps operate within the cell separator. One pumps blood into the centrifuge bowl, and the other controls the amount of anticoagulant added to the donor's whole blood as it flows into the tubing. Acid citrate dextrose (ACD) is the preferred anticoagulant-preservative for use in cellular component collection, but citrate phosphate dextrose (CPD) can also be used.

cell separator/apheresis machine for collection of plasma, cellular blood components

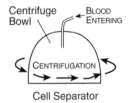

Cell Separator

Because each blood element has a different density, the desired component can be isolated and obtained from whole blood by adjusting the speed of centrifuge. It takes several hours to collect the desired amount of a component by apheresis. The small size of the centrifuge bowl and, in some cases, the low cell numbers of a component in circulation account for the collection time. The collected component remaining in the centrifuge bowl is then transferred to a collection bag and either discarded or used for transfusion.

Membrane Filtration

Plasma collection from healthy donors or for therapeutic removal of a diseased portion of plasma can be accomplished by membrane filtration. As blood is being collected it flows across a porous membrane. The pressure in the blood forces plasma through the pores of the membrane. The red and white cells as well as platelets are not removed whereas the plasma component is diverted into a collection bag.

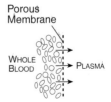

Membranes with different pore sizes are used to remove molecules of various sizes.

Adsorption

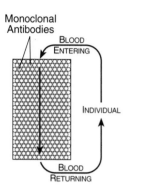

Monoclonal Antibodies

BLOOD ENTERING

INDIVIDUAL

BLOOD RETURNING

Adsorption is used to remove a diseased component from plasma, such as immune complexes, low-density lipoproteins, protein antigens, and antibodies, among others. Plasma is allowed to flow over or through a substance, such as monoclonal antibodies and polymers located in the adsorption chamber, and as it does the abnormal component sticks to the substance. The advantage to adsorption technology is that removal of the abnormal component usually does not require replacement fluid because such a small volume has been removed. Adsorption procedures are still largely experimental.

Plateletpheresis

Platelets are used for various medical situations and disease conditions. Individuals can receive them following heart surgery or for thrombocytopenia following chemotherapy. Those who receive many units of platelet or pooled platelet (from multiple donors) transfusions are exposed to many antigens. Such individuals oftentimes

refractory

become refractory, which means that they develop antibody against donor platelets, causing platelets to be rapidly cleared from the circulation after transfusion.

To decrease a recipient's exposure to multiple donors, platelets may be collected from a single donor by plateletpheresis. This procedure allows larger numbers of platelets (equal to 5 to 6 units) to be collected than can be collected from a unit of whole blood. For recipients who have developed HLA antibodies, platelets can be collected by plateletpheresis from donors whose HLA type matches the recipient's.

Collection

Before platelet collection begins, donor blood must be subjected to ABO and Rh grouping, antibody screening, and transmissible disease testing. Cross matching is not required for platelets if the amount of red cell contamination is less than 5 mL. However, if the platelet concentrate contains more than this amount, compatibility should be determined between donor and recipient blood.

Platelet donors can donate more often than whole blood donors, but time between platelet collection sessions should be a minimum of 48 hours. Donors who have had aspirin within 3 days of collection should be deferred because aspirin inhibits platelet function.

The minimum number of platelets to be obtained by apheresis is 3×10^{11} per unit. Platelets are usually collected in 200 to 250 mL of plasma in order to provide a liquid solution for transfusion. If donor plasma is incompatible with recipient red cells, most of the donor plasma may be removed. To prevent the introduction of contaminating white cells, leukocyte-depletion filters are used at the time of infusion.

3×10^{11} per unit

Irradiation   Platelets should be irradiated (2500 cGy) to destroy viable lymphocytes prior to transfusion if the platelets are donated by blood relatives, or if they are intended for neonates or immunosuppressed and immunodeficient patients.

destruction of viable lymphocytes

Storage   Platelets are stored at 20 to 24C with continuous gentle agitation to prevent aggregation. When platelets are prepared in an open system (not sealed off from room air), they can be stored for only 24 hours. When prepared in a closed system, their storage time is 5 days.

20 to 24C

Leukapheresis

Removal of white cells from a donor is called leukapheresis. White cells are usually removed for therapeutic reasons. For example, individuals with very high white cell counts due to leukemia can undergo this procedure. Granulocytes are collected by leukapheresis for transfusion purposes.

Granulocyte Collection

Although physicians disagree about the use of donor granulocytes, they have been successfully transfused in some recipients (mostly neonates) with bacterial infections who fail to respond to antibiotics. In order to increase the number of granulocytes available for transfusions, corticosteroids and/or hematopoietic growth factors can be given to a donor prior to apheresis. Due to their short life span, granulocytes should be used as soon as possible following collection.

destruction of viable lymphocytes

prevention of TAGVHD

Irradiation   Granulocytes designated for immuno-suppressed and immunodeficient recipients, neonates, or blood relatives of a donor should be irradiated with 2500 cGy (25 Gy) to destroy viable lymphocytes and prevent transfusion associated graft–versus–host disease (TAGVHD).

24 hours

Storage   Granulocytes can be stored for a maximum of 24 hours at room temperature.

Corticosteroids

increase white cell numbers

Corticosteroids are a class of steroids that have an effect on the immune system. The use of corticosteroids increases white cell numbers by stimulating the bone marrow to release additional granulocytes and by stopping the movement of white cells from circulation into body tissue spaces. A corticosteroid can be administered a day before collection and up to 2 hours before collection. A donor with ulcers, hypertension, or diabetes should be questioned about these conditions before receiving corticosteroids. Corticosteroids are given in pill form.

Hespan™

granulocytes

Hydroxyethyl starch (hetastarch; Hespan™) is a colloidal solution used to produce better yields of granulocytes during apheresis because it reduces the amount of red cell contamination in the granulocyte unit. Hespan is administered intravenously to an apheresis donor prior to collection. The amount of Hespan given is 500 mL. As blood enters the cell separator, Hespan causes red cells to aggregate at the base of the separator bowl. White cells and platelets form a buffy coat above this red cell aggregate, making it easier to separate them out for collection. The buffy coat is also known as the mononuclear cell fraction.

red cell aggregation

buffy coat

mononuclear cell fraction

Hespan Cautions Donors can experience adverse reactions to Hespan, usually in the form of a rash. Because Hespan is a volume expander, donors should be monitored to prevent fluid overload. The granulocyte concentration separated from whole blood requires that the recipient receiving the granulocyte unit be ABO and Rh compatible with the donor.

fluid overload

Hematopoietic Growth Factors

Given prior to apheresis, hematopoietic growth factors increase the numbers of circulating stem and progenitor cells. Growth factors include granulocyte-macrophage colony-stimulating factor (GM-CSF) and granulocyte colony-stimulating factor (G-CSF). Both growth factors promote increased granulocyte production within bone marrow. Once the marrow releases these granulocytes into circulation, they can be collected. Hematopoietic growth factors are usually administered subcutaneously (s.c.).

increase stem and progenitor cell numbers

promote granulocyte production

Peripheral Blood Progenitor Cell Apheresis

Peripheral blood progenitor cell apheresis refers to the collection of hematopoietic progenitor cells from the peripheral circulation of a recipient or donor (see Ch. 1, The Concept of Blood). Progenitor cells are infused into recipients whose bone marrow needs to reestablish blood cell production. Because hematopoietic progenitor cells are collected from the peripheral circulation, they are called peripheral blood progenitor cells (PBPCs). The collection procedure is known as cytapheresis.

PBPCs
cytapheresis

Uses A transfusion of PBPCs reestablishes blood cell lines and their components: red cells, white cells, and

PBPCs reestablish all blood cell types

platelets. It is becoming more common to use PBPCs alone to reestablish hematopoietic and lymphopoietic function. Studies conducted on autologous and allogeneic PBPCs show that they tend to engraft sooner than the bone marrow stem cells, with quicker recovery of white cells and platelets.

bone marrow rescue

Peripheral blood progenitor cells are used to rescue the bone marrow of patients receiving high-dose chemotherapy for malignancies such as leukemia, lymphoma, breast cancer, and Hodgkin's disease, among others. These cells are also used to decrease the incidence of neutropenia and thrombocytopenia in cancer patients. In other words, transfused PBPCs engraft in the bone marrow and reduce the time in which the individual is susceptible to infection and bleeding by hastening the growth of neutrophils and platelets. Neither autologous nor allogeneic PBPCs are infused through a blood filter.

more rapid neutrophil and platelet engraftment

Priming Normally the number of peripheral progenitor cells in circulation is low. A technique called priming is used to increase their numbers. Priming agents include: hematopoietic growth factors and certain chemotherapeutic agents, such as cyclophosphamide.

Autologous PBPCs Collection and Infusion

collected during remission

Autologous progenitor cells are collected while the individual is in remission because (1) the tumor burden is small, (2) the amount of chemotherapeutic drug is minimal, and (3) the progenitor cells have a better chance of engrafting. Collecting PBPCs by apheresis requires harvesting the buffy coat. Due to the low number of PBPCs in circulation, more than one collection session may be necessary. If collection is to be completed in one session, it can take 6 hours or more to harvest sufficient numbers of PBPCs.

DMSO

Once the buffy coat is collected, autologous PBPCs are mixed with dimethyl sulfoxide (DMSO), a cryoprotective agent, and frozen. They are stored frozen in liquid nitrogen at -196C. After a recipient receives high-dose chemotherapy and/or total body irradiation

(TBI), the unit of PBPCs is thawed at 37 to 40C and infused immediately because DMSO is toxic to progenitor cells at room temperature (25C). Thawed progenitor cells are infused without further treatment given to them. Peripheral blood progenitor cells are infused by methods identical to those of blood or bone marrow transfusion.

There are advantages to the collection of autologous PBPCs over autologous bone marrow stem cells. For example, there is a less likely chance of contamination by malignant cells, and it is simpler to collect autologous PBPCs than bone marrow stem cells.

Allogeneic PBPC Collection and Infusion

Until recently transfusions of PBPCs were autologous. Now a number of treatment centers have performed successful allogeneic PBPC collection for transplants. An infusion of PBPCs can be carried out in conjunction with an infusion of bone marrow stem cells. Allogeneic peripheral blood progenitor cell collection is the same as for autologous. However, allogeneic cells are not cryopreserved: they are infused immediately following collection.

Therapeutic Apheresis

In the therapeutic apheresis process, diseased platelets, white cells, plasma, or plasma components are removed from the individual's circulation. Therapeutic apheresis is usually only a palliative treatment, with positive effects lasting only a short time.

palliative treatment

Therapeutic Cytapheresis

This procedure is performed for some types of leukemia in which the white cell count is greater than $100 \times 10^9/L$. When leukocyte numbers reach these levels, stasis (decreased blood flow) in the brain or lungs

leukemia

thrombocythemia

can occur. Therapeutic cytapheresis is also performed for thrombocythemia when the platelet count is greater than 1000 x 10^9/L. Platelets are removed if there is evidence that an increased number of defective platelets is causing hemorrhage or clotting.

Plasmapheresis

removal of diseased or abnormal plasma or plasma components

This procedure is used to remove diseased or abnormal plasma or plasma components. Plasmapheresis is used to treat the following: hyperviscosity syndromes, myasthenia gravis, dysproteinemias, multiple myeloma, high levels of low-density lipoproteins, circulating antibodies (as in Waldenström's macroglobulinemia), and immune complexes. With some diseases, all plasma is removed from a patient and replaced with albumin or donor plasma. This procedure is called plasma exchange.

plasma exchange

Plasma or plasma components removed from circulation can be replaced by albumin, electrolyte solutions, or FFP. The amount of plasma removed and the amount of replacement fluid administered should be recorded accurately. Maintaining proper fluid balance within the individual is essential.

fluid balance

▪ QUESTIONS ▪

1. Explain plasmapheresis, plateletpheresis, and leukapheresis. How are they different from one another?

2. What is the purpose of therapeutic apheresis?

3. Identify four complications that can arise in a recipient during apheresis.

4. What are the symptoms of citrate toxicity?

5. Cellular components are separated from Whole Blood by centrifugation, membrane filtration, and adsorption. True or False?

6. Plasma collection can be accomplished by membrane filtration. Explain how this is done.

7. Adsorption is used to remove a diseased component from plasma. Give examples of these diseased components.

8. Single-donor platelets are preferable to those obtained from multiple donors. Explain why this is so.

9. When and why would a physician order Platelets to be irradiated before transfusion?

10. Give one example of why a physician would order leukapheresis.

11. Granulocytes have been successfully transfused in some recipients with bacterial infections who failed to respond to antibiotics. Why must granulocytes be used as soon after collection as possible?

12. Why may corticosteroids be given before a granulocyte collection?

13. Corticosteroids are administered in pill form. How are hematopoietic growth factors given to a donor prior to collection?

14. What is the mononuclear cell fraction?

15. Describe the procedure known as cytapheresis.

16. What type of cells are used to rescue the bone marrow of patients receiving high-dose chemotherapy?

17. When a bone marrow rescue is planned, why are autologous progenitor cells collected while the individual is in remission?

18. Why is it more advantageous to collect autologous PBPCs than to collect autologous bone marrow stem cells?

19. Why is therapeutic cytapheresis performed?

20. When is therapeutic cytapheresis performed?

21. List five conditions for which plasmapheresis is ordered.

CHAPTER **19**

Methods of Autologous Blood Recovery

Introduction

Autologous blood recovery is the collection of an individual's own blood prior to, during, or after surgery for reinfusion (transfusion) at a later time. Autotransfusion refers to the reinfusion of one's own blood. At the present time, there are four autologous blood recovery methods that allow patients to donate and receive units of their own blood during or following surgical procedures.

autotransfusion

(1) With preoperative predonation, patients donate blood weeks in advance of surgery.

preoperative
predonation

(2) With intraoperative hemodilution, patients donate blood immediately before surgery.

intraoperative
hemodilution

(3) With intraoperative blood salvage, a patient's blood is collected during surgery or processed from an extracorporeal circuit used during cardiopulmonary bypass surgery.

intraoperative
blood salvage

(4) With postoperative blood collection, a patient's blood is recovered from drains placed within the surgical site.

postoperative
blood collection

Written policies and guidelines regarding the collection and administration of autologous blood should be available for all personnel involved in autologous blood recovery procedures.

Some medical professionals feel that autologous blood is the safest blood—as long as collection and infusion guidelines are strictly adhered to. As with any transfusion there can be complications and adverse reactions associated with an autologous transfusion

319

that can cause harm and even death. Some physicians are conservative about using autologous blood for the disadvantages cited below.

Those who favor the use of autologous blood do so for the following reasons:

- It decreases the demand for allogeneic blood.
- It reduces or eliminates transfusion-transmitted disease.
- It prevents alloimmunization (development of alloantibodies to allogeneic blood).
- It eliminates some types of transfusion reactions, such as hemolytic reactions (ABO and Rh incompatibility) and transfusion-associated graft-versus-host disease (TAGVHD).
- It can be used in conjunction with allogeneic blood or blood components.
- It is a source of blood for individuals who have developed alloantibodies following multiple donor transfusions, transplants, or pregnancies.
- It is an acceptable form of transfusion for some religious sects.

Some disadvantages associated with autologous blood use include the following:

- Complications can occur as the result of the donation procedure. Some physicians feel that autologous donors do not meet the same stringent requirements for donation that volunteer donors do. For example, patients with indwelling catheters who would not be permitted to donate allogeneic units can donate autologous units.
- Equipment used for certain autologous collection and reinfusion procedures are occasionally implicated in adverse complications.
- Autologous blood units can become outdated due to delays or postponements in surgery.
- There is the chance that the recipient receives the wrong blood.
- Units may be administered out of sequence, as when an allogeneic unit is used before an autologous.

Complement Activation with Blood Collection Systems

Intraoperative and postoperative blood collection systems can reinfuse activated complement components to the individual being reinfused. Researchers are not sure why this is so, but it is believed that complement is activated by the surgical procedure itself. Usually, complement activation is directed against red cells and causes hemolysis. The recipient can have such problems as anemia or serious anaphylactoid reactions or immune reactions that cause capillary leakage, shock, and possibly death.

red cell hemolysis

Storage of Autologous Blood

Blood units collected by autologous recovery methods are stored at different temperatures. Predonated autologous blood is stored in a blood bank under the same conditions as allogeneic units (1 to 6C) but kept separate from them. Blood collected immediately prior to or during surgery can be kept either at room temperature (25C) for a period of 8 hours or at 1 to 6C for 24 hours provided it was refrigerated within 6 hours of collection. Blood collected postoperatively is reinfused right away and not usually stored. All autologous blood products should be filtered during reinfusion.

Preoperative Predonation

Predonated blood is used in surgical procedures in which the surgeon expects an individual to lose 2 to 3 units of blood during the operation. Vascular, orthopedic, urologic, and some cardiac procedures, for example, utilize predonated blood. Units of predonated autologous blood are held in reserve in a hospital blood bank in the event that the donor/patient needs a transfusion during or after the operation.

vascular, orthopedic, urologic, cardiac surgeries

Predonation Guidelines

The number of units an individual can predonate depends on the type of surgery and on his or her medical condition. In order to predonate blood, a surgical candidate must have a hematocrit (Hct) of 0.33 (33%) and a hemoglobin (Hgb) concentration of 11 g/dL (110 g/L). Predonation is not recommended if these blood levels are lower because anemia is indicated and blood collection at this time would accelerate this condition. To increase red blood cell production in individuals, iron supplements should be given during the predonation period.

Hct: 0.33

Hgb: 11 g/dL

Collection

A candidate for predonation gives a unit each week prior to surgery. As many as 4 units of autologous blood can be stored in reserve. The last donated unit should be collected prior to 72 hours before the surgical procedure so that blood volume can return to normal. The order of transfusing predonated units should be that the unit collected first is transfused first followed by units in the order of collection. In other words, the oldest unit should be transfused first.

first transfused unit/
first collected

Predonated blood can be collected at the hospital where surgery will take place or at an outside facility. If collected at the latter, the candidate must sign an informed consent contract agreeing that the donated blood be tested for certain transfusion-related diseases.

Testing

Every unit of predonated blood must undergo specific tests before it is available for use. It must be labeled with the individual's name, identification number, and ABO and Rh group. A unit of autologous blood should be clearly marked "For Autologous Use Only." If it has tested positive for disease, it must be labeled "Biohazard" for the safety of healthcare handlers. Some hospitals test autologous units for transfusion-related diseases, such as hepatitis B and C, HIV, HTLV-I/II, and syphilis.

Complications and Adverse Reactions

Individuals donating autologous blood can experience anemia, hypotension, diaphoresis (sweating), dizziness, syncope (loss of consciousness), decreased heart rate (bradycardia), rapid breathing, and the vasovagal response.

Adverse reactions associated with the administration of predonated autologous blood include: bacterial contamination of the unit, increased levels of cytokines in the unit, and circulatory overload. Bacterial contamination occurs when the patient/donor has a bacterial infection or bacteremia (bacteria in the blood) that is overlooked in the medical evaluation process. Individuals with leg or foot ulcers and patients with urinary and indwelling catheters should not donate autologous blood because of the chance of bacterial contamination. Autologous blood is likely to be older at the time of infusion and, therefore, has increased amounts of cytokines and biological response modifiers (BMRs), both of which are associated with febrile nonhemolytic transfusion reactions (FNHTRs). Circulatory overload occurs when physicians transfuse units of autologous blood simply because they are available.

bacterial contamination

cytokines and BMRs→FNHTRs
circulatory overload

Contraindications

There are some individuals for whom predonated autologous blood is not recommended. For example, collection of autologous blood from pregnant women remains a controversial issue. For the elderly, especially those 70 years or older, there are few if any benefits from autologous blood collection and use. Candidates with cardiac disease, such as aortic stenosis (tightness of aortic valve), left main coronary artery disease, unstable angina, cardiac failure, and recent myocardial infarction, among others, are poor risks for predonation and should be deferred from donating.

pregnant women
elderly

cardiac disease

Collection of predonated autologous blood is safe for pediatric patients, older children, and young adults who are less likely to be affected by the complications of predonation. For these individuals, autologous blood prevents alloimmunization.

Intraoperative Hemodilution

Intraoperative hemodilution is the withdrawal of whole blood from a candidate immediately before surgery, when a surgeon expects the individual to lose no more than 2 L of blood. Typically 2 L, which is the equivalent of 4 units, are removed and collected in anticoagulated blood bags. The individual receives either crystalloid or colloid solution to replace the blood withdrawn. Cardiac, orthopedic, vascular, and other major surgeries utilize intraoperative hemodilution.

cardiac, vascular, orthopedic, other major surgeries

Infusion of Crystalloids and Colloids

crystalloid infusion– 2:1 ratio

colloid infusion– 1:1 ratio

normovolemic anemia

Crystalloids are infused at a 2:1 ratio (2 parts crystalloid, 1 part blood) because they leave the vascular system more easily and are more readily removed by the kidneys. Colloids are usually infused at a 1:1 ratio. Due to their larger molecular size, colloids diffuse less easily through capillary pores, thus less colloid volume is needed to replace the blood withdrawn. Hemodilution with a crystalloid or colloid solution causes normovolemic anemia; that is, the individual's blood volume is maintained at a normal level but the number of red cells in circulation (Hct) is reduced. A small number of circulating red cells means fewer red blood cells are lost during the surgical procedure.

Benefits of Intraoperative Hemodilution

In the view of some medical personnel, hemodilution achieves specific benefits.

decreased blood viscosity

- Hemodiluted blood is less viscous and flows more easily, allowing more efficient delivery of oxygen to body tissues. Blood with decreased viscosity has a better chance of reaching all body cells.

elevated Hct

viable clotting proteins and platelets

- Reinfused blood elevates the candidate's Hct. Hemodiluted blood is kept at room temperature and therefore clotting proteins and platelets remain viable and possibly have some hemostatic effect when transfused within 8 hours of collection. If more time elapses before transfusion, the blood should be refrigerated.

- Intraoperative hemodilution has been shown to reduce significantly the use of allogeneic blood products and therefore the incidence of alloimmunization and transfusion transmitted diseases.

reduced use of allogeneic blood products

Infusion

Units of blood collected immediately before surgery, by the anesthesiologist, are usually kept in the operating suite. If a blood transfusion is needed during surgery, the units are reinfused in the reverse order from which they were withdrawn. The first unit removed is the last infused because it has not been hemodiluted and contains the greatest number of platelets and clotting proteins. It is infused after surgery when the individual is losing less blood and will therefore benefit the most from platelets and clotting proteins. Stored units must be used within 24 hours of storage.

first unit removed/ last infused

Donation Prerequisites

Candidates for intraoperative hemodilution should meet the following criteria:

- Hgb concentration greater than 12 g/dL (120 g/L)
- Absence of all clotting deficiencies
- Anticipated blood loss of no more than 2 L during surgery
- Absence of serious cardiac, kidney, hypertension, lung, or liver disease

These criteria are more stringent if hemodilution is to be instituted prior to cardiac surgery because patients with cardiac disease are apt to be volume-dependent.

Complications

The same complications and adverse reactions that occur with predonated autologous blood collection and use are also relevant to intraoperative hemodilution. These include bacterial contamination and circulatory overload. In the case of intraoperative hemodilution, cytokines usually do not present

bacterial contamination circulatory overload

problems because the blood is used before they have a chance to accumulate. Circulatory overload may be a problem for the same reason as in predonated blood use: blood is infused simply because it is available.

Intraoperative Blood Salvage

major surgeries

cardiac surgery

Intraoperative blood salvage is the collection and reinfusion of blood shed at the operative site during major surgeries or drained from the extracorporeal system used to provide cardiopulmonary support to individuals during cardiac surgery. Although rare, adverse events can occur with the use of intraoperative blood collection. They include: air embolism, hemolysis (increased plasma levels of Hgb can present problems for individuals with kidney disease), DIC, renal insufficiency, respiratory failure, and hemoglobinuria.

Contraindications

Intraoperative salvage is not recommended during procedures in which bacterial contamination (e.g., bladder and open bowel surgery), malignancy, other body fluids, such as amniotic fluid or urine, or sepsis is present. Reinfusion would expose the individual to possibly dangerous contaminants. Autologous collection is not recommended for individuals with sickle-cell disease because the quality of their red cells is not adequate.

Wash and Nonwash Collection Systems

wash system: washes blood and concentrates red cells

nonwash system: collects and reinfuses blood

Wash and nonwash collection systems are used in intraoperative salvage. A wash system collects and washes whole blood. It concentrates red cells by removing all other components. A nonwash system collects whole blood and reinfuses it without further processing. Wash and nonwash systems are used for different types of surgical procedures. Neither one, however, can be used for every surgical procedure. The decision to use a wash or nonwash system is made by the physician.

Both wash and nonwash collection systems require an anticoagulant to prevent blood from clotting. Heparin or ACD (acid-citrate-dextrose; similar to CPD) can be utilized as an anticoagulant for blood collected by wash systems. In nonwash systems the anticoagulant is ACD.

Wash Collection Systems

Wash systems remove almost all white cells, platelets, and plasma from whole blood except red cells. They are used exclusively for cardiac, certain liver, some orthopedic surgical procedures, and aortic aneurysm surgery due to the amount of debris generated, the drugs used, and the large quantity of blood shed. Wash systems are employed for many transplant and vascular procedures as well.

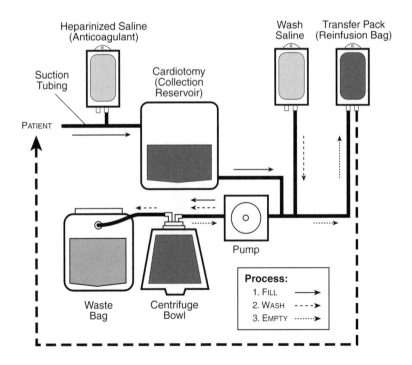

FIGURE 19.1 Schematic Representation of a Wash System

A wash system is used during certain surgical procedures to wash blood of debris and fluids and to concentrate red cells. During or after the procedure the red cells are reinfused into the patient.

ACD or heparin in
100 mL of 0.9% NS

Anticoagulants ACD or heparin mixed in 1000 mL of 0.9% normal saline are the anticoagulants used in wash systems. The ratio of anticoagulant-saline to blood flow is maintained between 1:5 and 1:10 (1 part anticoagulant is added to 5 to 10 parts of blood). The flow rate of the anticoagulant-saline solution can be adjusted to approximate the rate of blood collection. As blood is suctioned from the surgical site, the anticoagulant solution is mixed with the blood at the end of the suction aspirator.

1:5 to 1:10 ratio

Mechanical Operation Although easy to operate, wash systems are somewhat more complex than non-wash systems. The wash systems available for purchase are mostly computer controlled and fully automatic. A wash system has a cell processor/separator, a cardiotomy (collection canister), and a tubing set. A cell processor is basically a centrifuge device that spins and concentrates red cells by removing the white cells, platelets, and plasma. As the plasma is removed, the Hct increases and the red cells become packed. The more concentrated the blood is, the greater the Hct. A cardiotomy is a collection reservoir that holds any lost blood once it is suctioned from the surgical field. A tubing set contains the disposable parts of a wash system: the centrifuge bowl with integrated tubing, waste bag, and reinfusion bag.

wash system:
cell processor,
cardiotomy,
tubing set

The cell processor is set up prior to surgery. Lost blood suctioned from an individual during surgery and mixed with an anticoagulant is collected in the cardiotomy. When the cardiotomy is full, collected blood drains into the cell processor containing the spinning centrifuge bowl. The force of centrifugation pushes the red cells to the sides of the bowl. Plasma and any fluids used during surgery are spun off into the waste bag. When the centrifuge bowl is filled with red cells, the cell processor switches automatically to a wash cycle.

1500 mL of 0.9%
NS wash

The centrifuged red cells are washed with 1500 mL of 0.9% normal saline, which does not contain any anticoagulant. Contaminants, debris, and anticoagulant added during collection are transferred into the waste bag. The end product in the centrifuge bowl consists of red cells suspended in saline. The washed red cells are pumped from the centrifuge bowl into the reinfusion bag, also known as the transfer pack. The transfer pack is disconnected from the tubing set. All air in the bag must be expelled and the bag is passed to the anesthetist (CRNA) or anesthesiologist (MD) who administers the reinfusion. This blood is never infused under pressure because of the likelihood of air entering the patient and causing an embolus. An air embolus can be fatal.

A filter with a small pore is placed in the I.V. line and the patient reinfused with approximately 225 mL of red cells suspended in saline. The Hct of the reinfused blood is between 0.50 and 0.60 (50 and 60%).

Hct of reinfused blood: 0.50 to 0.60

Nonwash Collection Systems

Nonwash systems are used mainly during orthopedic surgeries that involve fracture repair and total knee procedures. These systems are not designed to collect the rapid or large blood loss that can occur during many major surgeries. Nonwash systems are most often utilized when blood loss is expected to be about 500 to 1000 mL (1 to 2 units of blood).

orthopedic surgeries

Mechanical Operation   Nonwash systems collect shed blood into a sterile canister. An anticoagulant, ACD, is added before or during blood collection. After the

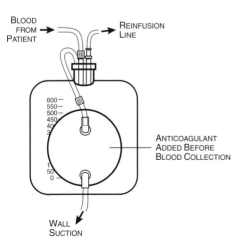

BLOOD FROM PATIENT →

→ REINFUSION LINE

600 —
550 —
500 —
450 —
40
3

ANTICOAGULANT ADDED BEFORE BLOOD COLLECTION

1
50 —
0 —

WALL SUCTION

FIGURE 19.2 Schematic Representation of a Nonwash System

A nonwash system is composed of a sterile, plastic canister that collects blood for reinfusion into the patient. The device is easy to use and set up.

canister is full of blood it is passed to the anesthetist or anesthesiologist for reinfusion. Further processing of nonwashed blood is unnecessary.

Complications and Cautions   Nonwashed blood can contain substances that can cause complications for the individual, although rarely. Plasma-free Hgb, hemolyzed red cells, drugs, possible bone chips, activated platelets, plasma, various irrigating solutions used during surgery, activated coagulation factors, and fibrin split products are examples of surgical debris. Some physicians maintain that reinfusion of nonwashed blood does not pose risks to a patient. Others feel that reinfusion of substances in nonwashed blood can be harmful, especially to patients with kidney and liver disease. The use of nonwash systems remains controversial.

surgical debris

Individuals who receive many units of washed blood cells must be monitored for coagulation deficiencies because washed blood is deficient in clotting factors. After an individual has received 4 to 5 units of washed blood, coagulation tests should be performed.

coagulation deficiencies

Postoperative Blood Collection

Postoperative blood collection refers to the collection and reinfusion of an individual's blood from a wound following surgery. Oozing blood is collected postoperatively by wound drainage systems via suction tubes inserted in the wound. Both wash and nonwash systems are also used to collect postoperative wound blood. Postoperative wound blood is collected following cardiac, thoracic (chest), and orthopedic procedures. Blood loss from cardiac or thoracic surgery is referred to as shed mediastinal blood.

cardiac, thoracic, orthopedic surgeries

Like other autologous recovery methods, postoperative blood collection helps reduce the need and use of allogeneic blood in transfusions following surgery. In the past, blood from wound drainage was discarded and the individual was transfused with allogeneic blood.

Complications   Postoperative shed blood can become contaminated with bacteria; therefore, it should be reinfused within 6 hours of collection or discarded. Postoperative blood is subject to clotting and subsequent clot lysis. Large amounts of reinfused blood containing fibrin split products can interfere with blood coagulation. Given the potential problems associated with increased fibrin split products, some hospitals limit the number of units of intraoperative or postoperative autologous blood that a person can receive.

fibrin split products

■ **QUESTIONS** ■

1. What is autologous blood recovery?

2. There are four autologous blood recovery methods for surgical patients. Identify them.

3. Why do some medical professionals feel that autologous blood is the safest?

4. There are disadvantages associated with the use of autologous blood. List four of these.

5. Red cell hemolysis can be associated with the infusion of autologous blood. Explain why this is so.

6. How is autologous blood stored?

7. When is predonated blood used in a surgical procedure?

8. What are the hematocrit (Hct) and hemoglobin (Hgb) guidelines for predonated blood?

9. As many as 10 units of predonated autologous blood can be store in reserve. True or False.

10. Is the order of transfusing predonated units important? Explain.

11. When is a unit of autologous blood labeled as "Biohazard"?

12. Adverse reactions can be associated with the administration of autologous blood. List three of these.

13. There are some individuals for whom predonated autologous blood is not recommended. List three categories for whom this is true.

14. Is autologous blood collection safer for children or adults? Why?

15. During intraoperative hemodilution, the individual receives either crystalloid or colloid solution to replace the blood withdrawn. Explain why crystalloids are infused at a higher ratio to blood than colloids.

16. Define normovolemic anemia. Why is it allowed?

17. Why is intraoperative hemodilution deemed beneficial by some medical personnel?

18. How much blood loss during surgery is anticipated for those individuals undergoing hemodilution?

19. List three donation prerequisites for intraoperative hemodilution.

20. Cytokines usually do not present a problem in intraoperative hemodilution. Why is this so?

21. Explain the term intraoperative blood salvage.

22. When is intraoperative blood salvage contraindicated?

23. Mr. Johnson has sickle-cell disease. How many units of autologous blood can be stored for him?

24. Describe two types of intraoperative blood salvage collection systems. When is one used and not the other?

25. Both wash and nonwash collection systems require an anticoagulant to prevent blood from clotting. Which ones are used for which systems?

26. Define cardiotomy and explain its use.

27. Who reinfuses the blood during an intraoperative blood salvage? and what major precaution must be taken?

28. After an individual has received 4 to 5 units of washed blood, what laboratory tests must be performed?

29. Which collection system is used for postoperative blood drained from a surgical site (wound)?

30. What is shed mediastinal blood?

CHAPTER 20

Bone Marrow Transplantation

Introduction

Bone marrow transplantation (BMT) refers to the restoration of an individual's hematopoietic and immune systems with the infusion and engraftment of stem cells from healthy bone marrow and/or progenitor cells harvested from the peripheral circulation or umbilical cord. This procedure is an accepted form of therapy for both fatal and nonfatal diseases. In conjunction with high-dose chemotherapy and total body irradiation (TBI), BMT is an effective therapy for treating many types of hematologic malignancies, such as leukemia; certain solid organ tumors, such as breast; nonmalignant disorders, such as thalassemias; and immunologic deficiencies, such as severe combined immune deficiency syndrome (SCIDS).

Stem and Progenitor Cells

Stem cells are primitive (undifferentiated) cells found in the hematopoietic marrow that give rise to all blood cells (see Ch. 1, The Concept of Blood). They are harvested from bone marrow. Progenitor cells are stem cells found in the circulation that give rise to mature blood cells. They are found and collected outside the bone marrow, that is, in the peripheral circulation and umbilical cord blood. Progenitor cells collected from the peripheral circulation are called peripheral blood progenitor cells (PBPCs). Cord blood progenitor cells (CBPCs) are collected from umbilical cord blood.

PBPCs
CBPCs

The terms stem cell and progenitor cell are often used interchangeably in reference to blood cell precursors infused in a bone marrow transplant. Both kinds of cells

blood cell precursors:
stem cell/progenitor cell

335

bone marrow
stem cell

are capable of restoring bone marrow function following a transplant procedure. The term bone marrow stem cell is used interchangeably with the terms stem cell, peripheral blood progenitor cell, and cord blood progenitor cell.

Peripheral Blood Progenitor Cells

faster engraftment
and recovery of
granulocytes

The use of PBPCs is becoming increasingly popular as a means of restoring hematopoietic function following high-dose chemotherapy and TBI, which destroys an individual's hematopoietic marrow. Because PBPCs are more mature than bone marrow stem cells, engraftment in the bone marrow may occur sooner, with faster recovery of granulocytes occurring within 2.5 weeks and platelets within 4 weeks. For individuals who have received pelvic irradiation and are unable to donate bone marrow, PBPCs may be the only source of stem cells. Peripheral blood progenitor cells are administered alone or in conjunction with bone marrow stem cells to enhance engraftment.

Cord Blood Progenitor Cells

The most recent alternative to stem cell and PBPC collection is the use of CBPCs. The incidence of graft-versus-host disease (GVHD), a complication of BMT, is fewer with CBPCs than with stem cells or PBPCs. Researchers believe this is because cord blood cells are less mature and, therefore, the T lymphocytes do not generate a strong immune response. At the present time, CBPCs have only been used in pediatric stem cell transplants, for conditions such as Fanconi anemia, some leukemias, and aplastic anemia, among others. CBPCs are being studied for possible use in adult transplants.

Sources of Stem and Progenitor Cells

harvested from live
donor

There are three sources of stem cells used for BMT: autologous, allogeneic, and syngeneic. Each must be harvested from a live donor. Like blood donors, stem cell donors must have their blood tested for infectious disease markers. When cord blood stem cells are used the mother's blood must be tested within two days before or following delivery for infectious disease markers, such as HBsAg, anti-HCV, anti-HIV 1/2, HIV-1-Ag, anti-HTLV I/II, and a serologic test for syphilis.

Autologous Sources Autologous stem cells are harvested from bone marrow or the peripheral circulation and administered to the individual who donated them, but they cannot be taken from someone with a stem cell disease or disorder. Autologous stem cell transplant is associated with fewer complications than allogeneic transplant. The risk of graft rejection and GVHD is virtually nonexistent because the body usually does not reject or react to its own tissue. However, a transient autoimmunelike reaction resembling GVHD can develop with an autologous transplant and cause symptoms of GVHD. Physicians are not sure why this happens. Autologous marrow transplants are rarely done on individuals over 60 years of age.

harvested from bone marrow or peripheral circulation

Examples of disease states treated with autologous stem cells include: some leukemias, some lymphomas, Hodgkin's disease, myeloma, and some solid organ tumors, such as breast, certain brain, and germ cell (testicular and ovarian) tumors.

Allogeneic Sources Allogeneic bone marrow stem cells, PBPCs, and CBPCs are harvested from either a (1) HLA-matched sibling or (2) a mismatched-HLA donor. The chances for engraftment of bone marrow are good for recipients who are mismatched for only one HLA gene. Recipients who are mismatched for two or more genes have a poor prognosis, with an increased incidence of graft rejection and GVHD, among other complications.

harvested from HLA-matched sibling or mismatched donor

There are greater HLA genetic differences within the general population than within families. Therefore there is a reduced chance of finding an HLA-matched donor from this pool. Siblings are the preferred source of allogeneic stem cells because their HLA molecules have the highest potential (25%) for being matched with those of the recipient. Allogeneic transplant is the most problematic because development of GVHD or graft

preferred source: siblings

rejection is directly related to the degree of HLA histocompatibility between donor and recipient. Allogeneic stem and progenitor cell transplants are usually confined to patients under 50 years of age.

harvested from
identical twin

Syngeneic Sources   Syngeneic stem cells are harvested from an identical twin for transplantation into the other twin. The HLA molecules of these individuals are the same. Therefore the likelihood of graft rejection or GVHD is virtually nonexistent. Occasionally, GVHDlike symptoms follow a syngeneic marrow transplant. They are believed to be caused by minor histocompatibility differences that exist between identical twins. This GVHDlike reaction is similar to the transient autoimmunelike disorder that occurs in autologous BMT.

Examples of disease states treated with allogenic or syngeneic stem cells include: aplastic anemia, myelodysplasia, thalassemias, severe combined immune deficiency disease (SCIDS), sickle-cell anemia, some leukemias, and some lymphomas.

Hematopoietic Growth Factors

To increase the yield of stem or progenitor cells it is best to harvest them following chemotherapy, while the bone marrow is recovering (producing more stem cells) or following the administration of hematopoietic growth factors, such as GM-CSF or G-CSF. Growth factors are administered s.c. for several weeks before collection.

Candidates for Bone Marrow Transplantation

Candidates for bone marrow transplant include individuals with congenital (primary) disorders and acquired bone marrow failure. Congenital bone marrow disorders are treated with an infusion of allogeneic or syngeneic bone marrow stem cells, PBPCs, or CBPCs. Persons with these disorders have defective stem cells and therefore must be treated with

congential (primary)
disorders and
acquired bone
marrow failure

syngeneic or allogeneic cells and not autologous. Acquired disorders can be treated with autologous, allogeneic, or syngeneic stem or progenitor cells.

Congenital Disorders

Congenital bone marrow disorders (primary marrow failure) produce defective stem cells. Examples of congenital disorders include: (1) thalassemias, which produce abnormal hemoglobin molecules; (2) severe combined immunodeficiency disease (SCIDS), which is the absence of an immune system at birth; and (3) some types of aplastic anemia, which is the absence or minimal production of all types of blood cells.

defective stem cells

Acquired Bone Marrow Failure

In acquired bone marrow failure, healthy stem cells are produced, but at sometime during the process of cell differentiation, blood cells become malignant. Leukemia and multiple myeloma (B cell tumor) are examples of diseases that occur with acquired bone marrow failure. Acquired bone marrow failure can also occur in individuals who receive chemotherapy and radiation therapy.

malignant blood cells

chemotherapy
radiation therapy

High-Dose Chemotherapy and Bone Marrow Failure

Many hematologic malignancies and solid organ tumors, such as brain, breast, some lymphomas, and germ cell, can be destroyed with high-dose chemotherapy. However, the high-doses of chemotherapy needed to destroy malignant cells are highly toxic to all tissues, including blood cells. Toxicity causes destruction of mature blood cells and myelosuppression of bone marrow, which if not treated with BMT leads to death. Myelosuppression is the destruction of hematopoietic marrow whereby stem cells are prevented from regenerating and producing mature blood cells. The toxicity of chemotherapy to tissue limits the amount of chemotherapy that an individual can receive.

destruction of
mature blood cells
myelosuppression
of bone marrow

Bone marrow transplantation allows physicians to treat individuals with high-dose chemotherapy and TBI and at the same time rescue them from death. Treating individuals with a BMT is a means of eradicating malignancies as well as restoring the hematopoietic and immune systems.

HLA Compatibility in Bone Marrow Transplantation

histocompatibility

MLA class I and class II molecules

Histocompatibility refers to the genetic similarity, or parity (likeness), between donor and recipient HLA class I and class II molecules (see Ch. 8, The Major Histocompatibility Molecules). Class I and II molecules are cell surface glycoproteins that are necessary for an individual to generate an immune response to foreign matter. For bone marrow transplantation the degree of HLA similarity between donor and recipient is essential to reduce the incidence of graft rejection and GVHD. Transplantation other than from an identical twin stimulates a strong immune response in the recipient.

optimal graft survival: HLA match at 3 HLA loci

tissue typing/ histocompatibility testing

Before a BMT can be performed, both class I and II HLA molecules of a potential donor and recipient must be identified by tissue typing to determine whether an HLA match exists. Donors and recipients for BMT are tested for the following HLA antigens at loci HLA-A, HLA-B, and HLA-DR. Physicians always prefer a precise match at these loci for optimal graft survival. A mismatch for 1 or 2 loci is sometimes accepted. Tissue typing is also known as histo-compatibility testing.

slightly mismatched donor stem cells

autologous marrow

Other Donor Sources If an HLA-matched donor cannot be found, other sources are considered for reconstituting a patient's hematopoietic system. Slightly mismatched donor stem cells can be administered, which means that there is some degree of difference between donor and recipient HLA molecules. Autologous marrow is another source, as long as the patient's stem cells are healthy.

Histocompatibility Testing Assays

There are several assays available for determining the compatibility of HLA class I and II molecules (see Ch. 8, The Major Histocompatibility Molecules). Some of these same assays are also used to determine whether the recipient has antibodies against donor HLA molecules. Antibodies do not usually cause complications with BMT, and the reason is not completely understood.

Categories of histocompatibility tests include the following:

- The serologic assay (using serum) determines class I and II HLA molecules and also the antibodies against HLA. This type of assay is called the microlymphocytotoxicity assay.

  microlympho-cytotoxicity assay

- The cellular assay (using cells), called the mixed lymphocyte culture (MLC) or mixed lymphocyte reaction (MLR), determines similarity between donor and recipient class II HLA molecules.

  mixed lymphocyte culture (MLC) or mixed lymphocyte reaction (MLR)

- Molecular assays (using DNA) test for class II HLA molecules. One assay is the polymerase chain reaction (PCR).

  molecular assays

Tests that type and match body tissues can be difficult to understand. Moreover, research is constantly being conducted to improve methods for identifying HLA molecules. Institutions that carry out organ and bone marrow transplantations have preferred tests for determining HLA compatibility.

The Transplantation Procedure

Harvesting Stem Cells

A bone marrow donor, either allogeneic or autologous, receives either general or epidural (spinal) anesthesia during the collection procedure. Following anesthesia, the physician inserts an aspiration needle into the iliac crests of the pelvis and withdraws the bone marrow. The aliquot (amount) of marrow that can be extracted

iliac crests of pelvis

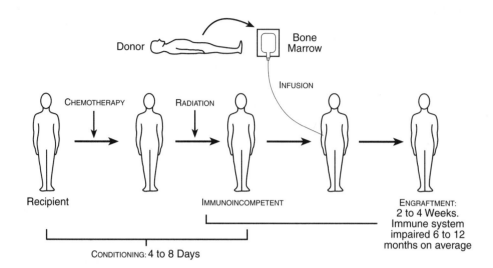

FIGURE 20.1 Allogeneic and Syngeneic Bone Marrow Transplant

After HLA histocompatibility testing has determined a compatible bone marrow donor, the recipient undergoes conditioning. Stem cells are infused within 24 hours following the conditioning program.

10 mL of marrow per kg of body weight

from a donor depends on the donor's body weight. Approximately 10 mL of marrow per kg of body weight can be withdrawn. (A kg equals 2.2 lbs.) To prevent clotting, marrow is harvested in heparinized syringes and mixed with a heparinized tissue culture medium to maintain cell viability. The collected marrow and culture medium are filtered through a fine mesh screen to remove fat, bone chips, clots, and other debris before being placed in transfusion bags.

The Conditioning Protocol

conditioning/ ablative therapy

Once an HLA-compatible donor is found, the transplant recipient undergoes a conditioning program in preparation for the BMT procedure. Conditioning is also referred to as ablative therapy. Depending on the disease, the hematologist-oncologist, along with other specialists, determines a conditioning protocol (plan). The protocol specifies the radiation and chemotherapeutic drugs that destroy any remaining malignant cells and reduce the risk of graft rejection and organ failure. Ablative therapy also clears marrow spaces for stem cell engraftment.

radiation and chemotherapeutic drugs marrow spaces cleared for stem cell engraftment

A conditioning program lasts from 4 to 8 days. During conditioning, a BMT candidate receives high-dose chemotherapy and sometimes total body irradiation (TBI). High-dose chemotherapy destroys malignant cells and the host's immune system. Examples of chemotherapeutic drugs used in the conditioning protocol are Busulfan, Cyclophosphamide, and Carmustine, among others. TBI ensures that marrow spaces are fully cleared and any remaining immunocompetent T and B lymphocytes and malignant cells are destroyed. The amount of radiation administered in ablative therapy ranges from 750 to 1500 cGy (7.5 to 15 Gy). The TBI can be delivered as a single dose or delivered over a period of 3 to 5 days (fractioned), which reduces the impact of radiation on other organ systems, such as the heart, lungs, and liver.

4 to 8 days

TBI

Conditioning Side Effects

There are serious consequences and side effects from ablative therapy, such as blood cell toxicity, organ toxicity, and immunodeficiency leading to infections. An unavoidable consequence is blood cell toxicity, which renders the host with a nonfunctioning immune system, anemia, and thrombocytopenia. An immunoincompetent individual is highly susceptible to many infections, especially GVHD. The drugs and radiation used in ablative therapy are highly toxic and can cause chronic problems of the heart, liver, lungs, eyes, and gonads (sex organs). Examples of chronic conditions are venoocclusive disease of the liver, cataracts of the eyes, and failure to grow and develop sexually.

blood cell toxicity

Autologous Bone Marrow Transplant

Remission and Purging   In order to harvest stem cells for an autologous BMT, the individual must be in disease remission. A state of remission is when the fewest possible malignant cells are present in the

disease remission: fewest malignant cells

marrow or peripheral circulation. If malignant cells are detected in autologous marrow, they can be removed by purging (cleansing) at the time of collection and before the marrow is frozen. To purge bone marrow, stem cells are mixed with monoclonal antibodies specific for tumor antigens or with chemotherapeutic agents that destroy malignant cells in vitro. Monoclonal antibodies are specially prepared antibodies that bind tumor cells, which can then be removed from the stem cell mixture. After harvesting, autologous stem cells must be stored in a frozen state (cryopreserved) while the recipient undergoes a conditioning program to clear the marrow spaces throughout the body and kill any remaining malignant cells that may still be present.

purging (cleansing) of malignant cells

monoclonal antibodies

Storage Harvested autologous stem cells are mixed with dimethyl sulfoxide, a cryoprotective agent known as DMSO, and frozen in liquid nitrogen (-196C). Stem

DMSO

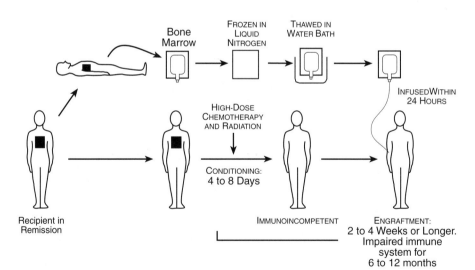

FIGURE 20.2 Autologous Bone Marrow Transplant

Marrow removed prior to ablative therapy is processed and frozen in liquid nitrogen. Within 24 hours following ablative therapy the stem cells are thawed in a water bath and quickly infused into the patient. PBSCs may be used in an autologous BMT to enhance engraftment.

cells can be stored in frozen state for 5 years. Because DMSO is toxic to stem cells at room temperature (25C), the frozen stem cells are thawed in a water bath and infused immediately to prevent damage to them.

Stem Cell Infusion

Following a conditioning program, stem cells are infused and engrafted in the recipient's bone marrow replacing defective or damaged stem cells. Engrafted stem cells begin to produce all elements of the hematopoietic system.

A stem cell infusion is a simple, straightforward procedure conducted exactly like a blood transfusion. Stem cells are transfused through a nonfiltered blood administration set via a peripheral or central venous line. In all BMT procedures, the stem cells are infused no later than 24 hours following ablative therapy, which allows time for chemotherapeutic drugs to be cleared from the body. Stem cells should be infused as rapidly as a patient can tolerate but not so quickly as to cause circulatory overload.

During a stem cell infusion, care must be taken to prevent circulatory overload, which is too much fluid in the vascular system. Recipients of autologous marrow may complain of a strong garlic taste caused by DMSO, but this disappears within a few minutes after the infusion. Hard candy or breath mints help counteract this garlic taste. Allogeneic stem cells are not frozen and therefore not stored in DMSO.

Engraftment of Stem Cells

A stem cell transplant is considered successful when engraftment takes place, that is, when the host accepts the graft. Engraftment typically occurs between 2 and 4 weeks after transplantation. The initial sign of stem cell engraftment is an increase in the white cell count, with monocytes being the first to appear in the host's circulation followed by neutrophils. All other blood cells—including granulocytes and lymphocytes, red cells, and platelets—appear in the following weeks and months.

2 to 4 weeks after transplantation

Immune Impairment

6 to 12 months

The host's immune system can remain severely impaired for 6 to 12 months and even longer due to the administration of immunosuppressive drugs or the presence of GVHD. Some patients' immune function recovers more slowly, even if they do not receive immunosuppressive drug therapy. Gradually, most immune function returns. The period of time that a recipient has a decreased white cell count, which makes the individual susceptible to many infections, can be shortened by the use of G-CSF and GM-CSF. PBPCs and CBPCs may also shorten the time an individual is leukopenic.

Immunosuppressive Drugs

Unlike solid organ recipients, stem cell recipients may not need to take immunosuppressive drugs for the rest of their lives to prevent graft rejection because their immune system and blood group eventually become that of the donor. If a BMT recipient has chronic GVHD, however, long-term immunosuppression is required. When GVHD is resolved, the individual can be taken off immunosuppressive drugs usually within 3 to 6 months.

Complications of Bone Marrow Transplantation

Bone marrow transplant therapy is not without risks, and there are many complications that can appear during and after the procedure. During infusion, the medical staff

fluid overload
emboli
allergic reactions

should monitor a recipient closely for fluid overload, emboli (clots) that may be in the infusion, and allergic reactions to donor white cell antigens.

immunodeficiency
infections

Complications occurring after the procedure include: immunodeficiency, and infections that develop because a BMT recipient is without an immune system (immunoincompetent) for an extended period of time, GVHD, graft rejection, graft failure, anemia, and thrombocytopenia. GVHD is the most common complication and the greatest threat to bone marrow engraftment. This disease causes many problems for the recipient, has a high mortality rate, and is responsible for most deaths following BMT.

serious and common complication: GVHD

Effects from Conditioning

There can be complications that are not obvious until a few days after the BMT procedure. These can result from ablative therapy or from infectious organisms. Effects from conditioning include: (1) organ toxicity, leading to pulmonary, cardiac, and liver complications; (2) hematologic toxicity, resulting in decreased blood cell counts, and (3) immunodeficiency and increased susceptibility to infections. Graft rejection, GVHD and reoccurrence of the underlying disease, such as leukemia, are other complications that can arise following BMT.

organ toxicity

hematologic toxicity
immunodeficiency
graft rejection
GVHD
disease reoccurrence

Immunodeficiency

Recipients of allogeneic stem cells suffer from severe immunodeficiency due to the very low numbers of functioning T and B lymphocytes. Actually, the number of lymphocytes returns to normal about 6 weeks post-transplant, but their immune function remains impaired for much longer. During the first 3 to 6 months immune recovery improves, but the individual is at high risk for contracting infections, among other problems. Immunodeficiency is characterized by an imbalance in the number of CD4+ helper and CD8+ cytotoxic T cells. Individuals who have experienced chronic GVHD are apt to have extended immunodeficiency.

imbalance in the number of CD4+ helper and CD8+ cytotoxic T cells

Individuals receiving autologous or syngeneic stem cells have a period of immunodeficiency, but it is much shorter and less severe than in allogeneic recipients. Also, the infections that attack these recipients are less severe than those that occur in allogeneic recipients.

Infections Associated with BMT

bacterial, fungal, viral, gastrointestinal infections

All BMT recipients are susceptible to many different pathogenic organisms that cause serious and life-threatening infections. Immediately following the transplant all recipients have few if any granulocytes in their system. Until their white cell count rises, immunoincompetent persons are very susceptible to bacterial and fungal infections. Some viruses, such as herpes simplex, and gastrointestinal complications caused by viral pathogens can also appear at this time.

Organisms that present the greatest threat initially are bacteria, fungi, and, later, viruses such as CMV. *Pneumocystis carinii* (protozoan) pneumonia and interstitial pneumonitis are two complications that arise in BMT recipients. *Pneumocystis carinii* occurs because of an incompetent immune system, whereas pneumonitis occurs because of the ablative therapy. Powerful, broad-spectrum antibiotics have reduced the incidence of such infections. The use of these antibiotics is discontinued once the white cell count returns to an adequate level, at which time the body can fight infection on its own.

opportunistic infections

interstitial pneumonitis

In Allogeneic Recipients Individuals who receive allogeneic transplants are very likely to contract opportunistic infections, such as *Pneumocystis carinii* pneumonia, that can seriously threaten life. The major complication following allogeneic transplant is interstitial pneumonitis, an inflammation or infection in the tissue spaces of the lungs. Conditions that increase the likelihood of developing interstitial pneumonitis include the following: age of the recipient, development of GVHD, immunodeficiency, and inflamed lung tissue caused by radiation or drugs. Individuals who have received high-dose therapies are more susceptible to developing interstitial pneumonitis.

In Autologous and Syngeneic Recipients These persons recover the function of their immune system faster than allogeneic recipients and therefore are less likely to have severe infections, although in some instances they develop *Pneumocystis carinii* pneumonia and cytomegalovirus infections in the post-transplant period.

Graft Failure and Graft Rejection

Graft failure is a major but rare complication, affecting less than 1% of all BMT recipients. It is a greater problem in solid organ transplantation. With a bone marrow transplant the first indication of graft failure is the inability of the grafted cells to function properly; blood cell production does not occur. When a host does not receive an adequate amount of stem cells, the donor marrow cannot reconstitute itself. Marrow spaces that are not fully cleared of bone marrow have no room for engrafting, another problem that can precipitate graft failure.

graft failure:
grafted cells
fail to function

Graft rejection occurs when recipient T cells have not been destroyed and recognize donor tissue cells as foreign and destroy them. Graft rejection is unlikely to occur in BMT because the recipient is immunoincompetent and therefore unable to mount an immune response.

graft rejection:
viable recipient T cells
destroy donor tissue cells

Anemia and Thrombocytopenia

Bone marrow transplant recipients are susceptible to anemia and thrombocytopenia. If these conditions develop, Packed Red Cell and Platelet transfusions are given to maintain normal levels of these blood components. All blood products, except from the stem cell donor, infused during this time must be irradiated to prevent TAGVHD. Irradiation destroys viable lymphocytes.

Graft-versus-host Disease

The results of GVHD are serious and sometimes fatal. GVHD is an immune response generated by immunocompetent donor T lymphocytes against the tissues of an immunoincompetent individual, such as the BMT recipient. This individual cannot mount a defensive immune response; therefore, donor T lymphocytes attack and destroy recipient tissue.

GVHD:
immunocompetent
donor T lymphocytes
against tissues of
immunoincompetent
individual

Phases

initiating phase:
donor helper CD4+
T lymphocytes
effector phase:
donor cytotoxic CD8+
T lymphocytes, etc.

GVHD occurs in two phases: an initiating phase and an effector phase. The initiating phase is usually carried out by donor helper CD4+ T lymphocytes that recognize foreign tissue and stimulate a GVHD response. The effector phase is carried out by donor cytotoxic CD8+ T lymphocytes, cytokines, and effector cells, such as macrophages and natural killer cells, that destroy host tissue.

Symptoms

Organs most affected in GVHD are the skin, liver, and gastrointestinal (GI) tract. The skin usually shows the first sign of GVHD. A slight rash appears and occasionally progresses to sloughing of skin layers. Liver symptoms include jaundice and hepatomegaly (enlarged liver), among others. GI symptoms involve a shedding of the inner lining (mucosa) of the bowel with bloody, watery diarrhea. Inflamed mucosa often provides an enticing site for bacterial or viral pathogens to enter the host.

Prevention

Preventing GVHD is a difficult but not impossible task. Prevention includes ongoing improvements in histocompatibility testing for closer HLA matching and use of drugs, such as methotrexate, cyclosporin, and steroids. These drugs inhibit donor T cells from recognizing recipient tissue as foreign. Better drugs and support measures, improved marrow manipulation techniques, and the use of autologous and allogeneic progenitor cells promote and advance patient care and therapeutic modalities.

Acute GVHD

1 to 4 weeks
following BMT

Acute GVHD is a common complication associated with BMT. In the first week to a month following a transplant, acute GVHD threatens many lives and is often fatal. It occurs in approximately 50% of all recipients, even in individuals who have received HLA-matched donor stem cells. The incidence of

GVHD increases with HLA-mismatched stem cells and in older recipients. Most patients recover from acute GVHD, but some develop chronic GVHD.

There are several factors that increase a recipient's chances of developing acute GVHD and they include: (1) the degree of genetic difference (HLA mismatch) between donor and recipient, (2) the age of the recipient, and (3) the level of toxicity of the conditioning program—the more toxic the greater the chances.

Causes The primary cause of acute GVHD is due to cytotoxic donor CD8+ T cells. These cells attach themselves to host tissue bearing foreign HLA class I molecules and lyse these cells.

cytotoxic donor CD8+ T cells attach to host HLA class I molecules

Signs and Symptoms The signs and symptoms of acute GVHD are fever, rash, usually on the hands, watery diarrhea, enlarged liver, elevated liver enzymes, and increased bilirubin level in blood. A confirmatory diagnosis of acute GVHD is made by skin biopsy.

Treatments The treatment for acute GVHD consists of corticosteroids and immunosuppressive therapy. Drugs such as methylprednisone, cyclosporin, and antithymocyte globulin are used to suppress the immune activity of donor cytotoxic CD8+ T cells. Some forms of acute GVHD do not respond to therapy and result in patient death.

corticosteroids and immunosuppressive therapy

Chronic GVHD

Chronic GVHD usually occurs later than 3 months following BMT and occurs in approximately 25% of recipients. This chronic immune response can develop even if acute GVHD has not developed first. Incidence of chronic GVHD increases as the individual's age increases. Both humoral (antibody) and cytotoxic T cell activity are responsible for this reaction. Chronic GVHD can be fatal, although rarely.

3 months following BMT

humoral and cytotoxic T cell activity

Chronic GVHD is similar to autoimmunelike disorders, such as progressive systemic sclerosis (scleroderma), which affects skin and organs. It is really a disease of impaired immunity, and patients are very susceptible to serious infections.

Signs and Symptoms   Signs and symptoms of chronic GVHD include: hand rash, fibrosis of the esophagus, obstructive lung disease, chronic anemia, leukopenia, thrombocytopenia, elevated liver enzymes, arthritis, and muscle inflammation (myositis). If symptoms are restricted to the skin and liver, prognosis is good. Prognosis is poor if symptoms are more widespread and nonresponsive to immunosuppressive therapy, such as corticosteroids, antithymocyte globulin, and methotrexate.

■   **QUESTIONS**   ■

1. List four categories of conditions for which bone marrow transplantation might be performed.

2. What types of cells are infused in a bone marrow transplant (BMT) to restore the hematopoietic and immune systems?

3. What types of cells are used in a BMT for individuals who have received pelvic irradiation?

4. Why do researchers believe the incidence of graft-versus-host disease (GVHD) is less with cord blood progenitor cells (CBPCs) than with peripheral blood progenitor cells (PBPCs)?

5. Identify the three sources of stem cells used for BMT.

6. Give at least three examples of diseases treated with autologous stem cells.

7. What is the preferred source of allogeneic stem cells? and why?

8. Explain the syngeneic source of stem cells.

9. When is the best time to harvest cells for a BMT?

10. Which group of candidates for BMT cannot be treated with an autologous source?

11. List three main categories of congenital bone marrow disorders.

12. Give two examples of diseases that occur with acquired bone marrow failure.

13. Define histocompatibility.

14. Why is a high degree of histocompatibility essential for a successful bone marrow transplantation?

15. Identify the three major categories of histocompatibility tests.

16. What determines the amount of marrow that can be extracted from a donor?

17. Describe a possible conditioning protocol planned for a BMT procedure.

18. What is ablative therapy?

19. What is the immediate, unavoidable side effect of the conditioning program?

20. When does a state of remission occur in a candidate for BMT?

21. How are autologous stem cells stored?

22. Recipients of autologous marrow may complain of a strong garlic taste. True or False? Explain your answer.

23. When is a stem cell transplant considered to be successful?

24. Solid organ transplant recipients must take immunosuppressive drugs for the rest of their lives. Why is this not true of BMT recipients?

25. BMT recipients must be monitored closely during infusion. Identify three immediate possible complications.

26. What is the most common complication of a BMT?

27. Which type of stem cell source is related to the greatest degree of immunodeficiency?

28. Interstitial pneumonitis is a major complication following allogeneic BMT. What factors are included in the likelihood of its development?

29. What is the percentage of BMT complicated by graft failure?

30. Packed Red Cells and Platelets are used for treating post-BMT anemia and thrombocytopenia. How are these blood products treated prior to infusion?

31. Define graft-versus-host disease (GVHD).

32. What is the first sign of GVHD?

33. How is acute GVHD treated?

34. What signs and symptoms indicate a good prognosis for chronic GVHD?

ANSWERS TO QUESTIONS

Chapter 1, The Concept of Blood, Page 13

1. Blood (a) acts as a transportation system, delivering oxygen, hormones, nutrients, and minerals to body cells and picking up waste products; (b) prevents blood loss and heals wounds through hemostasis; and (c) is the primary carrier of immunity.

2. Blood absorbs the digestive products used for cellular metabolism from the intestine, brings them to the liver, and then distributes them. Blood is also responsible for removing the waste products of cellular metabolism, such as carbon dioxide, and transporting them to the lungs, kidneys, and skin for excretion.

3. An average adult has 4 to 6 liters of blood.

4. Total blood volume refers to the amount of blood in the circulatory system.

5. Blood is made up of plasma, red cells, white cells, and platelets. Plasma is composed of water, proteins, carbohydrates, electrolytes, and vitamins, among other substances.

6. A cell in a microscopic structure that forms the tissue of an organism, including blood. A cell is surrounded by an outer membrane called the cell membrane or plasma membrane. Within this membrane are the cytoplasm, a jellylike substance that holds the cellular organelles. Organelles include such structures as the mitochondria, Golgi apparatus, ribosomes, and the nucleus, among others. Within the nucleus are the genes, the hereditary molecules made up of DNA, which are responsible for an individual's characteristics.

7. Unlike most cells of the body, red cells and platelets do not have a nucleus.

8. Hematopoiesis refers to the production of mature blood cells. These cells are formed from the primitive cells in the bone marrow called stem cells.

9. Each day, 1 trillion blood cells are produced in an individual to replace those past their life span.

10. Red blood cells increase in numbers in hypoxia; white blood cells are stimulated to increase by infection; and platelet production rises with blood loss.

11. A term sometimes used synonymously with stem cells is progenitor

355

cells. However, many medical professionals consider progenitor cells to be some what more mature precursor cells than stem cells. Progenitor cells are found in the circulation, outside bone marrow.

12. (a) Stem cells begin as pluripotential cells in the bone marrow where they give rise to the myeloid and lymphoid cell lines. (b) As they develop from multipotential to unipotential stem cells, the stem cells differentiate into red cells, white cells, platelets, and lymphocytes. (c) When fully differentiated, the cells are released into the circulation as mature blood cells.

13. Multipotential refers to the ability of stem cells to differentiate into any of the mature blood cell types. In hematopoiesis, once a multipotential stem cell becomes committed to the development of a particular blood cell type, it is referred to as a unipotential stem cell.

14. Colony-stimulating factors, interleukins, thrombopoietins, and erythropoietin along with vitamins, thyroid hormone, amino acids, and metals such as iron, magnesium and cobalt, are all necessary molecules for normal hematopoiesis.

15. There are thirteen interleukin molecules, numbered IL-1 to IL-13. Interleukins, such as IL-1 and IL-6, cause stem cells to produce precursors to red cells, granulocytes, lymphocytes, monocytes, and platelets.

16. Thrombopoietins are molecules responsible for the development of platelets from megakaryocytes.

17. The production of red cells is dependent on the renal hormone erythropoietin. This molecule is released by the peritubular cells of the kidneys.

18. Hematopoietic growth factors act on stem cells and progenitor cells, causing them either to undergo self-renewal or to differentiate further into mature functioning blood cells by binding to the receptors on the stem or progenitor cells. They are produced by a number of different cell types, such as endothelial cells, B cells, T cells, monocytes, fibroblasts, and kidney cells.

19. The following other molecules are necessary for blood cell development (a) vitamins, such as folic acid; (b) metals, such as iron; (c) amino acids; and (d) hormones.

20. Both types of marrow are composed of a spongy, fibrous matrix made up of endothelial cells, macrophages, fibroblasts, fat cells, and an extensive capillary network. yellow marrow is 96% fat and not involved with hematopoiesis. Hematopoietic marrow is where the

development of red cells, white cells, and platelets takes place.

21. Causes of adult extramedullary hematopoisis can include the following: tumor, disease, chemotherapies, ionizing radiation, and certain congenital disorders.

22. In the early embryo, blood cell development occurs in the blood islands of the yolk sac.

23. By the third month of fetal growth, blood cell development moves from the blood islands to the liver, spleen, and thymus. By the fourth month, it also occurs in the bone marrow where it continues throughout life.

24. At birth, the bone marrow becomes the site of hematopoiesis.

25. The cranium ceases producing blood cells in the elderly, and the cranium's hematopoietic marrow becomes gelatinous marrow.

26. Leukocytes, or white cells, protect the body against foreign matter. Erythrocytes, or red cells, transport oxygen and carbon dioxide throughout the body. Thrombocytes, or platelets, help prevent blood loss.

27. False. In persons with disease states, immature and abnormal blood cells can be present in greater than usual numbers.

28. Leukocytes include the following: granulocytes, which include neutrophils, basophils, and eosinophils; monocytes and macrophages; and the T and B lymphocytes.

Chapter 2, The Circulatory System, Page 28

1. The circulatory system is made up of two closed loops: the first, the major loop, delivers blood to body cells and returns it to the heart; and the second, the minor loop, delivers blood to the lungs before returning it to the heart. Together they may be said to from a closed-loop system.

2. Trauma can cause blood to be found outside the vascular space (or system).

3. Blood vessels include: arteries, arterioles, capillaries, venules, and veins.

4. All blood vessels and lymphatic vessels are lined with a layer of flat, endothelial cells called the endothelium. The heart is also lined with endothelium.

5. The aorta is the major artery.

6. Arteries carry blood away from the heart via the aorta, increasing in number and decreasing in size as they become arterioles, protected

and surrounded by muscle tissue, and branching into capillaries.

7. Arterioles are known as resistance vessels because of their small size and the increased muscle tissue surrounding them, which can constrict, thereby reducing blood flow.

8. The expansion and contraction of the aorta is called the Windkessel effect. It occurs when the left ventricle ejects blood into the aorta causing it to expand. Then as the aorta retracts to its normal size, the blood is propelled forward.

9. The arterial wall is made up of three tissue layers: the adventitia (outer), the media (middle), and the intima (inner). The media of large arteries has elastic tissue and very few muscle fibers. In arterioles, the media has little elastic tissue but many muscle fibers innervated (connected) with nerve fibers that cause blood vessels to constrict or dilate.

10. The action of nerve fibers on muscle fibers regulates the flow of blood within the body. When the muscle fibers in arterial vessels constrict, less blood flows through to the tissues. When these fibers dilate, more blood flows through to reach the tissues.

11. As the smallest blood vessels in the body, the capillaries are where the movement of substances between the blood and the tissues takes place. An individual capillary is only one cell thick, which allows for the easy exchange of these substances. Capillary networks exist in every organ and tissue and lie in close proximity to most body cells.

12. Interstitial fluid is composed of water, electrolytes, vitamins, and other substances that filter out of the plasma.

13. Interstitial fluid exists in the interstitial (extravascular) space, which is the microscopic area surrounding cells. It is filtered from the plasma through the capillary pores to where it constantly bathes the body cells, while allowing them to take up the vital substances needed for metabolism. Interstitial fluid also picks up the waste products of metabolism and returns them to the blood.

14. Due to their size, proteins cannot leave the vascular space. They are not usually found in the interstitial space.

15. Movement of fluid between the capillaries and the body cells is determined by hydrostatic and osmotic pressures. In the capillaries, blood is under hydrostatic (blood) pressure, which is greater than the osmotic pressure within the tissues. Therefore fluid is forced from the capillary into the interstitial space. Because proteins do not leave the vascular space, the protein concentration in plasma

increases and exerts osmotic pressure in capillary blood. Some fluid is pulled back into the vascular space. The rate of tissue fluid formation exceeds the capillary re-uptake. Maintaining fluid volume is very important to normal physiological processes.

16. The two major veins are the superior vena cava and the inferior vena cava.

17. Veins and venules work to return blood to the heart instead of distributing it to the tissues. They have thinner walls than arteries because they must expand to receive large volumes of blood from different organs. Veins are found throughout the body. Superficial veins lie beneath the skin and close to the surface, unlike arteries that are largely protected by muscle and other tissue. Deep veins lie within interior body tissues, accompanying the arteries with which they share their names.

18. Arterioles are known as resistance vessels because of their small size and the increased muscle tissue surrounding them. Veins are called capacitance vessels because they can expand their capacity to receive large volumes of blood. Working together, the resistance and capacitance vessels maintain a normal blood flow.

19. Varicose veins develop when the valves involved in venous return break down or become nonfunctional. These one-way valves prevent the backflow of blood that would occur in the lower extremities due to the pull of gravity. Along with the skeletal muscles of the lower extremities that contract with body movement, these valves are essential for returning blood to the heart.

20. The lymphatic system serves to maintain blood volume by assisting in the return of fluid in the interstitial space to the vascular system. It also plays a vital role in the body's immune system by carrying foreign matter to the lymph nodes that serve as small filtering stations for cell debris and antigen. It is not a closed-loop system because it originates as capillarylike vessels in the tissues and has no connecting point like the heart.

21. Edema occurs when abnormal amounts of fluid remain in the body tissues. The individual develops a swollen appearance. There are many causes of edema.

22. The cardiopulmonary system refers to the heart and lungs as they function together. The exchange of oxygen and carbon dioxide, the respiratory gases, occurs in the alveoli of the lungs. These are tiny air sacs that form grapelike clusters at the end of the very small airways of the lungs. Each alveolus is surrounded by a dense

network of capillaries. It is within the alveolar-capillary networks that O_2 from the outside environment is taken up by the blood and CO_2 is released to the outside via the act of breathing.

23. The lungs are large, pink, spongy organs within the rib cage of the chest.

24. There are approximately 300 million alveoli in the human lung.

25. When blood is returning from body organs and tissues it is deoxygenated, that is, low in O_2 and high in CO_2. This results in blood being a deep purple color. On its way to the lungs, deoxygenated blood enters the right atrium of the heart and flows through the right ventricle from where it is pumped into the pulmonary artery and into the lungs. In the alveolar-capillary network, CO_2 leaves and O_2 enters the bloodstream. The blood becomes bright red due to the increased saturation of Hbg by O_2.

26. After the exchange of CO_2 and O_2 takes place in the lungs, the pulmonary veins return the oxygen-rich blood to the left atrium of the heart through the mitral valve to the left ventricle. From there, blood is ejected into the aorta from where it is distributed to all organs and tissues via the arteries, arterioles, and capillaries.

27. The cardiopulmonary circulation and the peripheral circulation make up the vascular system. The former includes the heart and the great vessels: superior and inferior venae cavae, pulmonary arteries, and pulmonary veins, and aorta. The latter includes all vessels outside the chest cavity that are not part of the cardiopulmonary system.

Chapter 3, Special Circulations, Page 58

1. The heart is the pump for the entire circulation of the body. The kidneys cleanse the blood of impurities and produce urine. The liver detoxifies harmful substances in the blood and produces the majority of plasma proteins. All these functions are essential to normal physiology.

2. In fetal circulation, oxygenation of the blood takes place via the placenta, not in the fetal lungs.

3. The heart pumps, on the average, approximately 1800 gallons (7200L) of blood per day.

4. The heart is a four-chambered organ that lies within the chest cavity, about the size of a clenched fist. It is divided into two parts separated by a muscle wall called the septum. Each side has an upper (atrium) and lower (ventricle) chamber. The heart has three layers:

the outer layer (epicardium), the middle muscle layer (myocardium) and the inner layer (endocardium).

5. The right heart receives deoxygenated blood from the body via the superior and inferior venae cavae. This blood enters the right atrium and flows into the right ventricle where it is transported to the lungs via the pulmonary artery. The left heart receives the oxygenated blood from the lungs via the pulmonary veins to the left atrium from where it flows into the left ventricle. At this point it is pumped to all body tissues via the aorta.

6. The muscle wall of the left ventricle is three times thicker than that of the right ventricle because of the pumping demands of the former. The valve separating the two chambers on the right is called the tricuspid valve; that on the left, the mitral valve.

7. Atherosclerosis and thrombotic disorders are both associated with coronary circulation. When the diameter of the coronary vessels is altered, the blood flow is restricted and signs of ischemia are noted, including chest pain. Alteration can be caused by the buildup of atheroma on vessel walls or blockage caused by a thrombus (blood clot) within the coronary vessels.

8. The right coronary artery carries oxygenated blood to the myocardium of the right side of the heart; the left coronary artery carries oxygenated blood to the left side of the heart.

9. Other arteries involved in the coronary circulation include: the posterior descending artery (PDA), the left anterior descending (LAD) artery, the circumflex artery (Cx), and the conus artery.

10. Ostia are the openings of the coronary arteries in the wall of the aorta.

11. The cardiac veins return deoxygenated blood from the myocardium to both atria of the heart. The coronary venous system consists of the coronary sinus on the posterior surface of the heart and the anterior cardiac venous system. The former receives blood from the surface (superficial) veins of the heart and delivers it to the right atrium. The latter is made up of veins that originate in the antero-lateral surface of the right ventricle and empty into the left atrium.

12. The following are associated with CAD: genetics, hypertension, gender, diabetes mellitus, cholesterol level, diet, and smoking.

13. Atherosclerosis refers to the buildup of plaque (atheroma) along the walls of coronary arteries. This affects the diameter of the coronary arteries in particular and causes them to narrow which, in turn, affects the blood flow to the heart.

14. Atheroma is formed in coronary arteries when plaque is deposited on their endothelial surface. As the amount of plaque increases, blood flow through the artery decreases, because the vessel diameter has been narrowed. The section of heart muscle supplied by that artery and its tributaries receives less oxygen and fewer nutrients. With this restricted blood flow, the individual can develop ischemia (blood supply deficiency) and inadequate oxygen supply to the heart. Angina pectoris (chest pain) is a frequent sign of ischemia and indicates that the heart muscle is not receiving enough blood to meet its metabolic demands.

15. Cardiac output refers to the amount of blood pumped from the left ventricle per minute.

16. A myocardial infarction (MI) occurs when plaque ruptures within a coronary artery and forms a blood clot (thrombus). Blood flow distal to the clot is subsequently cut off. If the occlusion lasts for more than 15 to 20 minutes irreversible damage to the myocardium can occur as an infarct can cause scar tissue, or tissue necrosis, which will not allow for the transmission of electric impulses. As a result, normal muscle contraction does not occur and cardiac output decreases as does cardiac function.

17. If an individual is treated with thrombolytic drugs within 2 to 3 hours of the infarct, blood flow can be restored. Time is important in the prognosis as is the percentage of heart muscle hat has been destroyed. If the infarct size is greater than 40% of heart muscle, death is most likely.

18. CAD is first treated with medication. If this is not successful, angioplasty is the next treatment of choice. With a balloon catheter the size of the arterial lumen is increased and more blood reaches the ischemic area. Angioplasty is a temporary measure and is usually followed by a surgical procedure in which blood flow to the myocardium is reestablished by the grafting of healthy veins to bypass the obstruction.

19. Renal functions include the following: (a) blood filtration, (b) fluid balance regulation, (c) responding to the release of ADH and aldosterone, (d) erythropoietin release, (e) renin production, (f) maintenance of pH balance, and (g) electrolyte regulation.

20. The kidneys are two reddish-brown, bean-shaped organs located on either side of the spine in the retroperitoneum (flank area). Each kidney is about the size of a clenched fist and is covered by a smooth, tough, fibrous capsule. Within the capsule are two sepa-

rate and distinct regions: the outer cortex and the inner medulla. Within these are the functional filtering units called nephrons.

21. Nephrons are the filtering units of the kidneys. They are tubular structures consisting of several parts: the glomerulus, Bowman's capsule, renal corpuscle, renal tubule, and the peritubular capillaries.

22. In contrast to other organs, the capillary arrangement of the kidneys is structured "in series" (as opposed to "in parallel"). This means that one capillary network is followed by another. More specifically, blood flows from the capillary bed of the glomerulus to the peritubular capillaries.

23. Movement of fluid and substances in the renal circulation occurs as the result of all three processes: filtration; osmosis; and reabsorption. Filtration refers to the movement of fluid due to pressure, as when the water and solutes dissolved in the blood entering the glomerulus are filtered out into the Bowman's capsule. Osmosis refers to the movement of water from an area of low solute concentration to one of higher concentration. Reabsorption is the process of fluid return into the peritubular capillaries by filtration and osmosis. For example, when the body needs water, the kidneys reabsorb more water from the renal tubules. Low pressure and plasma proteins in these capillaries favor reabsorption.

24. Fluid remaining in the renal tubule that is not reabsorbed by the blood becomes urine, which is drained from the renal pelvis via the ureter to the bladder. It consists of water and solutes (waste) that are not needed by the body.

25. If the body is dehydrated (low in water or fluid volume), the kidneys reabsorb water from the renal tubule into the blood with the aid of tow hormones, ADH and aldosterone. Blood volume increases and dehydration abates.

26. Renal failure occurs when the kidneys are unable to cleanse the blood of its impurities. Waste products, excess water, acids, and electrolytes accumulate in the bloodstream and cause uremia, a form of blood poisoning that can lead to death.

27. Hemodialysis is the process by which an artificial kidney cleanses the blood. It is used in renal failure.

28. The liver is a unique organ, because it has a dual blood supply; is the largest organ in the abdominal cavity; and has more functions than any other organ.

29. The liver is responsible for the production of bile and plasma proteins.

30. Vitamins A, D, E, K, and B_{12} are stored in the liver.

31. The liver detoxifies drugs, alcohol, and waste products, (e.g., ammonia).

32. Fetal blood cells are produced in the liver.

33. The liver lies in the upper right quadrant of the abdomen just under the ribs and below the diaphragm. It is divided into left and right lobes. The right lobe is dome shaped and six times larger than the left lobe, which tapers to a point.

34. The functional unit of the liver is called a lobule. Each liver contains 50,000 to 100,000 lobules, which are made up of hepatocytes (liver cells).

35. Canaliculi are tiny tubes that transport bile and eventually merge with others to form the bile duct.

36. The liver receives blood via two distinct and separate sources. The hepatic artery, branching from the celiac artery, carries oxygenated blood to the liver. The portal vein delivers deoxygenated, nutrient-rich blood from the stomach, intestines, spleen, and pancreas to the liver.

37. The sinusoids are where blood from the hepatic artery and portal vein mix. They are lined with both epithelial cells and the Kupffer's cells which remove foreign matter such as bacteria. The sinusoids also provide storage for a large volume of blood.

38. The proteins in the hepatic capillaries are absorbed by the hepatocytes, where they are metabolized into simpler compounds called amino acids.

39. Plasma proteins produced by the liver include: albumin, coagulation factors (II, V, VII, VIII, IX, and X), antithrombin III, proteins C and S, and plasminogen.

40. Bilirubin, a breakdown product of hemoglobin, is excreted in the bile.

41. Hgb F is different from Hgb A in that the fetal hemoglobin molecule has a greater affinity for oxygen than the adult Hgb molecule.

42. The lungs of the fetus are deflated. Therefore they resist blood flow and are unable to exchange respiratory gases in utero. The fetus is supplied with oxygen from the maternal circulation via the placenta.

43. The foramen ovale and the ductus arteriosus are the two openings in the fetal ciruclation that allow blood flow to bypass the fetal lungs.

44. Fetal blood from the left atrium flows into the left ventricle and

out the aorta to circulate to the head and upper body. A developing brain is very dependent on a rich oxygen supply, and this is where the highest concentration of oxygen is.

45. At birth, breathing inflates the neonate's lungs, resistance to blood flow in the lungs decreases, and blood begins ciruclating through them. The openings in the fetal ciruclation either close or become dysfunctional.

46. Atrial septal defect (or patent foramen ovale) occurs when the foramen ovale remains open, decreasing the blood flow and oxygen to the newborn's tissues. It must be surgically corrected. Patent ductus arteriousus occurs when that opening does not close, thereby decreaseing the oxygen content and casuing the infant to become cyanotic. This congenital defect may be corrected with either medication or surgery, but it can be responsible for complications later in life.

Chapter 4, Red Blood Cells, Page 74

1. Erythrocytes.

2. Red cells are formed in the hematopoietic marrow; they have a life span of approximately 120 days.

3. The main functions of red blood cells are to take oxygen from the lungs to the different tissues of the body and then transport carbon dioxide from these tissues to the lungs.

4. True.

5. Erythropoiesis is the production of red cells in the hematopoietic marrow where erythropoietin (EPO), released by the kidneys, activates stem cells to produce erythrocytes.

6. The red cell is flexible biconcave disk. This shape allows for a maximum surface area for the transfer of respiratory gases in and out of the red cell. The flexibility of the erythrocytes enables these disks to change shape as they flow through the capillaries.

7. A red cell has a life span of approximately 120 days after it is released into the circulation. It is then removed from circulation by macrophages in the liver and spleen.

8. Erythrocytosis and polycythemia refer to an elevated red cell count.

9. Polycythemia refers to an extremely high blood count. The condition usually occurs in older patients and can present with night sweats, itching after a hot bath, splenomegaly, plethora, hemorrhage or thrombosis, blurred vision, or hypertension. It is treated by maintaining normal cell numbers through phlebotomy or cytotoxic drugs.

10. Anemia is a low red cell count and indicates a disease process somewhere in the body. It can present with dyspnea, weakness, pale mucous membranes, headaches, heart palpitations, and/or sluggishness. Older patients can experience cardiac failure, angina pectoris, confusion, and claudication. Anemia can be treated with the transfusion of red cells or the administration of recombinant erythropoietin.

11. Hemoglobin (Hgb) transports O_2 to the cells of the body, transports some CO_2, and buffers hydrogen ions, which prevents pH changes.

12. The respiratory gas O_2 binds Hgb at the heme molecule.

13. Because it contains an iron (Fe) atom, the heme molecule is responsible for the red color of blood. When the red color is brightest the red cells are saturated with O_2. The loss of O_2 to body tissues causes blood to take on a purplish color.

14. The percentage of Hgb that is bound to O_2 in arterial blood is called the oxygen saturation of arterial blood. The saturation is a measure of O_2 combined with Hgb and not the amount of Hgb in the blood.

15. The Bohr effect is the influence of pH and CO_2 on Hgb's affinity to bind and release O_2. When tissues have a decreased pH and an increased CO_2 concentration, Hgb has less affinity for O_2 and thus releases it into body tissues. In the lungs, where there is an increased pH and a decreased CO_2 concentration, Hgb binds O_2 more easily.

16. Hypoxia is a decreased concentration of O_2 in body tissues. When it occurs, it stimulates the kidneys to release erythropoietin, which increases the number of red cells.

17. The Hgb concentration in adult males is 13.5 to 18 g/dL; in females, 12 to 16 g/dL.

18. The Hgb concentration in newborns is greater than in adults, between 15 to 24 g/dL. Different types of Hgb molecules are produced during embryonic development with different polypeptide chains. Fetal Hgb molecules are designed to extract O_2 from maternal red cells at the placenta, and they have a greater affinity for O_2.

19. Sickle-cell anemia, a congenital disorder, results from Hgb S. When Hgb S releases O_2 into body tissues, it crystallizes and causes the red cell to take on a classic sickle shape. Distorted red cells become trapped in the microvasculature where they cause many problems, including joint pain, retinal degeneration, and infarctions of different organs, such as the liver and spleen.

20. Thalassemias are another genetic defect affecting Hgb. They are caused by the lack of one polypeptide chain or another. Patients with a thalassemia may experience fatigue, or they may be symptomless.

21. The 2,3-diphosphoglycerate molecule is produced within the red blood cell by the metabolic breakdown of glucose. It is bound to Hgb and allows it to release O_2 to the tissues more easily.

22. A storage lesion is damage incurred by blood in storage.

23. The hematocrit (Hct) is the percentage of whole blood occupied by red cells. As an index of red cell concentration, it is an indirect measure of the oxygen-carrying capacity of the blood.

24. In females the Hct ranges from 0.38 to 0.46, and in males from 0.42 to 0.54.

25. Hemolysis is the destruction of the red cell membrane and the release of Hgb into the plasma where it can no longer transport O_2. As a result, the ability of blood to oxygenate body tissues is decreased. In addition, remnants of the ruptured red cells (red cell stroma) can activate the clotting cascade, resulting in blood clots and stroma lodging in the microvasculature of such organs as the lungs and kidneys causing them to fail.

26. Hemolysis can be caused by the following: (a) an immune response, (b) sepsis, (c) a mechanical problem (e.g., with a hemodialysis machine), (d) medication or a toxin such as alcohol, (e) susceptible, aging red cells, (f) activation of the complement system, or (g) an enzyme deficiency.

27. A patient will have a high bilirubin level if the hemolysis is significant and it cannot be excreted fast enough by the liver. This will cause the skin and eyes to acquire a yellow color referred to as jaundice.

Chapter 5, Oxygen and Carbon Dioxide Transport, Page 90

1. Respiration refers to the exchange of respiratory gases (O_2 and CO_2) between the lungs and the body tissues. Ventilation is the process by which air moves in (inspiration) and out (expiration) of the lungs.

2. The intercostal muscles, the diaphragm, and the heart are essential to the respiratory process.

3. Diseases that involve diminished O_2 and CO_2 exchange include: emphysema, chronic obstructive pulmonary disease (COPD), congestive heart failure (CHF), and pneumonia.

4. a) O_2 combines with the Hgb molecule when inhaled from the atmosphere to ensure an adequate O_2 supply to body tissues. (b) Some CO_2 is also attached to the Hgb molecule and eventually exhaled into the atmosphere. (c) Hgb is also essential for the buffering of hydrogen ions.

5. Diffusion occurs when atoms or molecules move through a semipermeable membrane from an area of higher partial pressure (concentration) to an area of lower partial pressure.

6. The individual pressure exerted by each gas in the atmosphere is called the partial pressure.

7. The difference in partial pressures between two areas is referred to as the diffusion gradient.

8. Barometric pressure is the combined partial pressures of the gases of the atmosphere. It is greatest at sea level and becomes progressively less higher in the atmosphere.

9. Atmospheric (or barometric) pressure is determined by the following equation:

$$\text{Atmospheric pressure} = PN_2 + PO_2 + P \text{ (other trace gases)}$$

10. PO_2 is the driving force that moves O_2 from the lungs into red cells during external respiration and then from the red cells to the tissue cells during internal respiration. PCO_2 is responsible for moving CO_2 between tissue cells and blood and between blood and alveoli.

11. The loading and unloading of O_2 on and off the Hgb molecule is described by the oxyhemoglobin dissociation curve. O_2 is loaded on to Hgb in the lungs where the PO_2 is greater (association portion of curve). In the body tissues, oxygen is unloaded from the Hgb where the PO_2 is lower (dissociation portion of curve).

12. Hgb does not release all of its O_2 to the body tissues. It has the ability to save some for when needed, for example, during heavy exertion. This is called a physiologic advantage.

13. P50 is the partial pressure at which 50% of the Hgb is saturated. The normal P50 for PO_2 is approximately 26 mm Hg.

14. The affinity of O_2 for Hgb is affected by (a) the hydrogen ion concentration (pH); (b) PCO_2; (c) temperature; and (d) the amount of 2,3–DPG in the red cells.

15. In alkalosis (increased pH), O_2 has an increased affinity for Hgb, and the oxyhemoglobin dissociation curve shifts to the left; less O_2 is released to the tissues. In acidemia (decreased pH), O_2 has less affinity for Hgb and O_2 release to the tissues is enhanced; the curve

shifts to the right.

16. In external respiration, O_2 moves from the pulmonary alveoli into the red cells of the pulmonary capillaries, and CO_2 is diffused from the pulmonary capillary blood into the alveoli. In internal respiration, O_2 moves from the red cells in the capillaries into body tissue cells as CO_2 is diffused from the tissues into the blood. All of this activity takes place within a fraction of a second and happens simultaneously.

17. Because O_2 "combines reversibly" with Hgb in red cells, it can be released from Hgb when the blood reaches the body cells. O_2 is carried by Hgb; it does not react with it.

18. The amount of O_2 that body tissues receive is dependent on (a) the amount of blood flow in the tissues, (b) the Hgb concentration in the blood, and (c) the affinity of Hgb for O_2.

19. Cellular metabolism, the breakdown of proteins, carbohydrates, and lipids, causes CO_2 to form in the cells of body tissues.

20. (a) After CO_2 diffuses into the plasma, 5% of it dissolves in the plasma. (b) Thirty percent of this CO_2 enters the red cells where it binds to certain amino acids in the Hgb molecule. (c) Sixty-five percent is transported as bicarbonate ions (HCO_3^-) via plasma to the lungs.

21. Carbonic anhydrase (CA) is present when CO_2 combines with H_2O in the red cells to form carbonic acid (H_2CO_3) which dissociates into bicarbonate (HCO_3^-) and hydrogen (H^+) ions.

22. The pH refers to the concentration of hydrogen ions (H^+) in a solution. Any change in the blood pH affects the enzyme-dependent reactions of the body and can alter normal physiology.

23. The normal body pH ranges from 7.35 to 7.45; it is slightly basic.

24. The main buffers in the blood are Hgb and bicarbonate ions (HCO_3^-). They remove excess hydrogen (H^+) ions by "soaking them up," thereby preventing changes in blood pH.

25. The chloride shift occurs when HCO_3^- leaves the red cells to diffuse into the plasma and the chloride ion (Cl^-) in the plasma moves into the red cells. The chloride shift maintains the electrical neutrality between the red cells and the plasma as one negative ion (HCO_3^-) is exchanged for another (Cl^-).

26. Carbon dioxide is released by the red cells when (a) HCO_3^- diffuses from the plasma back into the red cells during the chloride shift; (b) Hgb molecules release H^+; and (c) H^+ and HCO_3^- rejoin to form H_2CO_3, which forms CO_2 and H_2O in the presence of

carbonic anhydrase (CA). The CO_2 enters the alveoli and is exhaled; the H_2O stays in the red cells.

Chapter 6, White Blood Cells, Page 112

1. For the purpose of this book, all nonself material (foreign matter) is referred to as antigen. Antigen includes bacteria, viruses, fungi, parasites, transfused or transplanted allogenic cells (cells from a genetically dissimilar individual), infected cells, and tumor cells.

2. In the body the immune response is activated by white cells, antibody, and complement proteins.

3. Cytokines are glycoprotein molecules that provide a highly complex communication network for white cells.

4. White cells circulate within the vascular and lymphatic channels, and some reside in the body tissues.

5. False. An increase in white cells is called leukocytosis.

6. Both infection and leukemia can cause an increased white cell count.

7. White cell production is decreased within the bone marrow in certain stem cell disorders, chemotherapy, or radiation therapy. In addition, white cells are destroyed in hypersplenism, certain autoimmune disorders, and with certain drugs.

8. (a) Granulocytes are a major group of white cells and include neutrophils, eosinophils, and basophils. (b) Monocytes are another group that mature into macrophages. (c) The third group are lymphocytes, which include T cells and B cells.

9. Diapedesis refers to the migration of neutrophils and monocytes through capillary pores into body tissues in response to antigen. Chemotaxis is the release of cytokines, complement proteins, and bacterial toxins that stimulate white cells to move (diapedesis) into the area of antigen invasion.

10. Systemic lupus erythematosus affects the skin, kidneys, and other organs and is associated with defective chemotaxis.

11. Phagocytosis, the ongoing process by which phagocytic cells engulf antigens, occurs as follows: (a) the antigen attaches to the receptor on the white cell membrane; (b) it is then ingested by the phagocytic white cell; and (c) finally it is killed and digested via enzyme activity.

12. Opsonization does not interfere with phagocytosis. It enhances the process by coating the antigen with antibody and complement proteins that make it more palatable to the phagocytic white cells.

13. The myeloid line of white cells which consists of monocytes, macrophages, and granulocytes, provides the first line of cellular defense against antigen. Myeloid cells are nonspecific and attack any and all antigen. Cells of the lymphoid lineage (lymphocytes) include T cells and B cells, which direct the body's response to antigen by generating a specific response. These cells mature as they are exposed to different antigens.

14. Granulocytes are divided into neutrophils, eosinophils, and basophils. They are named for the numerous enzyme-containing granules within their cytoplasm.

15. Neutrophils act quickly in response to inflammation and infection. They are strongly phagocytic. Once they have fulfilled their function in an area of antigenic invasion, they die and release chemicals that lead to pus formation.

16. A white cell count in which bands are detected is called a "shift to the left." Bands are immature neutrophils in the circulation. They are called bands because their nuclei are rectangular and nonsegmented. It is thought by some that their presence is a sign of infection.

17. In the body 50% of the neutrophils are found adhering to the endothelial lining of the capillaries, an event called margination. From the endothelium they can more quickly move into body tissues.

18. Neutrophilia, an increase in the number of neutrophils, can be caused by bacterial infections, heavy exercise, inflammation, malignancies, hemorrhage, hemolysis, myeloproliferative disorders, chronic granulocytic leukemia, hematopoietic factors, metabolic disorders, corticosteroid and epinephrine injections, seizures, pain, nausea, and vomiting.

19. Major basic protein, or MBP, is found in the eosinophil's cytoplasmic granules. It binds to antigen and lyses the antigen's membrane. It is toxic to all antigen, especially against parasitic worms (helminths).

20. Basophils release histamine and heparin.

21. If blood clots in an infected area, phagocytes cannot reach the antigen to destroy it. The infected tissue can die. The heparin released from the basophils helps prevent this.

22. Neutrophils are the most abundant and compose about 70% of the body's white cells. Eosinophils make up 2 to 5% and will increase under certain conditions. Basophils are the least common of the white cells (less than 0.5%).

23. After being released from the bone marrow at an immature stage, monocytes circulate for a day or two and then move into the tissue spaces where they mature into tissue macrophages (histiocytes).

24. Macrophages are the most important of the phagocytic white cells. They reside in the body for years and not only engulf antigen but also release chemicals needed for antigen destruction, such as cytokines.

25. In the liver they are called Kupffer's cells; in the lungs, alveolar macrophages. In the brain, they are called microglial cells; in the spleen, spleen macrophages. In the bone marrow these macrophages are referred to as dendritic cells, and in the GI tract, they are found in Peyer's patches and called peritoneal macrophages.

26. Endothelial cells, dendritic cells, B lymphocytes, and Langerhans' cells can function as antigen-presenting cells (APCs).

27. Lymphocytes are the most complex of the white cells. Like macrophages and granulocytes they help prevent disease and infection. However, they add specificity to the attack on antigen by directing the immune response. They can recognize, respond to, and retain memory for individual antigens. Their ability to distinguish self-tissue from nonself tissue is the basis of both cell-mediated and humoral immunity.

28. Both leukemia and Hodgkin's disease can cause lymphocytosis.

29. The response to antigen by T cells is called cell-mediated immunity.

30. False. T cells mature in the thymus. Lymph nodes are conglomerations of lymphatic tissue found throughout the body. They are where the T cells first encounter antigen.

31. CD stands for "cluster of differentiation," the protein molecule that distinguishes one type of T cell from another. For example, CD8+ T cells have the CD8 protein as their cell surface marker, and CD4+ T cells have the CD4 protein as their marker.

32. Helper T cells assist or activate other white cells in response to antigen. Cytotoxic T cells release lytic molecules that rupture target cells. Suppressor T cells are activated to stop the immune response, because if it is not suppressed it would destroy normal tissue. Finally, memory T cells remain after an infection and retain a memory for the offending antigen. They survive for many years in the lymph nodes and respond more rapidly on subsequent exposure to antigens to which they have been immunized.

33. The second exposure of memory T cells to antigen is called the anamnestic response. It is a more rapid immune response than the

primary response, which is known as immunization or sensitization.

34. In humoral immunity, antibodies opsonize microorganisms, tumor cells, and allogeneic cells leading to their destruction. Production of antibody is called humoral immunity and is associated with B cells.

35. B cells mature in the bone marrow. When released, they reside mainly in the lymph nodes but are also found in the vascular and lymphatic systems where they lie in wait for antigen. Once activated by antigen, they undergo rapid proliferation and differentiate into plasma cells that produce antibody.

36. With an autoimmune disease the body does not recognize and protect its own cells. T and B cells that destroy self-tissue are responsible. This phenomenon is called loss of self-tolerance. Rheumatoid arthritis (RA) and multiple sclerosis (MS) are examples of autoimmune disease.

Chapter 7, Antigen, Antibody, and Complement, Page 129

1. Antigen (Ag) refers to any foreign matter that enters the body and can bind to antibody and/or can bind to a T or B cell receptor molecule. An immunogen is any substance that can generate an immune response. All immunogens are antigenic, but not all antigens are immunogens. A pathogen refers to an antigen that can cause a disease, a microorganism or a toxin, for example.

2. Target cells are cells that are destined to be destroyed by the immune system.

3. Examples of antigen include: (a) microorganisms such as bacteria, viruses, parasites, fungi, and yeasts; (b) allogeneic cells (cells from a genetically dissimilar individual); (c) malignant cells; and (d) infected cells (cells inhabited by certain viruses, bacteria, or parasites).

4. Before a protein antigen can generate an immune response, it must be presented to CD4+ T cells with a class II MHC (major histocompatibility) molecule by an APC.

5. Lipid and carbohydrate antigens can be recognized directly by B cells; they do not need the help of CD4+ T helper cells. B cells/plasma cells produce antibodies in response to antigen invasion.

6. The epitope is the specific region of an antigen recognized by an antibody or lymphocyte receptor molecule.

7. Once an invading microorganism enters a cell it is safe from the immune response, because antibody molecules cannot penetrate cell membranes.

8. Antibody (a) opsonizes (coats) antigen and (b) activates the comple-ment cascade. Opsonization of antigen provides attachment points that phagocytic white cells can stick to so they can eventually engulf antigen. Complement proteins can work independently of antibody to destroy antigen, through opsonization and lysis, but are more effective when assisted by antibody.

9. Phagocytic white cells have surface molecules called receptors that allow antigen opsonized by antibody and/or complement to become attached to these white cells. The Fc receptor is the point on the phagocyte's membrane that binds antibody, and the C3 receptor is the point that binds complement.

10. True.

11. All antibody molecules have the same basic molecular arrangement: four chains of amino acids (two identical light and two identical heavy) held together by chemical bonds. Within each chain are two separate and distinct regions, the variable and the constant. The variable region is unique to each antibody, allowing it to bind to a specific antigen's epitope.

12. Antibody, produced after a body's first exposure to an antigen (sensitization), takes approximately 14 days to reach full power. Antibody produced after an anamnestic response (reexposure to the same antigen) takes only 5 to 7 days. In the anamnestic response, memory T and B cells mount a quicker attack. Antibody is produced in larger quantities, responds to lower concentrations of antigen, and has a higher affinity for the antigen.

13. Antibody destroys antigen in four main ways: (a) opsonization, (b) lysis of the antigen's membrane by complement proteins activat-ed by antibody, (c) antibody-dependent, cell-mediated cytotoxicity, and (d) neutralization.

14. An antibody's class—IgG, IgM, IgD, IgA, and IgE—is determined by the amino acid arrangements of its heavy and light chains. All members of a given class have the same amino acid arrangement in the constant regions of their protein chains.

15. The IgG antibody is the only immunoglobulin that can cross the placenta from the mother into the fetus. It can, therefore, provide immunologic protection to the newborn until its own immune system begins working.

16. IgM is the first antibody produced by the fetus. An increased level at birth indicates infection in the newborn.

17. IgA immunoglobulin occurs in tears, breast milk, bronchiole secretions, and saliva.

18. IgE is the causative agent in asthma, hay fever, and many allergic reactions. When IgE is released it binds to basophils and mast cells stimulating them to release histamine, which causes edema, sinus inflammation, itching, bronchiole constriction, and other allergic symptoms.

19. Anaphylactic reactions occur only in hypersensitive individuals and within seconds to minutes after an individual is exposed to a sensitizing substance.

20. Complement proteins are most effective in destroying antigen when they are assisted by antibody.

21. When the C3 molecule is activated, it splits into two fragments: C3a and C3b. C3a is an anaphylatoxin and is responsible for causing inflammation. C3b is the opsonizing fragment that enhances phagocytosis.

22. If complement proteins and phagocytic white cells cannot completely destroy invading antigen, other immune functions are initiated. T and B cells become active and amplify the immune response by producing antibody and/or cytotoxic T cells.

23. Complement proteins work within the immune system by (a) causing inflammation, (b) serving as chemotactic factors, (c) increasing vascular permeability, (d) opsonizing antigen to promote phagocytosis, (e) binding with antigen to form the membrane attack complex (MAC), and (f) causing adherence of antigen-antibody to surfaces, such as capillary endothelium, whereupon the antigen-antibody complex can be phagocytized.

24. True. Complement proteins function in a sequence of chemical chain reactions via either the classical or alternative pathway. Different types of antigen activate the proteins in the two pathways.

25. Three activated complement proteins of the classical pathway can be potent causes of anaphylactoid reactions. Activated protein components, C3a, C4a, and C5a, are called anaphylatoxins. Anaphylatoxins stimulate mast cells and basophils to release histamine, which can cause capillary leakage, edema, smooth muscle contraction, bronchiole constriction, a feeling of doom, and tachycardia as well as other symptoms. Anaphylatoxins are also chemotactic agents and function in the inflammatory response.

26. Individuals with deficiencies or defects in complement proteins endure frequent infections. One example is hereditary angioedema in which a defective chemical inhibitor blocks the classical pathway and causes tissue and vascular (angioedema) edema.

27. The complement system can be activated by the tubing used in hemodialysis when an individual's blood is exposed to foreign surfaces. When the complement system is activated by foreign surfaces, complement proteins attack an individual's own cells, and they are either phagocytized or lysed.

Chapter 8, The Major Histocompatibility Complex Molecules, Page 140

1. MHC molecules allow T cells to recognize protein antigen. T cells are unable to do so on their own. Once a T cell recognizes protein antigen, it can then direct the destruction of that antigen. The MHC molecules perform this task by presenting an antigenic peptide to a T cell.

2. In the blood, MHC molecules are found on white cells and platelets. They are not present on red cells.

3. In humans, MHC molecules are referred to as human leukocyte antigens (HLA) because they were discovered on white cell membranes and they stimulated antibody production following transfusion or transplantation..

4. The exception to the uniqueness of HLA occurs only in identical twins.

5. Alloimmunization is the production of alloantibody following exposure to alloantigen. Alloantigens are molecules in certain individuals that generate the formation of alloantibodies in other members of the same species. The terms immunization, antigen, and antibody are often used as shorthand for the terms alloimmunization, alloantigen, and antibody.

6. MHC molecules are divided into three classes: I, II, and III. Classes I and II are essential for the presentation of antigenic peptides to T cells for generation of the immune response. Class III MHC molecules are involved with the production of complement proteins and certain cytokines, such as tumor necrosis factors (TNFs).

7. Class I and class II MHC molecules differ in their molecular structure and are found on different body cells. Also, they present different types of antigen to either CD4+ or CD8+ T cells.

8. Class III molecules are involved with the production of comple-

ment proteins and also with certain cytokines, such as tumor necrosis factors (TNFs).

9. Leprosy and tuberculosis are caused by certain intracellular bacteria. Class I MHC molecules are required for the recognition and destruction of cells infected by these endogenous antigen.

10. HLA alloantigens and alloantibodies are implicated in the following transfusion reactions: febrile nonhemolytic transfusion reactions (FNHTRs), platelet refractoriness, transfusion-related acute lung injury (TRALI), and transfusion-associated graft-versus-host disease (TAGVHD).

11. The use of leukocyte-reduction filers can help prevent alloimmunization to HLA by removing white cells.

12. MHC molecules are referred to as HLA (human leukocyte antigens) because (a) they were discovered on leukocyte membranes, and (b) they induce alloantibody formation and CD8+ cytotoxic T cell activity in the recipient.

13. Individuals receiving a platelet transfusion will develop alloantibodies to the HLA on the donor platelets and to any leukocytes in the unit. During a subsequent transfusion, HLA antibodies formed during primary immunization can attach themselves to transfused platelets bearing complementary HLA. This results in a loss of platelet function called platelet refractoriness.

14. The major obstacle to successful organ transplantation is the reaction generated by the recipient's acquired immune system against donor tissue, that is, cells bearing foreign HLA. In allogeneic transplants, graft rejection occurs when, first, recipient CD4+ helper T cells recognize HLA on donor graft tissue as foreign. Recipient CD4+ T cells then activate CD8+ cytotoxic T cells. Finally, these T cells will lyse donor tissue, and graft rejection follows.

15. True. Precise HLA matches can be found only in donors who are siblings or in an identical twin, but even in these cases, rejection can occur due to minor differences in histocompatibility.

16. HLA similarity between donor and recipient is referred to as histocompatibility, whereas HLA dissimilarity is called histoincompatibility.

17. Improvements in immunosuppressive therapy are chiefly responsible for the growing success of solid organ transplantations.

18. Whether a BMT recipient accepts or rejects the graft or develops GVHD is directly related to the degree of HLA similarity existing between donor and recipient. BMT recipients will violently reject donor marrow that is not an HLA match.

19. Unlike the majority of genes, MHC genes are codominant, which means that neither allele is dominant or recessive. Instead, each allele shares equal expression in the MHC molecules produced. It is believed that there are approximately 100 million alleles for MHC. This makes MHC the most polymorphic of genes known in humans. The polymorphism associated with MHC makes it difficult to find an MHC match within the general population.

20. The transplant team identifies the best donor–recipient match through histocompatibility testing, antibody screening, and cross matching.

21. The lymphocytoxicity test is a serological assay that identifies class I and certain class II HLA and antibodies to HLA. Once recipient HLA are identified, the physician knows the HLA to look for in the prospective donor that will constitute a match.

22. A mixed lymphocyte culture is a cellular assay that identifies the degree of similarity between donor and recipient HLA class II DP, DQ, and DR. The degree of similarity is indicated by the amount of proliferation of recipient lymphocytes caused by donor HLA. The greater the difference between donor and recipient HLA, the more cellular proliferation there is. If no proliferation of lymphocytes occurs, a strong similarity between donor and recipient HLA is indicated, and this donor can be used for this recipient.

23. Fragments of DNA are used in molecular testing to identify the HLA gene itself. These molecular assays are very specific and highly sensitive. At the present time, only class II MHC molecules are determined by these methods.

24. In antibody screening the amount of alloimmunization in the recipient is determined by mixing recipient serum (containing antibodies) with a panel of cells containing lymphocytes with known HLA. the total percentage of lymphocytes destroyed by the recipient's antibodies is called the panel reactive antibody (PRA). A high PRA indicates extensive alloimmunization and will make it more difficult to find a donor within the general population for this recipient.

25. If a recipient has preformed antibodies against donor HLA, transplantation is contraindicated because the antibodies will provoke a strong immune response, which in turn will lead to graft rejection. This is prevented by antibody screening and cross matching to determine alloimmunization.

26. Cross matching determines if the recipient is alloimmunized to donor HLA. Recipient serum is mixed with prospective donor

lymphocytes. If the recipient has preformed antibodies against donor HLA, organ and bone marrow transplantation from this donor is contraindicated, as the antibodies will provoke a strong immune response leading to graft rejection.

Chapter 9, The Immune System, Page 160

1. The immune system is one of the most difficult systems of the body to understand. Highly complex cellular and chemical interactions take place continuously. New discoveries with new understandings are taking place so rapidly that many immunologists find themselves in disagreement.

2. Antigenic invaders can penetrate the body through (a) the skin; (b) mucous membranes of the mouth, intestine, bladder, vagina, and nose; (c) ciliated epithelia of the respiratory system; and (d) acids and chemicals of the gastrointestinal tract.

3. Edema, soreness, heat, and redness are all signs of inflammation at the site of antigenic invasion.

4. True. Acquired immunity is obtained and developed as one is exposed to antigen. The greater the variety of antigen to which one is exposed, the more developed acquired immunity becomes.

5. Acquired immunity is characterized mainly by (a) specificity, (b) diversity, (c) memory, (d) self-regulation, and (e) self-tolerance.

6. Cytokines, a class of glycoproteins, have major roles in hematopoiesis, the immune response, inflammation, and wound healing. Those released from macrophages are called monokines; those released from lymphocytes, lymphokines.

7. Cytokines allow white cells to communicate among themselves and with other cells in response to inflammation and infection. Interleukins (ILs) are important in cellular communication among various white cells. Interferons (INFs) help provide immunity against viruses, and tumor necrosis factors (TNFs), yet another cytokine, help provide immunity against tumor cells.

8. T cells direct cell-mediated immunity. When T cells respond to an antigen the response is referred to as cell-mediated. Helper T cells and cytotoxic T cells have specific roles in immunity leading to antigen destruction. B cells are involved in humoral immunity, which involves the production of antibody in response to antigen. B cells/plasma cells, after encountering antigen, produce antibodies in secondary lymphatic tissue (lymph nodes and spleen). Once antibody is released, it can leave the lymphatic system and encounter antigen that may have escaped into the bloodstream.

9. Immmunoincompetence is the absence of a competent immune system; in other words, the body cannot generate an immune response. Another term for immunoincompetence is anergy.

10. The immune response occurs in three steps or phases. (a) In the cognitive phase, the antigen-MHC complex binds to the T cell receptor. (b) In the second phase, the activator phase, T cells respond to bound antigen and release cytokines that cause a proliferation of T and B cells that then mount an attack against the antigen that stimulated them. (c) Finally, in the effector phase, granulocytes, macrophages, and complement are activated to opsonize and engulf antigen.

11. Exotoxins are those released from bacterial membranes, and endo-toxins are produced within bacterial cells and released when the bacteria are destroyed. Bacteria are microorganisms that act as antigen.

12. Viruses are nonliving microorganisms that attack cells from the inside. To make copies of themselves they must enter cells, and once inside they take over cell function. They cannot be destroyed by antibody or complement because once inside the cell they cannot be opsonized.

13. Malignant cells elicit humoral and cell-mediated immune responses and can be destroyed by the following: cytokines (e.g., tumor necrosis factor), antibody, cytotoxic T cells, killer cells through antibody-dependent cell-mediated cytoxicity (ADCC), macrophages, and/or a combination of any of these.

14. The spleen, tonsils, mucosa-associated lymphatic tissue and lymph nodes are all secondary lymphatic tissue.

15. When blood enters the spleen through the splenic artery, it flows through arterioles heavily endowed with T cells and macrophages. As blood filters through the spleen, these cells can destroy antigen before it can spread farther.

16. Vaccine is made up of weakened fragments of a pathogenic microorganism. After it is administered, the body becomes sensitized and produces antibody and memory T and B cells. If an individual becomes infected by the organism later on, these cells are able to destroy it before it has a chance to take hold. Vaccine solutions, such as the polio vaccine or the hepatitis B vaccine, are administered in 2 to 3 doses by mouth or by injection.

17. Antibody generated in response to vaccination is called active immunity, and the antibody is produced within the individual.

Passive immunity occurs when the antibody used to fight infection is produced within another individual or animal. An individual receives a concentrated solution of antibody in serum (antiserum) removed from a human or animal previously exposed. Tetanus toxoid is one example.

18. Disorders of the immune system are divided into (a) hypersensitivity, or allergic, reactions; (b) autoimmune diseases; and (c) immune deficiency disorders.

19. Anaphylaxis is a type I hypersensitivity reaction. It is a true medical emergency, because the individual can die if immediate medical attention is not available. It occurs when a person has developed IgE antibody to a sensitizing event in the past. When subsequently exposed to the same allergen the allergen attaches to the previously formed IgE causing mast cells and basophils to release histamine and other potent molecules. Bronchiole constriction, capillary leakage, increased secretions from mucosal surfaces, hemorrhage, laryngeal edema, and myocardial ischemia all can occur.

20. Antibody-dependent, cell-mediated cytotoxicity (ADCC) is a type II hypersensitivity reaction in which IgG or IgM opsonizes target cells that are then lysed by natural killer cells and/or macrophages. Hemolytic disease of the newborn is one example of ADCC.

21. Rheumatic fever is an example of type III hypersensitivity. In this kind of immune disorder, antigen-antibody complexes deposit themselves in body tissues where they have the ability, in some cases, to activate cytokines and complement that destroy tissue.

22. Graft rejection is a type IV hypersensitivity reaction that is mediated by T cells. Tissue damage is caused when helper T cells release cytokines that attract macrophages. Cytokines, macrophages, and cytotoxic T cells all play a role in tissue damage.

23. Solid organ graft rejection occurs through one of the following mechanisms: hyperacute rejection, which is antibody-mediated; acute rejection, which is both antibody- and cell-mediated; and chronic rejection, which is T cell-mediated.

24. In GVHD, donor CD4+ helper and CD8+ cytotoxic T cells attack the tissue of the recipient bearing both class I and II HLA molecules. Donor cytotoxic T cells destroy recipient tissues via lysis. This is another example of a cell-mediated type IV hypersensitivity reaction.

25. When self-tolerance is lost, an individual is susceptible to autoimmune disease wherein an abnormal immune response against an individual's own cells is produced.

26. Among diseases attributable to autoimmune disorders are some types of hemolytic anemia, arthritis, multiple sclerosis, insulin-dependent diabetes mellitus, and scleroderma.

27. Primary immune deficiency disorders are congenital defects in one's own immune system. When the defects are acquired disorders, the condition is a secondary immune deficiency disorder.

Chapter 10, Plasma, Page 174

1. Plasma, the liquid portion of the blood, performs the function of transporting blood cells and other solutes to and from tissue cells.

2. The following solutes are dissolved in plasma: proteins, carbohydrates, lipids, vitamins, electrolytes, and hormones.

3. True.

4. Large molecular weight proteins and lipids are the exception.

5. Plasma is made up mostly of water and normally is a straw-colored liquid. But depending on the condition and health of an individual, it can appear reddish, cloudy, or milky. It has a viscous sticky consistency due to the proteins dissolved in it.

6. Plasma provides much valuable information about what is happening in the body because it travels throughout the entire organism and provides a window to its chemical environment.

7. The term serum is sometimes used interchangeably with plasma, but the fluids are not the same. When a tube of blood is allowed to stand, the formed elements (blood cells) and coagulation factors in the sample will clot on the bottom of the tube, while the serum, a straw-colored fluid, rises to the top. Serum is plasma minus fibrinogen (a coagulation factor).

8. The three mechanisms that help maintain a balanced blood volume throughout the body are (a) vascular integrity, (b) osmotic pressure, and (c) the lymphatic system, which is responsible for returning interstitial fluid to the vascular system.

9. Congestive heart failure and pulmonary edema are complications associated with fluid imbalances.

10. Plasma proteins are essential in maintaining blood volume throughout the body, because they exert the osmotic pressure in the vasculature that helps maintain fluid balance.

11. The three main classes of proteins found in plasma are albumin, globulins, and fibrinogen.

12. (a) Albumin is essential for maintaining blood volume; it maintains

the osmotic pressure between blood and body tissues and acts as a major transport protein of other molecules (hormones and lipids) in the plasma. (b) Globulins are responsible for humoral immunity, act as enzymes in many metabolic processes, and also serve as transport molecules for heme, hormones, and metals in the body. (c) Finally, fibrinogen is a clotting protein.

13. Hypoproteinemia, or protein deficiency, can be caused by (a) decreased intake of protein (malnutrition); (b) decreased production of protein (cirrhosis); (c) decreased absorption (malabsorption syndrome); (d) excretion of proteins (nephrotic syndrome); or (e) hemodilution of blood in surgery.

14. Protein deficiencies can interfere with (a) the acid–base balance, (b) clotting mechanisms, (c) enzyme-dependent reactions, (d) fluid balance, and (e) the transport of substances such as hormones and nutrients to body tissues and organs.

15. A paraprotein is an abnormal immunoglobulin produced in response to certain malignancies of the spleen, liver, and bone marrow.

16. If the plasma concentration of an electrolyte is increased or decreased, fluid shifts, abnormal heart rhythms, clotting disorders, abnormal nerve conduction and other problems can occur.

17. Hyperviscosity is caused by an excess of immunoglobulins (proteins) in the plasma causing it to thicken and thereby slow blood flow. This condition is caused by such diseases as multiple-myeloma and Waldenström's macroglobulinemia. It is treated with plasmapheresis (the removal of plasma) and the suppression of paraproteins.

18. Electrolytes, lipids, carbohydrates, and vitamins are all nonprotein solutes found in plasma. They must be taken in with the diet as they are not synthesized in the body.

19. The five main electrolytes are calcium, chloride, potassium, sodium, and magnesium.

20. Normal concentrations of electrolytes are necessary for such processes as nerve conduction, blood clotting, and muscle contraction.

21. Bicarbonate assists in maintaining an acid-base balance within the body by acting as a buffer that helps control the acidity or alkalinity of the blood, maintaining a pH between 7.35 and 7.45.

22. Water and solutes filter through the very porous capillary membranes into the interstitial space. Unlike plasma, interstitial fluid contains very few proteins.

23. Reabsorption is an ongoing function that occurs when waste products are excreted from the tissue cells and reabsorbed into the vascular and lymphatic capillaries to be transported to various organs for excretion from the body.

24. Blood enters the capillary with a pressure imparted to it from the force of the heart contracting, called hydrostatic or capillary blood pressure, which forces water and solutes into the interstitial space. Osmotic pressure pulls the fluid back from the interstitial spaces into the vasculature; it is determined by the protein concentration in the plasma.

Chapter 11, Platelets, Page 189

1. Platelets are also called thrombocytes.

2. True. Platelets are one of the formed elements in the blood. They are enucleated (lacking a nucleus).

3. Platelets play a vital role in preventing blood loss from damaged blood vessels, a function known as hemostasis. They cover the injured site, forming a platelet plug, which helps reduce further blood loss until a fibrin clot is established.

4. Platelets change from a flat shape to a spherical one when forming the platelet plug. This structural change aids in their adhesion to damaged endothelium.

5. After platelets are released from the bone marrow into the circulation, they migrate to the spleen where they spend time before returning to the bloodstream. The retention of platelets in the spleen is called sequestration. About one-third of platelets are sequestered there at any one time.

6. Thrombocytosis occurs when the increase in the number of platelets rises above 450×10^9/L. Thrombocytopenia occurs when the number of platelets decreases to 150×10^9/L or below. Both disorders can result from congenital and acquired conditions, such as thrombasthenia, gray platelet syndrome, chronic infections, malignancies, and blood diseases, such as iron deficiency anemia.

7. Vascular integrity exists when there are no mechanical breaks in any of the blood vessel walls.

8. The hemostatic process begins with a vascular spasm. This is followed by platelet plug formation and coagulation protein activation, which leads to clot formation. Finally, clot lysis, the breakdown of a fibrin clot, occurs.

9. When vascular damage occurs the endothelial lining plays an

important role in hemostasis. Vessel walls release molecules that (a) attach themselves to activated platelets, (b) assist in fibrin clot formation, and (c) are involved with clot dissolution. Endothelial cells also produce anticoagulants, vasodilators, clot inhibitors, and fibrinolytics.

10. In platelet plug formation the first step involves contact between the platelets and damaged endothelium, which releases molecules that attach to platelet membrane receptors. The second step involves adhesion of the platelets to the damaged endothelial surface. In the third step, spreading, the platelets change their shape. The fourth step involves ADP release, which stimulates platelet aggregation. Finally, the fifth step occurs when the aggregated platelets form the platelet plug at the site of injury. This plug is then anchored in place by a fibrin clot.

11. A platelet plug is sometimes called a white thrombus.

12. The molecules that regulate the amount of ADP released by the platelets are called prostaglandins, including thromboxane A_2 (TXA_2) and prostacyclin (PGI_2).

13. Doctors often prescribe aspirin "to thin the blood," but actually aspirin serves to help reduce the formation of blood clots. It blocks the action of TXA_2 and prevents the release of ADP and, thereby, platelet aggregation.

14. All foreign substances can initiate platelet aggregation and inappropriate clot formation.

15. There are three types of thrombocytosis that cause an increase in the platelet count: transitory, reactive, and primary, also called essential thrombocythemia. The first occurs following exercise, physical stress, or the administration of epinephrine. The second, reactive thrombocytosis, results from increased platelet production in the bone marrow. Finally, primary thrombocytosis is a myeloproliferative disorder of stem cells.

16. Bleeding is likely to occur in thrombocytopenia when platelet numbers are low.

17. A low platelet count can be caused by any of the following: thrombasthenia, storage pool disease; some types of surgery, radiation, chemotherapy, transfusion reactions, certain malignancies, hypersplenism, DIC, and alcoholism.

18. Drugs that affect platelet function include: aspirin and ibuprofen, exogenous heparin, protamine, Dextran, some antibiotics, such as penicillin, and some anesthetics, such as halothane.

19. The platelet count indicates the number of platelets, and the bleeding time indicates the quality of the platelets.

Chapter 12, Coagulation, Page 209

1. The coagulation process is initiated by any vascular injury to the body or when blood is exposed to a foreign surface.

2. Fibrin is the end product of coagulation. It forms a net, or meshwork, over a platelet plug, stabilizes it, and anchors it in place.

3. Primary hemostasis consists of vascular spasm and platelet plug formation. Secondary hemostasis is responsible for coagulation, the prevention of further blood loss, and assisting in the repair of the endothelial lining.

4. The term extrinsic indicates the tissue factor that activates the extrinsic pathway. It is not normally found in the blood but comes from outside the blood. The term intrinsic indicates that all components necessary for coagulation are found within the blood.

5. The chemical components required to form a stable fibrin clot include: (a) coagulation factors (or coagulation proteins), (b) tissue factor (or tissue thromboplastin), (c) PF-3 (or platelet membrane phospholipid), and (c) calcium ions.

6. True. Coagulation factors are synthesized by hepatocytes within the liver.

7. Factor III is typically referred to as tissue factor, and factor IV is referred to as calcium.

8. Calcium assists in fibrin clot formation. It is needed to form a chemical bridge between a coagulation factor and PF-3 during the coagulation process.

9. Factor VIII, or antihemophilic factor, is deficient in classic hemophilia.

10. Mr. Jackson has von Willebrand's disease, a bleeding disorder with deficient or low levels of von Willebrand factor (vWF).

11. Fibrinogen, or factor I, is the inactive form, or precursor, of fibrin. It is a soluble plasma protein produced in the liver. To generate fibrin, fibrinogen is split (cleaved) by the enzyme thrombin.

12. A deficiency of factor XIII, or fibrin stabilizing factor, can lead to increased bleeding, poor wound healing, and/or an increased incidence of abortion.

13. Factor XII, or Hageman factor, has no function in in vivo coagulation. It is activated only when blood comes into contact with foreign surfaces.

14. The prothrombin time (PT) monitors the extrinsic pathway. The activated partial thromboplastin time (aPTT) and the partial thromboplastin time (PTT) monitor the intrinsic pathway.

15. Clot retraction is the contraction, or firming up of, the platelet plug forming the hard clot. As the protein fibers and microtubules in the platelet membrane shorten, the wound edges of the damaged vessel come closer together. As the vessel(s) heals, the fibrin clot is slowly broken down (lysed) by plasmin, allowing the blood flow to resume through the vessel. Vascular integrity is restored when endothelial damage is repaired and the blood flow resumed.

16. Coagulation controls the formation of fibrin and the fibrin clot to stop bleeding immediately after vascular damage. Fibrinolysis controls the eventual breakdown of fibrin. Both processes work together to restore endothelium and blood flow.

17. Plasmin is a protein, a serine protease, that regulates clot lysis or fibrinolysis. It circulates in its inactive form called plasminogen.

18. Tissue plasminogen activators are molecules released by tissue cells. They include tissue plasminogen activator (tPA) and urokinase. Streptokinase is a plasminogen activator produced by the bacteria beta-hemolytic streptococci. TPAs are used to dissolve blood clots.

19. Antithrombin III (AT-III), protein C, and protein S are natural anti-coagulants. They help prevent thrombosis within the vasculature by destroying any thrombin that forms. They also neutralize activated clotting factors such as Va, VIIIa, and Xa. They do this by maintaining fibrin formation at the site of vascular damage and preventing its occurrence elsewhere.

20. Vitamin K is found in green leafy vegetables, vegetable oils, and tomatoes.

21. Coumadin™ is a synthetic anticoagulant that can be obtained only by prescription. It blocks the action of vitamin K by inhibiting a step in the synthesis of vitamin K-dependent clotting proteins.

22. When a fibrin clot dissolves, small pieces of fibrin, called fibrin split products (FSPs), are released into circulation. They must be removed by the reticuloendothelial system (RES) of the liver.

23. If fibrin split products (FSPs) are not removed from circulation, they become potent inhibitors of coagulation by preventing fibrin threads from crosslinking and platelets from adhering to damaged endothelium.

24. Hemorrhagic disorders manifest themselves by bleeding, and include abnormalities of the vascular system or platelets or coagulation

factors. Thrombotic disorders manifest themselves through inappropriate clot formation within a blood vessel. This leads to interference with blood flow and to tissue necrosis. Both defects are either acquired or congenital.

25. Many clotting disorders are caused by liver disease, because the liver synthesizes most coagulation proteins.

26. Vascular disorders and defects are characterized by ecchymoses (bruising; black and blue spots), both of which indicate bleeding into the skin. Bleeding can also occur from the mucous membranes of the intestines, mouth, and nasopharynx.

27. Hemorrhagic telangiectasia is an hereditary disorder. It causes microvascular swelling, most commonly in the blood vessels of the skin, mucous membranes, and internal organs.

28. Von Willebrand's disease results from a deficiency of von Willebrand factor (vWF). It affects both platelet aggregation and clot formation. Platelet aggregation does not occur, and there are decreased levels of factor VIII in the blood. It can be due to either congenital or acquired defects.

29. Hemophilia A is a congenital hemostatic disorder that causes bleeding, because the body cannot form a fibrin clot. It is due to a deficiency of coagulation factor VIII or the presence of inhibitors against factor VIII. Hemophilia B, also known as Christmas disease, is due to a deficiency of factor IX or the presence of inhibitors against it.

30. Inappropriate clot formation within arteries is responsible for such conditions as myocardial infarction (MI), cerebral vascular accident (CVA, or stroke), and pulmonary embolus (PE).

31. Venous stasis occurs due to decreased or slowed blood flow through the vessel, usually after long periods of immobility. It does not usually lead to tissue necrosis. One example of venous occlusion is deep vein thrombosis (DVT), which can occur, for example, from prolonged sitting in one position, as on an airplane flight.

32. In DIC, both abnormal bleeding and clotting as well as clot lysis occur.

33. In children, DIC is most often caused by burns, infection, and trauma. Adults usually develop DIC in association with malignancies and infections.

34. Triggering events for DIC include any of the following: (a) obstetrical complications; (b) malignancies; (c) infectious organisms; (d) widespread tissue damage associated with burns and crush

injuries; (e) vascular defects; (f) immunological disorders; (g) toxins; (h) pieces of particulate matter, such as stroma; and (i) snake and spider venoms.

35. Excessive bleeding in DIC is caused by the consumption of coagulation proteins and platelets and increased levels of FSPs.

36. To restore hemostasis in DIC, the blood products Cryo, Platelets, and FFP are administered to replenish depleted clotting factors and platelets. Heparin and fibrinolytics are used, but use of them remains controversial.

Chapter 13, ABO and Rh Blood Group Systems, Page 221

1. The ABO blood group system is important in transfusion medicine because differences in ABO groups cause immediate immune reactions.

2. The most prominent Rh antigen is now referred to as the D antigen.

3. The ABO blood groups can be identified by the A and B antigens on the surface of the red cell and the anti-A and anti-B antibodies in the serum.

4. The AB blood group is associated with the A and B antigens; the A blood group with the A antigen; and the B blood group with the B antigen.

5. Group O blood has neither the A nor the B antigen. It can be transfused to all other blood groups in an emergency.

6. Antibodies of the ABO blood group are called isoagglutinins because they cause agglutination of red cells. Group A and group O individuals have anti-B antibodies; group B and O have anti-A antibodies; group AB have no antibodies; and group O have both antibodies. The prefix "iso" means the same; therefore, isoagglutinins refer to the antibodies in the blood of members of the same species.

7. In blood transfusion therapy, donor and recipient blood must be compatible; both individuals must have the same blood group. However, in an emergency, group A individuals can receive A or O Packed Red Cells; group B can receive B or O; group AB can receive A, B, AB, or O; but group O can receive only O.

8. Packed Red Cells are used in transfusion therapy. The plasma has been removed, and the red cells are concentrated.

9. In an ABO-incompatible transfusion an acute hemolytic transfusion reaction (AHTR) occurs. Antibodies in a recipient's plasma attach themselves to the donor red cell antigens and stimulate complement activation. Complement then attaches to the antigen-antibody

complex and causes lysis of the red cells. Lysis (or destruction) of the red blood cells can lead to clot formation in the microvasculature and, eventually, to anemia.

10. Symptoms of an acute hemolytic transfusion reaction include: shock, chills, fever, chest pain, dyspnea, back pain, and disseminated intravascular coagulation (DIC).

11. ABO compatibility between donor and recipient is required for organ transplantation procedures because a mismatch results in hyperacute graft rejection.

12. Rh antigens are protein molecules found on red cell membranes. The most prominent, the D antigen, occurs in approximately 85% of the population. However, a D- individual will produce anti-D antibody only after being exposed, or alloimmunized, to D antigen following transfusion, transplant, or pregnancy. D+ blood is preferentially given to a D+ individual. D- blood can be given to either a D- or D+ recipient.

13. If an Rh- (D-) individual receives a second transfusion of Rh+ (D+) blood, antibody developed from the first transfusion will destroy the newly transfused red cells. The individual will have antibody formed during the first exposure that have since reached a titer high enough to cause a severe antigen-antibody reaction (immune response) that can lead to hemolysis of the recipient's red cells and to anemia.

14. HDN (hemolytic disease of the newborn) is a form of isoimmune hemolytic anemia that results from an antigen–antibody response between incompatible fetal antigen and maternal antibody of the IgG type.

15. Fetal red cells can enter maternal circulation during an induced abortion, amniocentesis, ectopic pregnancy, spontaneous abortion (miscarriage), cesarean section, or vaginal delivery.

16. Symptoms associated with mild forms of HDN can go undetected or include mild jaundice or mild hepatomegaly. Severe forms of HDN can seriously compromise the fetus's health with anemia, heart disease, hypoxia, poor liver function, severe jaundice, DIC, kernicterus, and hydrops fetalis.

17. Hemolytic disease of the newborn (HDN) begins during fetal life and can progress into the early neonatal period. The level of hemolysis is greatest at birth because the fetus has been continuously exposed to maternal antibodies. It diminishes over time as does the number of maternal antibodies.

18. HDN can be treated with either intrauterine or exchange transfusion. The first is done in utero, when blood is injected into the abdominal cavity of the fetus or through the umbilical vein. This blood must meet specific requirements for fetal transfusion. The second, an exchange transfusion, is performed during the neonatal period when all fetal blood is replaced with that of a donor. It is usually reserved for the most severe cases of HDN.

19. The O, Rh- blood group is used for intrauterine transfusion therapy.

20. RhoGAM™ is one of several commercial drug preparations of Rh immune globulin (RhIG). It has greatly reduced the incidence of HDN when it is administered to a D- (Rh-) mother within 72 hours following sensitization by the D+ antigen. The drug prevents her from forming antibodies against the D antigen.

21. ABO HDN is less severe than Rh HDN and often requires no treatment. It occurs when a group A or B fetus is carried by a group O mother and may require phototherapy (UV light) to assist in breaking down bilirubin in a jaundiced newborn.

Chapter 14, Blood Transfusion, Page 235

1. Blood transfusions are ordered to (a) replace blood loss; (b) treat anemia, hemophilia, or internal bleeding; or (c) replace a specific blood component destroyed by disease or chemotherapy.

2. After collection, Whole Blood is usually separated into components—Packed Red Cells, Platelets, and Plasma.

3. An eligible adult can donate around 10% of his or her total blood volume. This comes to approximately one pint once every 8 weeks.

4. After the screening criteria have been met, blood is usually withdrawn from the veins in the antecubital fossa (at the bend of the elbow). A tourniquet is tightened around the upper arm to cause the vein to bulge and make insertion of the large-bore needle easier. The needle is connected to a plastic bag containing an anticoagulant-preservative solution. The collection should take no longer than 10 minutes.

5. Permanent preclusions for blood donation include: a history of hepatitis, heart disease, HIV infection, homosexual activity, and I.V. drug use.

6. Donated blood products are also tested for hepatitis B and C, human T cell lymphotropic virus I/II, and the human immunodeficiency virus 1/2.

392 Answers: Chapter 14

7. The four major components of anticoagulants-preservatives are citrate, phosphate, dextrose, and adenine. Citrate prevents clotting by binding calcium ions in plasma. Phosphate helps control the pH of the blood and maintain ATP levels. Dextrose helps maintain the viability of red cells. Adenine helps maintain levels of ATP.

8. Platelets are used for patients actively bleeding due to thrombocytopenia, and plasma derivatives are used for patients with coagulation disorders.

9. The maximum storage shelf life for Packed Red Cells is 42 days if stored in an additive system.. They must be maintained at 1 to 6C.

10. Certain storage lesions such as levels of 2,3-DPG and ATP are reversible. Labile clotting factors and hemolyzed red cells are not.

11. Identification of donor and recipient by ABO and Rh blood groups is called blood grouping.

12. True.

13. The two grouping tests are forward, or front, and reverse, or back. The first utilizes red cells and determines the presence or absence of A and B antigens on the cell membranes. The second determines the antibodies present in serum when they are mixed with reagent red cells known to have the A and B antigens. Both grouping tests must agree with one another in order for the blood group to be determined.

14. Agglutination indicates that the recipient has antibodies against the red cell antigens of the donor; this indicates incompatibility between the donor and recipient.

15. Leukocyte-depletion filters are used to remove white cells from blood and blood components, because these cells can cause transfusion reactions. They are usually used at the bedside as the individual is receiving the unit.

16. Use of a leukocyte-adsorption (or leukocyte-depletion) filter will lessen an individual's chance of contracting CMV.

17. To assure the safety of blood products and decrease the possibility of transfusion reactions, blood donors are carefully screened; the product is safely stored; the blood group is correctly identified; cross matching is accomplished; and the product is delivered with a filter via sterile technique. Vital signs are monitored during the actual transfusion.

18. Normal saline (0.9%) is used to decrease the viscosity of the blood cells. It does not damage red cells as other crystalloid I.V. solutions do. It is also used to prime the tubing for the actual transfusion.

19. Patients requiring a large volume of blood and premature infants should be infused with blood that has been warmed.

Chapter 15, Adverse Events in Transfusion, Page 260

1. Adverse events are transfusion complications and reactions that occur within the body during or following the infusion of blood or blood components. A transfusion reaction occurs when the adverse effect is due to an immune response, whereas a complication is a nonimmune response.

2. Adverse events are considered acute when they occur during or shortly after infusion, whereas delayed adverse events occur after 24 hours. Complications, such as rashes and welts, can be localized to the infusion site, while systemic adverse events occurring throughout the body, such as hypotension and shock, are usually more serious.

3. Adverse events caused by antigen that binds antibody (an immune response) include: hemolytic, allergic, anaphylactic, transfusion-related acute lung injury, transfusion-associated graft-versus-host disease, and post-transfusion purpura.

4. A hemolytic transfusion reaction (HTR) occurs when the antibodies of the recipient react with the antigens of the donor's red cells and red cells are hemolyzed or removed from circulation at an increased rate.

5. An HTR may be classified as acute or delayed and as occurring intravascularly or extravascularly (e.g., in the spleen).

6. AHTRs (or acute hemolytic transfusion reactions) usually occur as the result of a clerical error in the identification of the correct ABO blood group.

7. The most diffiuclt adverse event to manage in an AHTR is renal failure. It involves the following: intravascular hemolysis, DIC, complement activation, cytokine release, hypotension, renal vasoconstriction, and the formation of intravascular thrombi, all of which can lead to uremia and death. Dialysis is required if the kidneys cannot function.

8. The first step taken in a transfusion reaction is to stop the transfusion immediately.

9. One type of delayed hemolytic transfusion reaction is caused by primary immunization when an individual is first exposed to an antigen. It occurs within 2 weeks of the transfusion as antibody titers (levels) increase and cause extravascular hemolysis of any

donor red cells still in circulation. The second type occurs in individuals previously sensitized as an anamnestic (secondary) response to the sensitizing antigen, usually 3 to 7 days after the transfusion.

10. Hives (welts) and itching are the usual signs of an allergic transfusion reaction. Usually mild, the reaction can become more serious and lead to wheezing and stridor.

11. Stop the transfusion. Antihistamines are effective in the treatment of an allergic transfusion reaction; once they are administered the transfusion can be restarted.

12. Anaphylactic transfusion reactions are sometimes fatal unless immediate medical therapy is initiated. They occur after hypersensitive individuals, those who have developed IgE antibody following primary immunization, are reexposed to the sensitizing antigen.

13. Anaphylactoid reactions can be caused by certain nonsteroidal anti-inflammatory drugs, certain narcotics, some blood products, muscle relaxants such as curare, and exercise.

14. For either an anaphylactic or an anaphylactoid reaction the transfusion must be stopped immediately. An I.V. line with normal saline should be kept open and such drugs as epinephrine (adrenaline) should be readily available for quick administration as well as intubation equipment. The latter will be necessary if the patient develops severe laryngeal edema.

15. A vasovagal response is a reaction caused by stress or pain. It is manifested by decreased heart rate and blood pressure and possible loss of consciousness.

16. Hypersensitive individuals are at greatest risk for an anaphylactic reaction. These individuals have developed antibody in response to a previous exposure to an allergen. Hypersensitivity develops only after a sensitizing event.

17. Traditionally, an FNHTR has been defined as an increase in body temperature of 1C or higher following a blood transfusion.

18. Febrile nonhemolytic transfusion reactions occur most often in those individuals who have been sensitized to numerous leukocyte alloantigens following multiple transfusions or in women who have had multiple pregnancies.

19. Biological response modifiers (BRMs) are active molecules such as cytokines, complement proteins, and lipids. They accumulate during storage and are dependent on the number of leukocytes in a transfusion unit.

20. The causes of FNHTRs are (a) red cell-related or (b) platelet-

related. If red-cell units are leukocyte-reduced, the incidence of FNHTR is reduced. If an FNHTR occurs, the recipient is treated with antipyretics. If the FNHTR is platelet-related, additional filtering for BRMs is used. However, filtering platelets activates complement, which can precipitate an FNHTR. Plasmapheresis removes most BMRs and reduces the chances of an FNHTR.

21. False. TRALI occurs within 1 to 6 hours following the administration of a plasma-containing blood product.

22. The most obvious sign of transfusion-related acute lung injury, or TRALI, is acute pulmonary edema with no evidence of myocardial damage or volume overload. Release of fluid from the vascular system into the lung tissue causes severe respiratory distress. Other symptoms include: fever, cyanosis, tachycardia, hypotension, and hypoxemia.

23. Pulmonary vascular damage can be induced by (a) agglutinins, (b) HLA antibodies, or (c) white cells that aggregate and settle in the small vessels of the pulmonary vasculature and cause endothelial cell damage.

24. The treatment for TRALI usually consists of steroid administration to curb the immune response along with mechanical ventilation and oxygen therapy for respiratory support.

25. Transfusion-associated graft-versus-host disease (TAGVHD) occurs (a) in immunocompetent individuals, (b) in individuals receiving blood transfusion from a blood relative, and (c) in unrelated donors who share an HLA haplotype.

26. The most serious symptom of TAGVHD is bone marrow aplasia and resultant pancytopenia (a decrease in the number of all blood cells). The mortality rate is as high as 90% due to infections and hemorrhage resulting from the ensuing granulocytopenia (decreased white cells) and thrombocytopenia (decreased platelets). There is no known treatment.

27. If donor blood components are irradiated prior to infusion, TAGVHD can be prevented in susceptible individuals.

28. In an individual who has had multiple platelet transfusions and is now showing signs of bleeding, one would suspect post-transfusion purpura.

29. Post-transfusion purpura is treated with corticosteroids, which lessen the immune response; plasmapheresis, which removes antibodies that destroy donor platelets; and/or intravenous gamma-globulin (IVGG), which provides already-formed antibodies.

30. The following transfusion reactions are not prompted by an immune response: acute nonimmune hemolytic reactions, circulatory overload, hemosiderosis, and infections associated with blood transfusions.

31. An acute nonimmune hemolytic transfusion reaction may result when blood is hemolyzed in any of the following situations: the infusion of blood that has been improperly warmed, infusion of a hypotonic normal saline solution, infusion through a small-bore needle, or the infusion of a contaminated product containing bacterial endotoxins.

32. Ms. Hayes was suffering from circulatory overload. Her transfusion added more fluid to her circulatory system than it could accommodate.

33. Hemosiderosis is treated with a chelating agent known as desferrioxamine, which binds excess iron and removes it from the body.

Chapter 16, Transfusion and Disease Transmission, Page 280

1. Since the 1980s, disease transmission via blood transfusion has been reduced because of (a) newly developed blood tests that are 99% accurate, (b) more stringent donor standards, and (c) the ability of donors to exclude themselves anonymously.

2. Hepatitis and AIDS are the two diseases of greatest concern; they are both viral diseases.

3. False. Blood banking standards and transfusion policies are set by the American Association of Blood Banks (AABB) and the FDA.

4. Other transfusion-transmissible diseases include: syphilis; malaria; babesiosis; cytomegalovirus (CMV); and Epstein-Barr virus (EBV).

5. No. Ms. Carter-Jones' blood contains antibody and/or antigen to an infectious agent. She is not an appropriate blood donor.

6. The seven hepatitis viruses are hepatitis A (HAV); hepatitis B (HBV); hepatitis C (HCV), which was formerly called non-A non-B; hepatitis D (HDV), formerly known as delta; hepatitis E (HEV); hepatitis F; and hepatitis G. The identities of the latter two are still being established.

7. The major signs and symptoms of hepatitis are jaundice, fatigue, weight loss, and loss of appetite, among others.

8. The most serious form of hepatitis is hepatitis B. Individuals infected with this virus usually experience liver damage and are at an increased risk for liver cancer in later life. It is transmitted

by coming into contact with blood or body secretions or sexual intercourse.

9. True. Seemingly healthy individuals can be carriers and transmitters of HBV.

10. Hepatitis B vaccine provides protection against HBV. It is strongly recommended for health care workers and other persons routinely in contact with blood and body fluids.

11. HBV vaccine is recommended for newborns, because it stimulates an individual's immune system to produce antibody against HBV. If exposed to the virus, the individual mounts an immune response before it can do any damage.

12. Any health care worker exposed to the blood or body fluids of an HBV-infected individual should receive hepatitis B immune globulin (HBIG) as soon as possible or within 7 days of the time of exposure.

13. Hepatitis C is also a blood-borne virus but is apt to be a milder infection than hepatitis B. The majority of HCV-positive individuals are asymptomatic and become chronic carriers. The incubation period for HBV is from 6 to 8 weeks, whereas that for HCV is anywhere from 2 to 26 weeks. There are approximately 300,000 new cases of HBV in the U.S. each year as compared with approximately 170,000 of HCV.

14. There are many routes for the transmission of HIV virus, including blood transfusion; contaminated needles; sperm, vaginal secretions, menstrual blood, breast milk, or other body fluids passed directly from infected individuals to recipients.

15. (a) The enzyme-linked immunosorbent assay (ELISA) is the initial screening test for antibody to HIV. If it is positive, the Western blot is used to confirm the presence of the virus. (c) Also, the FDA requires that all blood and blood components be tested by the HIV-1 antigen test, known as HIV-1-Ag.

16. HIV destroys communication among cells in the immune response. It replicates and destroys CD4+ T cells and macrophages; therefore, they can no longer alert other cells—phagocytes, cytotoxic T cells, B cells—to mount an immune response. Antigen recognition, conversion of T cells to become cytotoxic cells, and antibody production cannot take place. As the number of CD4+ T cells declines, infections become more prevalent and also more difficult to treat.

17. The standards indicating that an individual has progressed from being HIV-positive to having AIDS have been determined by

the Centers for Disease Control and Prevention (CDC). They are based on the number of CD4+ T lymphocytes and the absence or presence of an opportunistic infection.

18. Along with decreased number of CD4+ T cells, AIDS is clinically defined by the presence of such diseases as Kaposi's sarcoma; *Pneumocystis carinii* pneumonia; toxoplasmosis; and candidiasis.

19. Classic symptoms of AIDS include: fever; night sweats; fatigue; infections; and tumors such as Kaposi's sarcoma. Infections include *Pneumocystis carinii* pneumonia caused by an ubiquitous protozoan microorganism and thrush, a fungal infection. Lymphadenopathy (enlarged lymph nodes) is another complication.

20. At present, there is no cure for AIDS. Drugs like AZT (azidothymidine) can prolong its onset, but such drugs cause many side effects. Treatment may cause chronic problems such as anemia, liver damage, thrombocytopenia, neutropenia, and other blood disorders. Drugs known as protease inhibitors show promise in decreasing the amount of virus in the blood.

21. Like other retroviruses, the HTLV-I/II can lie dormant in cells for years. For this reason they are said to have a long latency (present, but hidden) period between the time of infection and the actual signs of disease.

22. HTLV-associated myelopathy (HAM) is a neurologic condition once called tropical spastic paraparesis. It is caused by HTLV-I and has been seen most frequently in Japan and the Caribbean. HAM attacks and damages an individual's spinal cord.

23. Syphilis is caused by the bacterium *Treponema pallidum*, which enters the body through the mucous membranes of the genitourinary tract or any other contact site. It is also transmitted by contact with contaminated material, blood transfusion, and from mother to fetus.

24. There are three stages associated with syphilis. (a) The primary stage is characterized by chancres which appear on the skin of the penis and vulva approximately 2 weeks following exposure. (b) In the secondary stage, about 6 weeks after the appearance of the primary lesions, other lesions appear on the skin and mucous membranes along with possible fever, headache, rashes, and generalized malaria. (c) When the disease reaches the tertiary stage the blood vessels, heart, and nervous system are affected. Paralysis and psychoses may also occur.

25. Approximately 30 to 60% of the adult population have been exposed to CMV. However, less than 10% of adults are infective.

The virus can survive indefinitely and become reactivated in individuals whose immune systems are suppressed or compromised. Like other herpetic viruses, it has DNA as its genetic material and has the ability to infect many different types of cells.

26. Immunoassay, immunofluorescence, and hemagglutination are among the tests used to detect the presence of CMV in blood and body tissue. These tests determine the presence of antibody to CMV.

27. The most serious effects of CMV are seen in immunoincompetent individuals who can develop pneumonitis, retinitis, gastritis, and other inflammatory conditions. In immunocompromised individuals (e.g., those undergoing transplant surgery or chemotherapy), a CMV infection can cause rejection of an allogenic graft or superinfection. In some cases, the latter contributes significant morbidity and mortality.

28. Transfusion or transplant candidates susceptible to CMV who should receive CMV-safe (seronegative, donated from an individual who has no antibody to CMV) blood are newborns weighing less than 3 pounds; pregnant women who are seronegative and require an intravenous or intrauterine transfusion; seronegative individuals who are to receive a bone marrow or organ transplant from a seronegative donor; recipients of autologous bone marrow who are seronegative; and seronegative individuals with AIDS.

29. It is thought that most bacterial contamination of blood comes from the donor via either of two ways: (a) improper cleansing of the venipuncture site or (b) from an undiagnosed bacteremia, such as might occur following dental extraction, sigmoidoscopy, or barium enema.

30. A recipient's reaction to bacterially contaminated blood includes: an elevated temperature, bright red flushing of the face, abdominal cramping, a feeling of warmth, vomiting, diarrhea, and possibly shock. DIC may also occur.

31. There are three major techniques used as standard precautions in transfusion therapy. (a) First, each unit of blood product should be examined for such signs as blood clots, gas bubbles, or a dark appearance of the plasma due to the extensive destruction of red cells. (b) Second, special care must be taken to prepare the venipuncture site, ensuring its sterility and compliance with AABB and FDA standards. (c) Third, a unit of Packed Red Cells must be infused within 4 hours from the time the transfusion is initiated and should not remain at room temperature any longer than necessary.

Chapter 17, Component Therapy, Page 304

1. With component therapy, individual blood components processed from Whole Blood are used to treat many conditions and diseases. For example, Packed Red Cells can be used to treat anemia, platelets for treating thrombocytopenia, and plasma for various coagulation defects.

2. Volume expanders are crystalloid or colloid solutions that can be given to maintain blood volume.

3. A unit of Whole Blood has a volume of 450 ml (+/- 45 ml). Its hematocrit (Hct) is typically between 0.36 and 0.44 (36 and 44%).

4. True. Although Whole Blood is rarely used in transfusion therapy (it is considered wasteful and may be harmful), it can be justified for an individual who has suffered massive blood loss, usually greater than 25% of total blood volume.

5. For certain transfusion recipients white cells are removed to prevent: (a) the transmission of such diseases as CMV; (b) FNHTRs; and (c) alloimmunization to human leukocyte (HLA) antigens, also known as major histocompatibility complex (MHC) molecules.

6. Fresh frozen plasma (FFP) is the blood component created after red cells and platelets have been removed.

7. None. Additive solutions are used only for Packed Red Cells.

8. Packed Red Cells are collected in one of three anticoagulant-preservatives—CPD, CP2D, or CPDA-1.

9. Washing of frozen red cells is called deglycerolization. Before a unit can be transfused it must be washed with a series of saline solutions to remove glycerol.

10. Excessive platelet destruction occurs in idiopathic thrombocytopenia (ITP). Platelets are destroyed faster than they can be replaced and therefore an infusion of platelets would not be able to stop the bleeding.

11. Although ABO compatibility is preferable in a platelet transfusion, it is not necessary because of the small number of red cells present in platelet concentrates.

12. The volume of platelets obtained from a unit of whole blood is much less than that of red cells. Recipients usually need many units. Therefore the platelets are pooled (mixed together). Pooled platelets must be transfused within 4 hours if they are prepared in an open system shortly before use.

13. Pooled platelets increase a recipient's exposure to numerous donor antigens and to transmissible disease.

14. Components that can be derived from plasma are cryoprecipitate, liquid plasma, coagulation factor concentrates, albumin, plasma protein fraction, immune serum globulins, and antiprotease concentrates.

15. If fresh frozen plasma (FFP) is separated from whole blood within 8 hours following collection and quickly frozen, clotting factors V and VIII will retain most of their effectiveness (clotting activity).

16. FFP can be stored up to 1 year at -18C or lower.

17. Liquid plasma is used to treat clotting factor deficiencies for which there is no specific concentrate available, such as factors XI and XII.

18. Cryoprecipitate, often referred to as Cryo, is a 20 to 50 ml concentrated solution of coagulation proteins. In order to produce it, a unit of FFP is thawed. During the thawing process, a white precipitate is formed. The plasma is removed, the cryoprecipitate is resuspended in a much smaller volume of plasma, and then it is refrozen.

19. Cryo is primarily used to treat congenital and acquired fibrinogen and factor XIII deficiencies. It is also used, uncommonly, to treat Willebrand's disease and hemophilia A.

20. Fibrin glue is prepared by mixing Cryo and bovine (cow) thrombin. It is applied topically to stop bleeding that cannot be controlled by any other means. For example, it can be used surgically in an area where sutures cannot control the bleeding.

21. Antihemophilic factor (AHF) is used to treat hemophilia A, a congenital disorder in which an individual has little if any factor VIII. Factor IX concentrate is used to treat hemophilia B (Christmas disease), another congenital disorder affecting the production of factor IX.

22. An infusion of factor IX concentrate can cause thrombosis. Recently a factor IX concentrate has been produced containing minimal amounts of factors II, VII, and X. It offers a decreased chance of causing thrombosis.

23. Immune serum globulins are concentrated solutions of antibodies (immunoglobulins) prepared from plasma. They are also called gammaglobulins.

24. There are three types of immune serum globulins that can be prepared from plasma: (a) intravenous immune globulin (IVIG)

used to treat immune deficiency disorders; (b) hyperimmune globulins used to provide passive immunity to individuals exposed to such diseases as hepatitis B or tetanus; and (c) immune globulins prepared for intramuscular (IM) administration. The latter contains antibodies against a variety of infectious organisms, such as measles and hepatitis A.

25. C1-esterase inhibitors are antiprotease concentrates prepared from plasma. They are used to treat defects in the complement system that cause hereditary angioedema which, if untreated, leads to urticaria and edema of the skin and mucous membranes.

26. Vitamin K is a fat-soluble vitamin necessary for complete synthesis of certain clotting proteins, including factors II, VII, IX, X, and proteins C and S.

27. Granulocyte transfusion may be indicated to treat (a) neutropenia, (b) patients with bacterial sepsis unresponsive to antibiotics, and (c) individuals with defective white cell production.

28. If blood volume is inadequate (hypovolemia) many organ systems, especially the heart, brain, and kidneys, do not function properly. This situation can present serious problems and possibly lead to death.

29. Normal saline (NS) is an ideal I.V. solution because it is easily removed by the kidneys. It is infused with Packed Red Cells and other components because it decreases blood viscosity and does not hemolyze red cells.

30. Lactated Ringer's is a widely used volume expander similar to NS that contains added calcium and magnesium. It cannot be infused with blood products because calcium can induce clotting. Dextrose, a simple sugar solution, cannot be used in blood transfusions because it causes red cell hemolysis.

31. There are two types of colloid volume expanders: (a) natural colloids like albumin and plasma protein fraction (PPF) and (b) synthetic colloids such as dextran and hydroxyethyl starch. Colloids are useful in maintaining blood volume especially in burn patients and in patients in shock from bleeding. Because of their protein concentration they are effective in maintaining osmotic pressure.

32. Albumin is used mainly to treat individuals with liver disease or those who have lost large volumes of blood due to burns, trauma, surgery, or plasma exchange. It is also used to treat neonatal hyperbilirubinemia.

33. PPF is likely to cause hypotension (decreased blood pressure) when infused and, therefore, is used less often than albumin.

34. Dextran and Hespan™ are two synthetic plasma volume expanders. Because of its molecular size and shape, dextran stays within the vasculature for approximately 6 hours. Hespan can remain in the vasculature for up to 24 hours. Both are used to replace lost blood volume due to burns, surgery, or sepsis. Both can cause hypersensitivity reactions. Rash, dyspnea, decreased blood pressure, and nasal congestion have been related to dextran. Fever, chills, rash, nausea and vomiting have been associated with Hespan. Both can interfere with hemostasis. Dextran can also interfere with blood grouping and cross matching tests. Hespan is also used in the collection of granulocytes by apheresis.

35. Hematopoietic growth factors were discovered through recombinant DNA technology. They are found to stimulate the growth and differentiation of stem and progenitor cells into mature blood cells.

36. Following the initiation of recombinant erythropoietin (rEPO) therapy it takes approximately 2 weeks before red cell production increases, and 2 to 3 months before an individual's Hct reaches the desired level.

37. Before the discovery of rEPO end-stage renal disease patients were given Packed Red Cells for anemia. Fluid overload was a hazard. Recombinant EPO has almost eliminated the need for blood transfusions in these individuals. It is also used for some anemias in patients with AIDS or certain malignancies as well as preoperatively.

Chapter 18, Apheresis, Page 317

1. Apheresis is the removal of whole blood from a donor/recipient for the purpose of isolating a specific component or components. It is most often performed to collect plasma and is called plasmapheresis. When used to collect platelets, it is called plateletpheresis, and for collecting granulocytes, it is called leukapheresis.

2. Therapeutic apheresis is used to remove a diseased or defective component from an individual's blood. Depending on the condition treated, the component may or may not be replaced. For example, diseased plasma can be removed and replaced with albumin, crystalloids, or FFP.

3. Complications that can arise in a recipient during apheresis include: hemolysis, infectious disease transmission, bacterial infection, allergic reaction, pulmonary complications, and citrate toxicity.

4. The symptoms of citrate toxicity during apheresis are numbness and tingling around the mouth and extremities and muscle cramps. At times, individuals can also experience chest pain, vomiting, nausea, chills, or fever.

5. False. Cellular components are separated by centrifugation only.

6. Membrane filtration can be used for the therapeutic removal of a diseased portion of plasma. As blood is being collected, it flows across a porous membrane. The pressure in the blood forces the plasma through the pores of the membrane. The red and white cells as well as the platelets are not removed. The plasma component is directed into a collection bag.

7. The following are examples of diseased components to be removed from plasma via adsorption: immune complexes, low-density lipoproteins, protein antigens, and antibodies.

8. Those individuals who receive platelets from multiple donors are exposed to many antigens. Often they become refractory, which means they develop antibodies against the donor platelets, causing them to be rapidly cleared from circulation after the transfusion. The use of single-donor platelets decreases a recipient's exposure to multiple donors.

9. Platelets should be irradiated to destroy viable lymphocytes prior to transfusion if the platelets are donated by blood relatives, or if they are intended for neonates or immunosuppressed and immunodeficient patients.

10. Leukapheresis, the removal of white cells from a donor, may be ordered in the case of an individual with a very high white cell count due to leukemia.

11. Granulocytes should be transfused as soon as possible after they are collected because of their short life span.

12. Corticosteroids increase white cell numbers by stimulating the bone marrow to release additional granulocytes and by stopping the movement of white cells from circulation into body tissue spaces. They are given to a donor prior to leukapheresis.

13. Hematopoietic growth factors are usually administered subcutaneously.

14. Hydroxyethyl starch, or Hespan™, is a colloidal solution used to produce better yields of granulocytes during apheresis. It causes red cells to aggregate at the base of the separator bowl. White cells and platelets form a buffy coat above this red cell aggregate, which

makes it easier to separate them out for collection. The buffy coat is also known as the mononuclear cell fraction.

15. Cytapheresis is a collection procedure whereby hematopoietic progenitor cells are collected from the peripheral circulation where they are called peripheral blood progenitor cells (PBPCs). The procedure is used to reestablish hematopoietic and lymphopoietic functions.

16. Peripheral blood progenitor cells (PBPCs) are used to rescue the individual's bone marrow.

17. Autologous progenitor cells are collected while the individual is in remission because (a) the tumor burden is small, (b) the amount of chemotherapeutic drug is minimal, and (3) the progenitor cells have a better chance of engrafting.

18. The collection of autologous PBPCs is somewhat more advantageous than that of autologous bone marrow stem cells because there is a less likely chance of contamination by malignant cells, and it is simpler to collect autologous PBPCs than bone marrow stem cells.

19. Therapeutic cytapheresis is considered a palliative treatment because its positive effects last only a short time.

20. Therapeutic cytapheresis is performed for some types of leukemia is which the white cell count is greater than $100 \times 10^9/L$. It is also performed for thrombocytopenia, when the platelet count is greater than $1000 \times 10^9/L$.

21. Plasmapheresis is used to treat the following: hyperviscosity syndromes, myasthenia gravis, dysproteinemias, multiple myeloma, high levels of low-density lipoproteins, circulating antibodies (as in Waldenström's macroglobulinemia), and immune complexes.

Chapter 19, Methods of Autologous Blood Recovery, Page 332

1. Autologous blood recovery is the collection of an individual's own blood prior to, during, or after surgery for reinfusion.

2. The four methods of autologous blood recovery that allow patients to donate and receive units of their own blood during surgical procedures include: (a) preoperative predonation, for which patients donate blood weeks in advance of surgery: (b) intraoperative hemodilution, for which patients donate blood immediately before surgery; (c) intraoperative blood salvage, for which the patient's blood is collected during surgery or processed from an extracorpo-

real circuit used during cardiopulmonary bypass surgery; and (d) postoperative wound collection, for which a patient's blood is recovered from drains placed within the surgical site.

3. They feel that autologous blood is the safest for some of the following reasons. It reduces or eliminates transfusion-transmitted disease. It prevents alloimmunization and eliminates some types of transfusion reactions and TAGVHD. It can be used in conjunction with allogeneic blood. It is a source of blood for those individuals who have developed alloantibodies following multiple transfusions, transplants, or pregnancies. Finally, it is acceptable to some religious sects that might object to allogeneic transfusion.

4. Autologous donors are not subjected to the same stringent requirements for donation that volunteer donors are, and therefore, complications can occur as a result of the donation procedure. Second, equipment used is occasionally implicated in adverse reactions. Third, there is always the possibility that autologous units can be outdated due to delays or postponements in surgery. Finally, there is chance the recipient can receive the wrong blood or that units can be given out of sequence, i.e., an allogeneic unit is given before an autologous one.

5. Intraoperative and postoperative blood collection systems can reinfuse activated complement components to the recipient. Usually complement activation is directed against red cells and causes hemolysis.

6. Autologous blood is stored at different temperatures. Predonated autologous blood is stored in the same way as allogeneic units (1 to 6C) but kept separate from them. Blood collected immediately prior to or during surgery can be kept at room temperature for up to 8 hours or at 1 to 6C for 24 hours if it is refrigerated within 6 hours of collection. Blood collected postoperatively is usually reinfused right away and not usually stored.

7. Predonated blood is used in surgical procedures when the individual is expected to lose 2 to 3 units of blood.

8. For predonated blood the Hct should be 0.33 and the Hgb 11 g/dL.

9. False. As many as 4 units of predonated autologous blood can be stored in reserve.

10. Yes. The order should be that the unit collected first is transfused first, followed by units in the order of collection.

11. Autologous blood receives the "Biohazard" if it has tested positive for disease. This is done for the safety of health care handlers.

12. Adverse reactions associated with the administration of predonated autologous blood include: bacterial contamination of the unit, increased levels of cytokines in the unit, and circulatory overload.

13. The use of autologous blood is contraindicated for pregnant women, those 70 years or older, and individuals with certain cardiac diseases, such as CAD, angina, or recent MI.

14. Collection of predonated autologous blood is safer for children, because they are less likely to be affected by the complications of predonation. For these individuals, autologous blood prevents alloimmunization.

15. Crystalloids are infused at a higher ratio because they leave the vascular system more easily and are readily removed by the kidneys. Colloids have a larger molecular size and diffuse less easily through capillary pores. Therefore less colloid volume is need to replace the blood withdrawn.

16. Normovolemic anemia occurs when an individual's blood volume is maintained at a normal level, but the number of red cells is reduced. A small number of circulating red cells means that fewer red cells are lost during surgery.

17. There are three main reasons why intraoperative hemodilution is considered beneficial. First, hemodiluted blood is less viscous and flows more easily than regular blood. As a result, it has a better chance of reaching all body cells. Second, hemodiluted blood, at room temperature, allows the clotting proteins and platelets to remain viable. Finally, hemodilution reduces the need for allogeneic blood products, thereby decreasing the incidence of alloimmunization and transfusion transmitted diseases.

18. For candidates for intraoperative hemodilution, anticipated blood loss during surgery should be no more than 2L.

19. Candidates for intraoperative hemodilution should meet these criteria: Hgb greater than 12g/dL; absence of all clotting deficiencies; anticipated blood loss of no more than 2L; and the absence of hypertension and serious cardiac, kidney, lung, or liver disease.

20. Cytokines do not usually present problems because the blood is used before they have a chance to accumulate.

21. Intraoperative blood salvage is the collection and reinfusion of blood shed at the operative site during major surgeries or drained from the extracorporeal system used to provide support to individuals during cardiac surgery.

22. Intraoperative blood salvage is contraindicated for those surgeries

in which bacterial contamination (bowel and bladder surgery), malignancy, other body fluids, such as amniotic fluid or urine, or sepsis is present. Reinfusion would expose the individual to possibly dangerous contaminants. It is also contraindicated for individuals with sickle-cell disease.

23. Autologous collection is not recommended for individuals with sickle-cell disease because the quality of their red cells is not adequate.

24. Wash and nonwash collection systems are used in intraoperative blood salvage. A wash system collects and washes whole blood. It concentrates red cells by removing all other components. It is used exclusively for cardiac, certain liver, and some orthopedic procedures as well as for aortic aneurysm and many transplant and vascular surgeries. A nonwash system collects whole blood and reinfuses it without further processing. It is used mainly during orthopedic surgeries that involve fracture repair and in total knee replacement.

25. Heparin, CPD, or ACD must be used as an anticoagulant for blood collected by wash systems. CPD or ACD must be used for nonwash systems.

26. A cardiotomy is a collection canister. It is used in intraoperative wash systems as a reservoir that holds any lost blood once it is suctioned from the surgical field.

27. The reinfusion of blood during intraoperative blood salvage is administered by an anesthetist (CNRA) or anesthesiologist (MD). Care is taken that the blood is never infused under pressure because of the likelihood of air entering the patient and causing an embolus.

28. After an individual has received 4 to 5 units of washed blood, coagulation tests should be performed, because washed blood is deficient in clotting factors.

29. Both wash and nonwash systems are used to collect postoperative wound blood.

30. Blood lost from the thoracic cavity is referred to as shed mediastinal blood.

Chapter 20, Bone Marrow Transplantation, Page 353

1. BMT is performed as an effective therapy for (a) many hematologic malignancies, (b) certain solid organ tumors, (c) nonmalignant disorders, such as the thalassemias, and (d) immunologic deficiencies, such as SCIDS.

2. Stem cells, which are found in the hematopoietic marrow, and progenitor cells, which are found in the circulation, are infused in a BMT. The cells can be used singly or in combination. (The term bone marrow stem cell is used interchangeably with the terms stem cell, peripheral blood progenitor cell, and cord blood progenitor cells.)

3. For individuals who have received pelvic irradiation and are unable to donate bone marrow, peripheral blood progenitor cells (PBPCs) may be the only source of stem cells.

4. Researchers believe the use of CBPCs correlates with a lower incidence of GVHD, because cord progenitor cells are less mature and, therefore, the T lymphocytes do not generate a strong immune response.

5. The three sources of stem cells used for BMT are autologous, allogeneic, and syngeneic.

6. Examples of disease treated with autologous stem cells include: some leukemias, some lymphomas, Hodgkin's disease, myeloma, and some solid organ tumors.

7. Siblings are the preferred source of allogeneic stem cells because their HLA molecules have the highest potential (25%) for being genetically matched with those of the recipient.

8. Syngeneic stem cells are harvested from an identical twin for transplantation into the other twin. The likelihood of graft rejection of GVHD for these individuals is virtually nonexistent, because the HLA molecules of the two are the same.

9. It is best to harvest stem or progenitor cells following chemotherapy while the bone marrow is recovering (producing more stem cells) or following the administration of hematopoietic growth factors.

10. Those individuals with congential (primary) bone marrow disorders cannot be treated with an autologous source. Their stem cells are defective, and these individuals must be treated with syngeneic or allogeneic cells.

11. Congenital bone marrow disorders include: the thalassemias, which produce abnormal hemoglobin molecules; SCIDS, which is the absence of an immune system at birth; and some types of aplastic anemia, which is the absence or minimal production of all types of blood cells.

12. Leukemia and multiple myeloma (B cell tumor) are examples of diseases that occur with acquired bone marrow failure.

13. Histocompatibility refers to the genetic similarity, or parity (likeness), between donor and recipient MHC class I and class II molecules.

14. For a successful BMT a high degree of histocompatibility is essential in order to reduce the incidence of graft rejection and/or GVHD.

15. Categories of histocompatible tests include: serologic (microlymphocytoxicity), cellular (mixed lymphocyte culture), and molecular (polymerase chain reaction) assays.

16. The amount of marrow that can be extracted from a donor depends on the donor's body weight.

17. The conditioning protocol for a BMT candidate lasts from 4 to 8 days. During this time the individual receives high-dose chemotherapy, which destroys malignant cells and the host's immune system. Sometimes the candidate also receives total body irradiation (TBI), which can be delivered as a single dose or fractioned over a period of 3 to 5 days.

18. The conditioning program is also referred to as ablative therapy.

19. An unavoidable consequence of ablative therapy is blood cell toxicity, which renders the host with a nonfunctioning immune system, anemia, and thrombocytopenia.

20. A state of remission is when the fewest possible malignant cells are present in the marrow or peripheral circulation.

21. Autologous stem cells are stored in a frozen state (cryopreserved). They are mixed with DMSO (dimethyl sulfoxide), a cryoprotective agent, and frozen in liquid nitrogen. They can remain frozen for 5 years.

22. True. DMSO used in the storage of autologous stems cells can cause a strong garlic taste in the recipient of autologous marrow. Hard candy or breath mints may counteract the taste.

23. A stem cell transplant is considered successful when engraftment takes place, that is, when the host accepts the graft, which typically occurs between 2 and 4 weeks after the procedure. The first sign of successful engraftment is an increase in the white cell count.

24. Stem cell recipients may not need to take immunosuppressive drugs for the rest of their lives to prevent graft rejection, because their immune system and blood group eventually become that of the donor.

25. During infusion of stem cells in a BMT procedure, the medical staff should monitor the recipient closely for fluid overload, emboli that may be in the infusion, and allergic reactions to donor white cell antigens.

26. Graft-versus-host disease (GVHD) is the most common complication and the greatest threat to bone marrow engraftment. The disease causes many problems for the host and has a high mortality rate.

27. Recipients of allogeneic stem cells suffer from severe immunodeficiency due to the very low numbers of functioning T and B lymphocytes. Those individuals receiving autologous or syngeneic stem cells have a period of immunodeficiency, but it is much shorter and less severe than in allogeneic recipients.

28. The development of post-BMT interstitial pneumonitis is related to the age of the recipient, the development of GVHD, immunodeficiency, and inflamed lung tissue caused by radiation or drugs.

29. Less than 1% of all BMT recipients suffer graft failure.

30. All blood products to be infused in BMT recipients with anemia or thrombocytopenia must be irradiated. The exception is for those products from the stem cell donor.

31. Graft-versus-host disease (GVHD) is an immune response generated by immunocompetent donor T lymphocytes against the tissues of an immunoincompetent individual, such as the BMT recipient. This individual cannot mount a defensive immune response. Therefore donor T lymphocytes recognize the host as foreign and destroy recipient tissue.

32. Organs most affected by GVHD are skin, liver, and the GI tract. The skin usually shows the first sign, with a slight rash that may progress to a sloughing of skin layers. Liver symptoms of jaundice and hepatomegaly follow. GI symptoms involve a shedding of the inner lining of the bowel resulting in bloody, watery diarrhea.

33. The treatment for acute GVHD consists of corticosteroids and immunosuppressive therapy. Drugs such as methylprednisone and cyclosporin are used to suppress the immune activity of donor cytotoxic CD8+ T cells.

34. If the signs and symptoms of chronic GVHD are restricted to the skin and liver, the prognosis is good.

GLOSSARY

A Blood Group One of four groups in the ABO blood classification system. The A antigen is present on the red cell membrane, and the plasma contains anti-B antibody. A group A individual can receive only group A or O Packed Red Cells.

AB Blood Group One of four groups in the ABO blood classification system. Both A and B antigens are present on the red cell membrane, and neither the anti-A nor the anti-B antibody is in the plasma. AB is the least common ABO group found in the U.S. population. A group AB individual can receive group A, B, AB, or O Packed Red Cells.

ABO Blood Group System The most important of several systems for classifying human blood for use in transfusion medicine.

Acetaminophen A synthetic, aspirinlike compound with antipyretic (antifever) and analgesic (pain killing) effects. An example is Tylenol™.

Acid-base Balance Refers to the equilibrium between acids and bases in the body. It is maintained by buffers, such as bicarbonate in plasma, and by the regulating activities of the lungs and kidneys in excreting waste products. These systems prevent the buildup of excessive acids or bases in the blood and tissues. Normally blood is slightly alkaline, or basic.

Acid Citrate Dextrose A citrate anticoagulant-preservative that can be used in the collection of blood during autologous blood recovery and apheresis.

Active Immunity A form of immunity in which the body provides its own antibody against disease-causing antigen. It occurs following infection or vaccination.

Acquired Immune Deficiency Syndrome (AIDS) A serious, usually fatal condition in which the immune system is destroyed by HIV and therefore cannot respond normally to infections. Individuals with AIDS often develop Kaposi's sarcoma and recurrent severe opportunistic infections such as *Pneumocystis carinii* pneumonia and fungal infections. It is the opportunistic infections that are usually fatal to the person with AIDS.

Additive System A solution consisting of dextrose, mannitol, saline, and adenine that is added only to Packed Red Cells for storage. These chemicals extend storage life from 35 to 42 days. No anticoagulative properties are associated with them. Another term is additive solution.

413

Adenosine   The chemical compound that is a major building block of many biologically active compounds, such as DNA, RNA, ADP, and ATP.

Adenosine Triphosphate (ATP)   A compound consisting of adenosine, the sugar ribose, and three phosphate molecules. It is involved in many reactions involving the storage and transfer of energy in cells.

Agammaglobulinemia   A congenital or acquired condition in which the production of antibody does not occur.

Agglutination   The clumping together of antigen-carrying cells or of microorganisms resulting from their interaction with antibody.

Alanine Aminotransferase (ALT)   A liver enzyme whose presence can be tested for in a sample of blood. An elevated level indicates liver damage due to diseases such as hepatitis, cirrhosis, or cancer. The measure of blood ALT is no longer required by the FDA prior to transfusion.

Albumin   The plasma protein synthesized in the greatest amount by the liver. It transports substances within the blood and assists in generating oncotic pressure.

Alleles   Pairs of genes that code for the same trait and located at the same loci on a pair of chromosomes. An example is the alleles on chromosome 6 that code for MHC molecules.

Allergen   Any chemical substance, such as a protein, that causes the symptoms of an allergy in a hypersensitive individual. Examples of allergens include: ragweed, pollen, fish, eggs, peanuts, dust, and parasites, among others.

Alloantibody   Antibody produced against alloantigen. Also referred to as isoantibody.

Alloantigen   Antigen found in members of a species that causes antibody production in other members of the same species. Also called isoantigen.

Allogeneic   A term that refers to the genetic differences between individuals of the same species. Most often used to denote cells taken from a donor and transfused or transplanted into a genetically nonidentical recipient. MHC molecules on the cell surfaces are responsible for genetic dissimilarity and make individuals different from one another immunologically.

Alloimmunization   The production of alloantibody in response to alloantigen. It occurs only in members of the same species.

Alveoli   Tiny saclike structures that form grapelike clusters at the end of the terminal airways located in the lungs. Oxygen and carbon dioxide transfer takes place between the blood and the atmosphere in the alveoli, which function in close proximity with the capillary network.

Amino Acid A chemical compound that is the basic building block of proteins. It contains an amino group (NH_2) and a carboxyl group (COOH).

Anamnestic Response The immune response generated on reexposure to the same antigen. The anamnestic response is more rapid than primary immunization, and IgG is the antibody predominantly produced.

Anaphylatoxins The complement components C3a, C4a, and C5a. When released into the blood they cause basophils and mast cells to release histamine from their intracellular granules. Anaphylatoxins can cause a reaction very similar to an anaphylactic reaction, but IgE is not produced.

Anaphylaxis A severe and sometimes fatal hypersensitivity reaction due to the injection or ingestion of a substance to which the individual has become sensitized by previous exposure. Symptoms include: weakness, shortness of breath, edema, cardiac and respiratory abnormalities, and hypotension. Death may occur within minutes of exposure.

Anemia A red cell count below $4.2 \times 10^3/\mu L$. Anemia indicates a disease process somewhere in the body.

Anergy The lack of a competent immune system. Also called immunoincompetence.

Angina Pectoris The chest pain associated with the decreased amount of blood that reaches the myocardium as the result of plaque buildup in the coronary arteries.

Antibody A complex protein molecule produced by B cells/plasma cells in response to the presence of antigen. It binds to antigen and in some cases causes the activation of complement components. Once bound by antibody the antigen is destined for destruction, usually by phagocytosis carried out by certain white cells.

Antibiotic A natural or synthetic substance that interferes with the growth of microorganisms, such as bacteria.

Anticoagulant-preservative A citrate solution added to blood to prevent clotting and to preserve red cell viability. To date, only CPD, CP2D, CPDA-1 and ACD are available for transfusion.

Antigen Any foreign protein, carbohydrate, or lipid molecule found on microorganisms, infected cells, foreign cells, or malignant cells that stimulate the immune response through (1) antibody release from B cells/plasma cells or (2) cytotoxic T cell activity. The majority of antigen is protein.

Antigen-antibody Reaction The process by which the immune system recognizes an antigen and causes the production of antibody specific to that antigen. Antibody binds to antigen, which is then destroyed.

Antigen-presenting Cell (APC) A white cell, such as a macrophage or other phagocytic cell, that is capable of internalizing antigen, breaking the antigen into small fragments called peptides (proteins), binding a peptide to an MHC molecule, and presenting that peptide to CD4+ T cells. APCs are needed by CD4+ T cells to respond to protein antigen.

Antigen-antibody Complex Antigen bound by antibody that is destined to be destroyed.

Antithrombin III (AT-III) The natural anticoagulant that attaches itself to activated coagulation factors in the plasma and removes them, thereby preventing inappropriate clot formation.

Antipyretics The term used to describe substances, such as aspirin, that reduce or lower fever.

Aorta The major artery that carries oxygenated blood from the left ventricle of the heart and delivers it to organs.

Aortic Valve The three-cusp valve that separates the aorta from the left ventricle of the heart.

Apheresis The process by which a specific component is removed (1) from the blood of an individual for whom the component is problematic or (2) for use in transfusion therapy. Cytapheresis, plateletpheresis, and plasmapheresis are types of apheresis procedures.

Arrhythmia An abnormal heart rhythm that can present serious problems for the individual.

Arteriole A small branch of any artery that leads to the capillary network.

Atheroma Plaque (fatty deposits) that builds up along the arterial wall.

Atherosclerosis The buildup of atheroma along the arterial wall that results in a decrease of blood flow.

Atmospheric Pressure Pressure generated by the gases within the atmosphere. The combination of the individual partial pressures makes up the atmospheric pressure. Also called barometric pressure.

Atrial Septal Defect The defect that occurs when there is a hole in the septum between the right and left atria of the heart.

Autologous Blood An individual's own blood. The term usually refers to the collection and administration of that blood. There are four ways an individual can donate blood for transfusion later.

Autologous Blood Transfusion The transfusion of one's own blood that is collected by predonation, hemodilution, intraoperative salvage, or postoperative wound drainage. Use of this blood eliminates certain transfusion-related diseases and certain transfusion reactions.

B Blood Group One of four groups in the ABO blood classification system. It has the B antigen on the red cell surface and anti-A antibody in the plasma. This group can receive either B or O group Packed Red Cells.

B Cell   The lymphocyte that on stimulation by antigen or CD+ T cells transforms itself into a plasma cell for secretion of antibody.

Babesiosis   A rare, sometimes fatal disease that can be transmitted through a blood transfusion. The organism that causes babesiosis is a protozoan parasite that resides inside the red cell.

Bacteremia   A bacterial infection in which antigen enters the circulatory system and spreads throughout the body.

Bacteria   Any of a large group of organisms found in soil, water, and air. Some cause disease in humans as well as other organisms. Generally classified as rod-shaped (bacillus), spherical-shaped (cocci), comma-shaped (vibrio), or spiral-shaped (spirochetes).

Basophil   A type of white cell that is normally about 1% of the total white cell count. Its main function is the release of histamine and heparin at the site of antigen invasion. A basophil that moves into the tissues is called a mast cell.

Bile   A chemical substance produced in the liver and stored in the gallbladder until it is needed for fat digestion within the small intestine.

Binding   The process whereby two or more molecules join in a chemical reaction. Binding may activate, inhibit, or neutralize the molecules in the reaction.

Blood Clot   Blood that has gone from a liquid state to a semisolid state. Clot formation requires interaction among platelets and certain molecules in the blood—Ca^{++}, phospholipids, and coagulation proteins. All of these molecules must be present for a clot to form.

Blood Grouping   A technique for determining a person's blood group. In grouping for the commonly used ABO groups, cells and serum are mixed with reagents to determine the blood group of the donor and/or recipient.

Blood Islands   Groups of primitive cells found in the yolk sac of the embryo that are the precursors to blood cells and constitute the early beginnings of the vascular system.

Blood Transfusion   The infusion of blood or blood components into an individual for the treatment of a medical condition, disease, or blood loss due to surgery or trauma. Transfused blood may be either allogeneic or autologous.

Blood Volume   The amount of blood circulating throughout the body in the vascular system. Normal blood volume in the adult is about 5 liters. Maintaining blood volume is essential for organ function, especially of the heart, brain, and kidneys.

Bone Marrow   A specialized, spongy, fibrous matrix in the center of bones. Hematopoietic marrow is involved in the production of blood cells. Yellow marrow is found in the long bones and is 96% fat.

Bronchi/Bronchioles The tubes, or airways, of the lungs that lead from the trachea, or windpipe, to the alveoli.

Bronchospasm The closing off of the bronchi and bronchioles caused by the release of histamine by basophils.

Budding The process whereby new viruses are released from an infected cell by rupturing the cell's membrane.

Buffer A chemical substance that prevents dramatic changes in the pH of a solution by binding (removing) hydrogen ion (H^+) or hydroxyl ion (OH^-) from the solution.

Capillaries The smallest blood vessels in the body. They connect arterioles and venules. Only one cell layer thick, the walls of capillaries allow for the transfer of oxygen and nutrients to the tissues and the transfer of waste products and carbon dioxide from the tissues to the blood.

Carbohydrates A broad class of molecules made up of carbon, hydrogen, and oxygen. Examples of carbohydrates include: sugars, starches, and some antigens. The most common carbohydrate is glucose.

Carbon Dioxide (CO_2) A color-less, odorless gas given off by the tissues into the blood, which carries carbon dioxide to the lungs for expiration. Carbon dioxide levels in the blood regulate the breathing rate. Carbon dioxide is transported to the lungs as bicarbonate ion.

Cardiac Output The amount of blood pumped by the left ventricle each minute.

CD4+ T Lymphocyte A subset of T cells that directs the immune response to protein antigen. Also called a helper T cell. A CD4+ T cell is MHC class II restricted. HIV attacks and destroys CD4+ T cells.

CD8+ T Lymphocyte A subset of T cells that destroys infected cells, allogeneic cells, and tumor cells by lysing them with toxins. Also referred to as a cytotoxic T cell. A CD8+ T cell is MHC class I restricted.

Cell-mediated Response The immune response brought about by a helper T cell when it recognizes a foreign invader and stimulates (1) the B cell to produce antibody or (2) other T cells to become cytotoxic.

Cell Membrane The outer perimeter of a cell that contains (holds in) the cytoplasm and cellular organelles.

Cell Separator The apparatus used in apheresis and autologous blood wash devices to separate blood components by centrifugation (high speed spinning).

Chemotaxis The movement by a cell or organism toward or away from a chemical stimulus.

Clotting Time The time required for blood to clot, usually determined by observing clot formation in a small sample of blood.

Coagulation The process by which liquid blood is changed into the semisolid mass referred to as a blood clot. Coagulation can occur in an intact vessel, but usually occurs with an injury to a vessel or when blood comes into contact with a foreign surface. Blood clots that form in the vasculature of the brain cause strokes.

Coagulation Factor Any one of numerous protein factors in the blood that are essential for fibrin formation. Most coagulation factors are serine proteases synthesized in the liver.

Colony-stimulating Factors A class of cytokine molecules that function as hematopoietic growth factors. They are essential to blood cell development.

Complement Fixation The attachment of complement to antigen or an antigen–antibody complex that leads to antigen destruction by lysis or phagocytosis.

Coumadin™ (Warfarin) A drug used as an anticoagulant in individuals with artificial heart valves or for those prone to strokes. It blocks the action of vitamin K, which is necessary for coagulation.

C3 Receptor The protein complex found on one of the constant regions of the antibody molecule and also on the cell membrane of neutrophils and macrophages. Complement bound to antigen attaches to this receptor/point.

Cross Matching The mixing of the red cells of a donor with the serum of a potential recipient to determine compatibility for transfusion. Clumping occurs when incompatible blood groups are mixed; it does not occur when compatible blood groups are mixed.

Cryoprecipitate The white layer of precipitate that forms in fresh frozen plasma (FFP) as it thaws. It is very rich in factors VIII, XIII, and fibrinogen. It is used to make fibrin glue. Also referred to as Cryo.

Cyanosis The blue color of skin that occurs when inadequate amounts of oxygen reach the tissues.

Cyclosporin A drug used to suppress the immune system to prevent graft rejection following organ and bone marrow transplantation.

Cytokines A broad class of glycoproteins that have many important functions within the body, such as acting as inflammatory molecules and hematopoietic growth factors, among others.

Cytomegalovirus A virus of the herpes family that can be transmitted through a blood transfusion. The virus usually presents problems only to individuals with deficient or defective immune systems, such as transplant recipients and neonates.

Cytoplasm The fluid or jellylike substance within the cell membrane in which cellular organelles are suspended.

Cytotoxic That which is toxic to a cell, such as chemotherapeutic agents or lytic molecules.

Degradative Enzymes Digestive enzymes in the granules and lysosomes of white cells that aid in antigen destruction.

Deoxygenated Blood Blood low in oxygen returning from body tissues to the heart for circulation through the lungs where blood becomes oxygenated.

Deoxyhemoglobin Hemoglobin that has released some of its oxygen to the tissues.

Dialysis The process whereby the blood is cleansed outside the body using a hemodialysis machine. Hemodialysis is primarily utilized for individuals suffering from end-stage kidney disease.

Diapedesis The movement, or passage, of white cells through the capillary pores in response to foreign organisms and chemotactic factors.

Differentiation The process of cellular maturation by which immature cells, such as stem cells, mature into fully differentiated blood cells.

Diffusion The movement of a substance from a region of greater concentration to a region of lower concentration, such as the diffusion of the respiratory gases between the blood and tissues.

Diphosphoglycerate Commonly known as 2,3-DPG, this molecule is found in the blood bound to the hemoglobin molecule. It functions by allowing hemoglobin more easily (1) to release oxygen to the tissues and (2) to pick up oxygen in the lungs.

Disseminated Intravascular Coagulation (DIC) A process in the body in which clot formation and clot lysis happen in a simultaneous, uncontrolled fashion. The treatment depends on the cause, but blood products such as Platelets, fresh frozen plasma, and Cryo are administered to replace components that are being consumed by the body.

Diuretic A drug that is administered to increase the production of urine in order to remove excess fluids from the body.

Donation Donating blood for one's own use or someone else's for the treatment of medical diseases and conditions.

Edema The swelling of tissue caused by the retention of fluid in the interstitial space.

Electrolyte An element or compound that when dissolved in a solution, such as plasma, produces ions. For example, when NaCl (sodium chloride) is placed in solution, it separates into Na⁺ ions (sodium) and Cl⁻ ions (chloride). Electrolytes are essential for normal physiological processes, such as muscle contraction and blood clotting.

Endogenous Antigen Antigen, such as viruses and certain bacteria, that destroy a cell from within and cannot be destroyed by antibody and/or complement.

Endothelium A layer of flat cells that lines blood vessels and the heart. A tear or rupture of it stimulates the coagulation system to form a clot.

Enzyme A protein molecule that accelerates the rate of a chemical reaction. If it were not for enzymes, most physiologic reactions would not occur or would occur too slowly.

Enzyme-linked Immunosorbent Assay (ELISA) An initial screening assay to determine whether or not blood has antibody to foreign organisms, such as HIV. If results are positive, further tests such as the Western blot are done to substantiate the results of the ELISA.

Eosinophil A type of white cell that normally makes up about 1 to 3% of the total white cell count. They are abundant in people with allergies and parasitic infections.

Epinephrine The hormone released by the adrenal gland following stimulation of the sympathetic nervous system. Epineph-

rine has been synthesized and one of its therapeutic uses is to treat anaphylactic reactions. Also called adrenaline.

Epitope The portion of an antigen, called an antigenic peptide, that can bind to either an antibody or the T cell receptor.

Erythema Also called polycythemia vera, erythema is a stem cell disorder that produces extremely high red cell numbers.

Erythrocyte A mature red cell that contains the hemoglobin molecule. The main function of this cell is to transport oxygen and carbon dioxide between the lungs and the tissues.

Erythropoiesis The process of red cell production that takes place in hematopoietic bone marrow and is controlled by the hormone erythropoietin.

Erythropoietin A hormone produced by the peritubular cells of the kidneys in response to the decrease in the partial pressure of oxygen in the blood passing through the kidneys. It increases production of red cells.

Exogenous Antigen Antigen that causes damage outside cells through the production of toxins, such as produced by the majority of bacteria. Exogenous antigen can be destroyed by antibody and/or complement.

Extramedullary Hematopoiesis The development of blood cells in organs other than bone marrow, usually the spleen or liver. In adults, this condition occurs only in individuals with certain disease states.

Extravascular   A term that describes the area outside the vascular system. Usually used in reference to fluid or blood that has left the circulatory system and is in the interstitial space.

Extravascular Hemolysis   Hemolysis (lysis of the red cell) that takes place outside the vascular system, such as in the spleen.

Fc Receptor   The protein complex found on one of the constant regions of the antibody molecule and also on the cell membrane of neutrophils and macrophages. The antibody-antigen complex attaches to this receptor/point.

Febrile   The term used to indicate fever.

Fetal Hemoglobin (Hgb F)   The hemoglobin molecule produced during fetal development. Hgb F has a stronger affinity for oxygen than adult hemoglobin, which allows it to remove oxygen from the mother's blood.

Fibrin   An insoluble protein in blood that along with platelets forms a stable blood clot. Fibrin is formed by the action of thrombin on fibrinogen, which is the inactive soluble form of fibrin.

Fibrin Glue   A product manufactured by mixing cryoprecipitate, thrombin, and calcium. Used almost exclusively in surgery, it is topically applied to bleeding surfaces that cannot be controlled by other means. It has the potential for transmitting bloodborne diseases.

Fibrin Split Products (FSPs)   Pieces of fibrin released into plasma when a fibrin clot is dissolved. They are potent inhibitors of coagulation if allowed to remain in the circulation.

Fibrinogen (Factor I)   A protein present in plasma that is essential to the process of blood coagulation. During the process of blood coagulation, factor I is converted into fibrin by thrombin in the presence of calcium ions and prothrombin 3 (PF-3).

Fibrinolysis   The dissolution of a clot in which fibrin is broken down into smaller pieces called fibrin split products (FSPs).

Fibrinolytics   Molecules in plasma that are activated by tissue enzymes, such as tPA, for the dissolution of a fibrin clot. Also used therapeutically to treat inappropriate blood clots within the vasculature.

Filtration   The movement of a substance, usually a liquid, through a semipermeable membrane that allows fluid to pass through while retaining the particles suspended in the fluid.

Fresh Frozen Plasma (FFP)   The liquid portion of blood that is removed from whole blood and frozen immediately. It is used in the treatment of bleeding disorders such as DIC.

Fungi A group of plantlike microorganisms that includes molds and yeasts. They have the potential to be pathogenic.

Gammaglobulin The fraction of serum that contains antibody. It provides the chief defense against bacteria, viruses, and toxins. Extracted from donor plasma and commercially processed, gammaglobulin is used in passive immunization.

Globin The protein portion of the hemoglobin molecule.

Globulin Any one of several simple proteins found in blood.

Graft Failure The failure of a transplanted organ or bone marrow to carry out its intended physiologic function.

Graft Rejection The rejection of solid organ or bone marrow following transplantation. It can occur when (1) the recipient's immune system mounts an attack against donor tissue or (2) donor lymphocytes attack recipient tissue.

Graft-versus-host Disease (GVHD) An immune response generated in a bone marrow transplant or blood transfusion recipient. GVHD is caused by donor lymphocytes that recognize the recipient as foreign and mount an attack against the recipient's cells. It usually occurs in recipients with a defective or deficient immune system.

Granulocyte A type of white cell characterized by the presence of granules in its cytoplasm. There are three types—neutrophils, eosinophils, and basophils.

Great Vessels Vessels directly attached to the heart. They are the superior and inferior venae cavae, pulmonary artery, pulmonary veins, and aorta.

Haplotype A group of closely linked genes, usually inherited as a block. An example of a haplotype is the block of MHC genes located on chromosome 6.

Hematocrit (Hct) The percentage of red cells in the total blood volume. It is also called the packed cell volume or crit.

Hematology The science and study of blood, blood-forming tissues, and blood diseases.

Hematopoiesis The process by which blood cells are produced in hematopoietic marrow.

Hematopoietic Growth Factors Molecules produced by various body cells that stimulate stem cells to produce specific blood cells. Growth factors include the interleukins, colony-stimulating factors, and the hormone erythropoietin.

Hematopoietic Marrow Marrow in the center of flat bones—the ribs, pelvis, sternum, and vertebrae—that is responsible for blood cell production in the adult. Hematopoietic marrow is found in different sites depending on the age of the individual.

Heme The molecule within each polypeptide chain of hemoglobin that is the binding site for oxygen. Heme is also responsible for the red color of blood.

Hemodilution A decrease in the concentration of blood cells in circulation with a concurrent increase in plasma volume. Hemodilution utilized before surgery to reduce blood loss is called intraoperative hemodilution. The amount of blood withdrawn is replaced with an equal volume of I.V. crystalloid or colloid solution. Hemodilution also occurs when large volumes of I.V. solutions are transfused.

Hemoglobin (Hgb) A complex protein found in red cells containing the iron pigment heme. It functions by transporting oxygen and carbon dioxide. In the high oxygen content of the lung, oxygen binds with Hgb to form oxyhemoglobin. After depositing oxygen in the tissues and combining with carbon dioxide, Hgb becomes carboxyhemoglobin.

Hemoglobinemia The presence of free hemoglobin in plasma. Like hemoglobinuria, hemoglobinemia occurs following red cell hemolysis.

Hemoglobinuria The presence of hemoglobin in the urine. It most often occurs following red cell hemolysis.

Hemolysis The breakdown of the red cell membrane and the release of hemoglobin into plasma. It occurs normally at the end of the red cell's life cycle and abnormally in certain antigen-antibody reactions on exposure to certain bacteria, during hemodialysis, and in other situations.

Hemolytic Disease of the Newborn (HDN) A condition arising during fetal life that is caused by an incompatibility between the mother's blood group and that of the fetus. The mother produces IgG antibody that crosses the placenta and attacks fetal red cells.

Hemophilia An inherited disease characterized by excessive bleeding. It occurs most often in males. There are two forms of the disease, A and B. With each form, one of the coagulation factors is missing, or a factor is produced at a reduced concentration, or the body produces an inhibitor to the factor that makes it inactive.

Hemorrhagic Disorder A disorder of the vascular and/or coagulation systems that causes inappropriate bleeding. An example is hemophilia.

Hemostasis The cessation of bleeding, naturally through coagulation, mechanically with surgical clamps and sutures, or chemically with drugs.

Heparin A molecule produced from beef lung or pork mucosa used to inhibit blood clot formation. Although heparin has no anticoagulant effect on its own, it enhances the action of antithrombin III (AT-III), which is the body's natural anticoagulant.

Hepatitis A serious disease that causes inflammation of the liver and can lead to cancer. It is most often caused by the *Hepadneviridae* family of viruses, certain ones of which can be transmitted by blood products. Bloodborne hepatitis, such as B and C, can be fatal. B and C hepatitis can remain in the blood for many years, making the individual a carrier and unable to donate blood. Hepatitis C accounts for the majority of all transfusion-related hepatitis.

Hepatitis B Immune Globulin (HBIG) An injectable product prepared from plasma containing antibody to hepatitis from an individual previously infected with the virus. HBIG should be administered within 7 days of a individual's coming into contact with infected blood.

Hepatitis B Vaccine A vaccine specifically designed to prevent an individual from contracting hepatitis B. The vaccine is administered in three injections. Vaccination should be mandatory for individuals likely to come into contact with infected blood.

Hepatomegaly A term that describes an enlarged liver, which is an early indicator of liver disease.

Histamine A molecule produced and released by basophils and mast cells (tissue basophils) in response to antigen, in allergic reactions, and in the inflammatory response. It causes vessels to dilate, decreases blood pressure, and is responsible for the effects of an anaphylactic reaction.

Histocompatibility The likeness, or parity, of MHC/HLA molecules between individuals. Histocompatible individuals will accept grafts from one another.

Histoincompatibility The difference, or disparity, of MHC/HLA molecules between individuals. Histoincompatible individuals will reject grafts from one another.

Homeostasis The balance of all body systems that provides the ideal environment for normal physiologic reactions.

Host–versus–graft Disease The immune response that arises in an organ transplant recipient. Drugs are administered to suppress the immune response and prevent the recipient's (host's) lymphocytes from attacking the donor's cells and causing organ rejection.

Human Immunodeficiency Virus (HIV) A virus responsible for the fatal disease AIDS and belonging to a class of viruses called retroviruses. Retroviruses have RNA as their genetic material and also contain reverse transcriptase, an enzyme that allows it to convert RNA to DNA and insert its DNA into the host cell. HIV mainly attacks the CD4+ helper T lymphocytes and macrophages, thereby destroying major cells of the immune system.

Human Leukocyte Antigen (HLA) Protein molecules found on the cell membrane of almost all body cells except red cells. HLA are also referred to as MHC or major histocompatibility complex molecules. HLA have an antigenic effect when transfused or transplanted into an individual other than an identical twin.

Humoral Immune Response The immune response to antigen that causes the production of antibody.

Hydrogen Ion (H⁺) The ion produced when an acid, such as HCl (hydrochloric acid), is placed in solutions, such as water or plasma. The H^+ ions that are set free increase the acidity of the solution. They must be picked up by a buffer, such as HCO_3^- ion (bicarbonate) or hemoglobin.

Hydrostatic Pressure Pressure formed within the capillaries due to blood pressure.

Hypersensitivity A term that refers to the abnormal response to an allergen, for example, asthma, and hay fever, among others.

Hypersplenism The condition that causes the spleen to remove increased numbers of blood cells from circulation.

Hyperviscosity The term used to describe plasma that is thickened due to increased amounts of plasma proteins. It occurs with diseases such as multiple myeloma.

Hypervolemia An increase in the volume of circulating fluid in the vascular system.

Hypogammaglobulinemia A deficiency of immunoglobulins within plasma. It may be caused by a hereditary or acquired disorder. Individuals deficient in immunoglobulins have a defective immune system and cannot generate a humoral immune response (antibody production).

Hypothermia The condition in which the body temperature is below 35C or 95F. It occurs most often in elderly and young children on exposure to cold temperatures. Hypothermia may be utilized in some types of surgery to reduce the metabolic requirements of the body thereby lowering oxygen demand.

Hypovolemia A decrease in the volume of fluid circulating in the vascular system. The patient should be treated with the appropriate fluids—blood products, cystalloids, or colloids.

Hypoxemia A decrease of oxygen in the blood.

Hypoxia A decrease of oxygen in the tissues. If the condition continues for any length of time, erythropoietin is released from the kidneys and red cell production takes place.

Immune Response The response generated by lymphocytes and other white cells, complement proteins, and antibody that leads to antigen destruction. Lymphocytes control the immune response.

Immune System The system of the body that protects humans from invasion by foreign matter. It is responsible for the immune response to antigen.

Immunocompetence The term used to indicate that someone has a functioning immune system.

Immunogen Any foreign matter capable of causing an immune response.

Immunoglobulins Chemically complex protein molecules produced by B cells/plasma cells in response to antigen. When immunoglobulins are secreted from B cells/plasma cells they are called antibodies. There are five classes of immunoglobulins.

Immunoincompetence The term used to indicate that someone has a nonfunctioning immune system. There are many causes, such as chemotherapeutic drugs, radiation, and bone marrow failure, among others.

Immunosuppression The suppression of the immune system following organ and bone marrow transplantation through the use of drugs such as cyclosporin.

Inferior Vena Cava The major vein of the body. It receives venous blood from organs and the lower extremities and returns it to the right atrium of the heart.

Inflammation The process that occurs when the physical and/or chemical barriers of the body are penetrated. It occurs following tissue injury and is evidenced by heat, pain, swelling, and redness in the inflamed tissue.

Inhibitors Molecules that inhibit the action of other molecules, such as the complement inhibitors that arrest the action of complement.

Interferons The class of cytokine molecules that plays a role in the destruction of virally infected cells.

Interleukins A class of cytokine molecules that has several functions, such as acting as hematopoietic growth factors and in inflammatory reactions.

Interstitial Space The space in tissues that separates body cells from one another.

Intravascular The term that describes anything located within the circulatory system, from blood to catheters.

Intravascular Hemolysis Hemolysis of red cells that occurs in the vascular system.

Ion An atom carrying an electric charge. Ions that carry a postive charge are called cations, for example, sodium (Na^+). Ions that carry a negative charge are called anions, for example, chloride (Cl^-).

Ionization The breakdown of substances, such as acids, bases, and salts, into their individual ions.

Ischemia The reduction in blood flow to tissue. It occurs with coronary artery disease, for example. Ischemia is evidenced by pain in the area of obstruction.

Isoantibody *See* Alloantibody.

Isoantigen *See* Alloantigen.

Jaundice A yellow color of the skin and whites of the eyes that indicates liver disease. The yellow color is due to bile seeping into the tissues.

Lactate Dehydrogenase A tissue enzyme released into the bloodstream following muscle damage. It is found following a myocardial infarction, for example.

Lag Period The time between exposure to an infectious organism and the appearance of antigen or antibody in the blood. Also called the window period.

Leukemia A disorder of the white cells in which increased numbers of immature cells are produced. The disease may be treated with chemotherapy and/or bone marrow transplantation. There are many types of leukemia.

Leukocyte A white cell. There are three types of white cells—neutrophils, basophils, and monocytes/macrophages. All types function in conjunction with the immune system to provide defense against foreign matter.

Leukocyte-reduced Blood A blood product or products that have had white cells removed by filtration to prevent transfusion reactions. There are several ways that white cells can be removed from whole blood. Filtering is the most efficient.

Lobule The functional unit of the liver. The lobule consists of several hepatocytes connected to a central vein and canaliculi.

Lymph Interstitial fluid that drains into the lymphatic channels. It has a clear-to-cloudy appearance.

Lymphadenopathy The swelling of lymph nodes that can occur for many reasons. The condition is usually due to viral infections and is prevalent in individuals with AIDS.

Lymphatic System A network of capillarylike vessels, ducts, nodes, and organs that helps maintain the fluid environment of the body. The lymphatic vessels have two large vessel—the thoracic duct and right lymphatic duct—that empty into veins in the upper chest and return fluid to the vascular system. The lymphatic system is also involved with immunity: antigen is presented to T and B cells within the lymph nodes.

Lymph Nodes Tissue that acts as filtering stations along the lymphatic channels. Lymph nodes are found throughout the body and are most obvious in the armpits, neck, and groin.

Lymphocyte A white cell that normally makes up about 25% of the total white cell count, but increases in the presence of infection. There are two groups of lymphocytes, T cells and B cells.

Lysis Destruction of the cell membrane, usually through the action of lytic molecules eating holes in the cell membrane.

Lysozyme A powerful digestive enzyme in the lysosomes of macrophages that aids in antigen destruction.

Macrophage A large white cell that phagocytizes and digests foreign matter and debris in the body. It exposes digested an antigenic peptide on its cell membrane and presents it a to T cell for destruction. Some macrophages are fixed in organs, such as the liver, spleen, and tissues, while others circulate in the blood.

Major Histocompatibility Complex (MHC) Molecules Molecules coded for by genes located on chromosome 6. Class I and class II molecules are essential for the presentation of a peptide fragment to T cells.

Malaria A blood disease endemic to many areas of the world. It can be transmitted through a blood transfusion or mosquito bite. The organism that causes malaria is a protozoan parasite that lives in the red cell. Infection permanently prohibits blood donation.

Margination The adherence of certain white cells to the endothelial lining of blood vessels, where they are available to enter the tissues when needed.

Mast Cell A basophil or basophil-like cell that leaves the vasculature and takes up residence in the tissues where it releases histamine and other molecules that play a role in antigen destruction.

Megakaryocyte A large cell found in hematopoietic marrow that is the precursor to platelets. A megakaryocyte fragments its cytoplasm to form platelets.

Membrane Attack Complex (MAC) A group of five complement components that attach to microorganisms and to the membranes of infected and allogeneic cells. They bore holes leading to antigen and cell destruction.

Metabolism The process whereby ingested food products are broken down into simpler molecules through a series of chemical reactions.

Monocyte A white cell that leaves the circulation and enters the tissue. On entering tissue, this cell matures into a macrophage.

Mononuclear Phagocytic System (MPS) Aggregates of macrophages found in various organs and tissues, such as the liver, spleen, and lung. Also referred to as the reticuloendothelial system (RES).

Mucus A viscous fluid secreted by mucous membranes that acts as a protective barrier over mucous membranes. A lubricant that consists chiefly of glycoproteins, particularly mucin.

Mucous Membrane The smooth lining of many organ systems of the body, such as the gut, bladder, and vagina, among others.

Myeloperoxidases One of several chemical substances found in the granules and lysosomes of neutrophils and macrophages that aid in antigen destruction.

Myeloproliferative Disorder The term used to define conditions that occur in bone marrow and interfere with the production of blood cells.

Myocardium The layer of the heart that is the heart muscle. It is responsible for heart contraction. This layer suffers damage following a heart attack, or myocardial infarction.

Necrosis The destruction of tissue due to decreased or absent blood flow. The arrest of blood flow is usually due to thrombus formation in the vasculature.

Nephron The functional unit of the kidneys responsible for filtering and cleansing the blood.

Neutrophil A granular white cell that phagocytizes and engulfs bacteria and debris. An increase of neutrophils occurs during acute infection.

Nonwash Device An autologous blood recovery system that collects whole blood shed during surgery. Once the collection reservoir is full, the collected blood is reinfused into the patient. No cleansing of the blood occurs.

Normovolemic A normal volume of circulating blood.

Nucleus A protoplasmic body in a cell that contains the hereditary material of the cell and controls the cell's metabolism, growth, and reproduction. Enucleated refers to the absence of a nucleus.

O Blood Group One of four groups of blood in the ABO classification system. Group O blood has no antigens on its membrane, and its plasma containsboth anti-A and anti-B antibodies. Individuals with group O blood can only receive group O Packed Red Cells.

Opportunistic Infection Any infection that attacks an individual with a compromised immune system, for example, someone with AIDS.

Opsonization The coating of antigen with antibody and/or complement components. Opsonization enhances phagocytosis and thereby aids in the destruction of antigen.

Organelles Bodies suspended in the cytoplasm of cells, such as the mitochondria, Golgi bodies, and ribosomes, among others.

Organ Rejection The rejection of a donor organ generated by the immune response following transplant. Organ rejection may be caused (1) by the recipient's immune system or (2) by donor lymphocytes in the transplanted organ.

Osmosis The movement of water against a concentration gradient. Water passes through a semipermeable membrane from a region of lower solute concentration to a region of higher solute concentration. Water movement stops when the concentrations are balanced.

Osmotic Pressure The pressure generated in the blood and tissues that depends on the concentration of proteins and other solutes, such as electrolytes.

Ostia The opening of blood vessels or other tubular structures.

Oxygen (O_2) A colorless, odorless gas that is essential to all cells of the body for cellular reactions, such as metabolism.

Oxygenated Blood Blood that has passed through the lungs and exchanged its carbon dioxide for oxygen. This blood is pumped from the left ventricle to the various organs and tissues.

Oxygen-free Radicals Atoms of oxygen in the lysosomes and granules of neutrophils and macrophages that aid in antigen destruction.

Oxyhemoglobin Hemoglobin saturated with oxygen.

Packed Red Cells A blood component derived from whole blood by removing most of the plasma. Now the most common blood product used in transfusion. It is the only component that can be stored in additive systems.

Parasite An organism that lives on or in the host deriving nourishment from it. Some parasites cause inflammation, while others cause infection and destroy tissue. Examples of human parasites include: fungi, yeast, bacteria, protozoa, worms, and viruses.

Passive Immunity Immunity provided by antibody produced in sources outside the body, for example, when cells or serum from an immunized individual are transferred into a nonimmunized individual. Used in young children to prevent the development of certain diseases such as diphtheria.

Pathogen Any microorganism that enters the body and causes a disease or infection.

Perfusion The movement of blood through the vasculature. Usually used in reference to capillary blood flow.

pH A logarithmic term that provides a close estimate of the hydrogen ion concentration [H^+] in solution. The pH describes the acidity or alkalinity of a solution. If the pH is low, the solution is acidic; if it is high, the solution is alkaline.

Phagocyte A white cell that surrounds and engulfs foreign organisms and cellular debris for destruction and removal from the body.

Phagocytosis The process by which certain blood and tissue cells (such as macrophages) engulf and digest organisms for destruction. Usually performed by white cells in response to foreign invaders.

Phospholipids   Molecules containing a nitrogenous base, phosphoric acid, and a fatty acid. They are found in many body cells and function in numerous important biological reactions, such as coagulation.

Plaque   The buildup of atheroma (fatty deposits) along the inner wall (endothelium) of blood vessels, usually within arteries, such as the coronary arteries.

Plasma   The straw-colored liquid portion of blood consisting of water, proteins, electrolytes, glucose, fats, vitamins, and hormones. The formed elements of blood are suspended in plasma.

Plasma Cell   A transformed B cell that produces antibody in response to antigen.

Plasma-free Hemoglobin   Hemoglobin that is released from damaged red cells. Released into the plasma, plasma-free hemoglobin is removed from the body by the kidneys. It may tinge urine a pink color.

Plasmin   The enzyme produced by the cleavage of plasminogen into plasmin for the dissolution of a fibrin clot.

Plasminogen   The inactive form of plasmin that circulates in blood until cleaved into plasmin by tissue plasminogen activator (tPA).

Platelet   A small, disk-shaped enucleated body in blood that is essential for hemostasis.

Pneumonia   A condition in the lungs that interferes with the exchange of oxygen and carbon dioxide between the blood and the lungs. It may be caused by either a bacterium or virus. If left untreated, it can be fatal, especially in the elderly and young.

Polycythemia   A serious, life-threatening condition characterized by too many red cells in the circulation. Blood flow through the capillaries becomes difficult. Patients often undergo chemotherapy to decrease the number of red cells.

Polymorphism   The condition of having a range of many similar forms within a species. For example, HLA genes code for similar yet many very different HLA molecules in humans.

Polypeptide   A polypeptide is a part of a protein molecule. Chains of amino acids attached together form a polypeptide molecule, or protein.

Pooled Platelets   Platelets collected from multiple donors and mixed together for use in transfusion. Multiple donors, however, increase the chance of disease transmission and transfusion reaction. Pooled platelets are often used after bypass surgery.

Pore Size   The size of the opening in a blood filter. Filters have different pore sizes depending on their intended use. Standard blood filters in administration sets have pore sizes of 150 to 270μ. They filter out large particles. Microaggregate filters have pore sizes that range from 20 to 40μ and can filter out very small particles.

Predonation A term that refers to the collection of autologous blood weeks before its anticipated use during surgery. The individual may donate up to 4 pints, depending on the estimated needs of the operation.

Progenitor Cells Stem cells found outside the bone marrow within the peripheral blood or umbilical cord that have the ability to produce more of themselves as well as mature blood cells. They are used to repopulate the bone marrow with blood cells following chemotherapy and/or radiation therapy.

Protease Inhibitors A relatively new group of drugs used to treat individuals with HIV. The drugs have shown much promise in reducing the viral load within the blood.

Protozoan A microorganism that is responsible for several diseases, including malaria, serum sickness, and *Pneumocystis carinii* pneumonia, among others.

Pseudopods The long armlike extensions formed by platelets when generating a platelet plug. The term pseudopod means "false foot."

Pulmonary Artery The artery that leaves the right ventricle of the heart and carries deoxygenated blood to the lungs for elimination of carbon dioxide and uptake of oxygen.

Pulmonary Edema The buildup of fluid in the lung tissue that leads to difficulty in breathing and if not treated, death.

Pulmonary Veins Vessels that carry oxygenated blood from the lungs to the right atrium of the heart.

Reagent In this book, reagent refers to commercially prepared products used to identify the presence of another substance. Examples are commercially prepared anti-A and anti-B antibodies used to identify the A and B antigens on the red cell.

Regeneration The process whereby cells, especially stem cells, produce more of themselves to replenish their numbers.

Renal Failure Also known as kidney failure, this condition occurs when the kidneys no longer cleanse the blood. There are many causes, one of which occurs following an incompatible transfusion reaction.

Respiration The exchange of the respiratory gases between the blood and lungs and the blood and tissues.

Reticuloendothelial System (RES) A unit of the body made up of phagocytic cells, including Kupffer's cells of the liver, splenic macrophages of the spleen, and dendritic cells of bone marrow. RES functions in the immune response by fighting infection and ridding the body of cellular debris. It is also called the mononuclear phagocytic system (MPS).·

Retrovirus A family of viruses equipped with both reverse transcriptase (enzyme that converts RNA into DNA) and RNA (its genetic material). Most organisms have DNA. HIV is a retrovirus.

Rh Antigen An antigen present on the red cells of about 85% of the population. Also known as the D antigen. It is the antigen responsible for hemolytic disease of the newborn (HDN). Individuals with the antigen are Rh positive (Rh-) and those lacking it are Rh negative (Rh-). Blood transfusion recipients are classified for Rh status as well as ABO status.

Right Lymphatic Duct The lymphatic duct that drains lymphatic fluid from the right side of the body and returns it to the circulatory system.

Self-Tolerance The ability of the body to recognize its own tissue and as a result not mount an immune response against it.

Sensitization The term used to indicate primary exposure to an antigen. Also referred to as immunization.

Septicemia The widespread destruction of tissue due to the presence of bacteria or their toxins in the blood. It can be the cause of DIC.

Sequestration The retention of platelets in the spleen. One-third of platelets are normally sequestered in the spleen.

Serine Proteases A term used to describe several of the coagulation factors. Serine proteases are enzymes that cleave coagulation factors. Cleavage confers activity on these factors.

Seroconversion Evidence of a disease process occurring in the body provided by testing that identifies the presence of antigen or antibody in serum.

Seronegative A term indicating that there is no evidence of disease in the blood. In other words, testing shows no antibody or antigen.

Seropositive A term indicating that there is evidence of disease in the blood. In other words, there are detectable antigen and/or antibody.

Serum Plasma minus fibrinogen. If left to stand, a sample of blood forms a clot at the bottom of the tube. The remaining straw-colored fluid portion that rises to the top is called serum.

Shock The condition that exists when inadequate blood flow is returned to the heart. Loss of consciousness often occurs.

Single-donor Apheresis A procedure whereby a specific component is removed from a donor's blood and used to treat a disease or condition in another individual.

Soluble Having the ability to dissolve in a solvent.

Solute That which is dissolved in a solvent.

Solvent The liquid part of a solution.

Stem Cell An immortal cell in hematopoietic bone marrow capable of producing all blood cells.

Stroma 1. The spongy fibrous matrix in the center of bones. 2. The remnants of cells that have been hemolyzed or lysed. Also known as ghosts.

Subcutaneous (s.c.) Under the skin. Usually used in reference to an injection.

Superior Vena Cava The major vein of the body that drains blood from the head and upper body and returns it to the right atrium of the heart.

Superoxides Molecules released from the granules and lysosomes of neutrophils and macrophages that aid in antigen destruction.

Systemic Throughout the body.

Target Cell In this book, target cell refers to any cell destined for destruction by the components of the immune system.

T Cell A small lymphocyte that matures in the thymus and is the chief agent in cell-mediated immunity. T cells stimulate (1) B cells to produce antibody and (2) other T cells to lyse antigen.

T Cell-dependent Antigen An antigen that must be presented to T cells for recognition and destruction. Protein antigen is a T cell-dependent antigen.

T Cell-independent Antigen Any nonprotein antigen. Non-protein antigen does not have to be presented to T cells for destruction. Carbohydrate and lipid antigens are T cell-independent antigens.

T Cell Receptor The protein complex on the T cell membrane that attaches to an antigen-MHC complex. Once the T cell has attached itself to the antigen-MHC complex, antigen recognition by the T cell occurs.

Thoracic Duct One of two major vessels of the lymphatic system. This vessel drains lymphatic fluid from the left side of the body and returns it to the circulatory system.

Thorax The chest cavity, which is separated from the abdominal cavity by the large flat muscle called the diaphragm.

Thrombin A coagulation factor found in plasma and formed from prothrombin, factor X, and calcium. It cleaves fibrinogen to fibrin and is necessary for clotting.

Thrombocyte A blood platelet.

Thrombocythemia A disease state usually caused by a disease of the stem cells and characterized by very high platelet numbers. The condition may cause increased bleeding or increased clot formation. Increased bleeding is more likely.

Thrombocytopenia A condition characterized by a lower than normal platelet count resulting in bleeding and easy bruising. Causes include drug use, the immune response, neoplastic diseases, and radiation, among others.

Thrombocytosis An increase of platelet numbers within the blood. There are several types of thrombocytosis. When it is a disease, it is referred to as thrombocythemia.

Thrombolysis The breakup or dissolution of a blood clot, either naturally or following thrombolytic therapy. The thrombolytic agent may be naturally occurring or synthetic.

Thrombopoietin Any growth factor that has an affect on the development of platelets.

Thrombosis The formation of a blood clot (thrombus) within the vasculature. It can occur, for example, in coronary artery disease.

Thrombotic Disorder An abnormality of the blood that causes increased blood clot formation within the vasculature. It may be caused by either an acquired or hereditary defect.

Tissue Factor (TF) The phospholipid released from damaged tissue that binds with calcium and

factor VII to produce factor VIIa. TF initiates the extrinsic pathway of coagulation.

Tissue Plasminogen Activator (tPA) A fibrinolytic agent produced by most body cells that causes lysis of a blood clot. It is prepared commercially for treating clot formation, such as those that occur in heart attacks.

Tissue Typing Testing done prior to organ and bone marrow transplantation that identifies HLA and antibody to HLA.

Total Blood Volume The amount of blood in the circulatory system. It is about 5 to 6 liters in an adult.

Toxins Molecules released by microorganisms that act by poisoning cells and causing disease.

Transfusion Reaction The reaction in the body to the infusion of blood or blood component(s). It may be mild or severe and in the latter can lead to death. A transfusion reaction occurs when antigen or antibody in donor blood react with antigen or antibody in recipient plasma.

Tumor Necrosis Factor A class of cytokines that plays an essential role in tumor immunology by helping to destroy malignant cells.

Urticaria An allergic reaction occurring in the skin and manifested by elevated patches of red skin that are very itchy.

Uremia The presence of urine in

the blood indicating renal disease. It is also known as blood poisoning.

Vaccine A weakened (attenuated) or killed virus that is administered by injection or by mouth to induce active immunity to a specific disease. An example is the polio vaccine.

Variable Region The region of the antibody molecule located at the ends of the "Y arms," which are the points where antigen binds to antibody.

Vascular Integrity When vessels of the body are intact and blood circulates in an uninterrupted fashion.

Vascular Space The area occupied by the vessels of the vascular system. A term used when referring to blood or fluid in circulation.

Vascular System Another name for the circulatory system.

Vasculature A broad term that refers to the vessels of the circulatory system.

Vasculitis An inflammation of the blood vessels that can lead to DIC.

Vasoconstriction The decrease in vessel lumen size following the release of certain molecules such as histamine. Blood flow is reduced through constricted vessels.

Vasodilators Chemicals that cause blood vessels to relax and increase the size of their lumen.

Vasovagal Response A response that occurs in the body following intense pain. It is characterized by many symptoms similar to those associated with an anaphylactic reaction.

Venous Stasis The cessation or slowing of blood flow through a vessel due to occlusion. Prolonged immobility, such as sitting, can be a cause.

Ventilation The movement of air into and out of the lungs. The movement of air into the lungs is inspiration and the movement of air out of the lungs is expiration.

Venules The smallest vessels associated with the venous system. They originate at the distal end of the capillary bed.

Viremia The presence of virus or viral particles in the blood.

Virus A protein-covered core of nucleic acid. Although it is not considered living, a virus can reproduce itself in the host cell. The protein coat is called a capsid.

Vitamin K A fat-soluble vitamin essential for blood coagulation and important in certain energy transfer reactions. It is found in green leafy vegetables, egg yoke, yogurt, and fish liver oils.

Von Willebrand Factor (vWF) A molecule released by platelets and endothelium that plays a role in hemostasis. It is bound to factor VIII and transports this factor in its inactive form.

Volume Overload The condition that occurs when the vascular system has too much fluid. Edema is very common following volume overload.

Warfarin A synthetic anticoagulant with the trade name Coumadin™. It prevents blood clots from forming by blocking the action of vitamin K.

Wash Devices Systems used during surgery to collect, wash, and reinfuse autologous blood. They are used in intraoperative blood salvage and in postoperative wound drainage collection. Only red cells and a small amount of saline are reinfused; all other components are washed into a waste bag.

Western Blot Test A more specific blood test for HIV than the ELISA. It detects the presence of antibody to HIV in a blood sample. The test is usually done following two positive results from an ELISA. A confirmatory result is indicative of an HIV infection.

Whole Blood Blood that has had no components removed from it. It is collected in an anticoagulant-preservative—CPD, CP2D, or CPDA-1. Whole blood is usually processed into its components for multiple uses.

Windkessel Effect The dilation and contraction of the aorta when blood from the left ventricle is ejected into the aorta. The expansion and contraction of the aorta forces blood forward.

Yellow Marrow The nonhematopoietic marrow in the center of long bones consisting mostly of fat.

Yolk Sac That part of the developing fetus and embryo used as a food source by the fetus and embyro.

BLOOD TESTS

Contents

Electrolytes

Other Tests

Preface

Blood, The Most Tested Tissue

The body tissue most often tested is blood. Blood tests provide "windows" on the health status of body systems and therefore of the individual. Test results and values are valuable diagnostic tools in modern medicine to assess patient health, determine clotting status pre- and post-operatively, monitor disease therapy, and conduct routine health exams. In this book, the term "value" is used when the test reports a number, and "result" is used when no number is reported. A test value indicates the normal range for the substance being tested. An assay is a test technique for determining the quantitative or qualitative presence of a substance. There are many types of assays, such as immunoassays, chemical, and biological. The clinical assessments and decisions made in treating a disease or condition are derived in large part from the values and results of blood tests. However, blood sudies give only part of the clinical picture and must be analyzed in conjunction with the physical signs and symptoms exhibited by the individual. Understanding blood test results and the conditions or diseases indicated by them is essential for the treatment and care of patients.

Components Used in Blood Testing

Blood tests utilize blood samples from whole blood, plasma, serum, or cellular components. Specimens used in whole blood and plasma studies must be collected in anticoagulated tubes; tests requiring serum do not need to be anticoagulated. In this book, the sample used is indicated beneath the test title.

Sampling Sites for Blood Tests

Most blood tests use a sample of venous blood. Venous samples are usually drawn from the veins in the antecubital fossa located in the bend of the elbow on the medial aspect (underside) of the forearm. They also may be drawn from central venous catheters, such as a central venous pressure (CVP) line or a Swan-Ganz line. Blood samples should not be drawn from an arm in which an I.V. is being administered because inaccurate results or values are likely.

Some blood tests utilize arterial samples (blood drawn from an artery). For example, blood gas analysis. Arterial samples are usually drawn from the radial artery located on the medial aspect (underside) of the wrist. They can also be withdrawn from an arterial line, which is a catheter placed in an artery. Very small samples of blood, such as capillary blood samples, can be obtained by doing a finger or ear lobe stick on an adult and a great toe or heel stick on an infant. Capillary samples are usually drawn into microcapillary tubes.

Blood collection tubes have color coded tops that identify the additive present in the blood tube. The color coded tops are red (no additive; for tests using serum samples), green (heparin; for tests using plasma samples), lavender (EDTA; ethylenediamine tetraacetate; for tests using whole blood), blue (citrate; for clotting studies using plasma samples), gray (oxalate; for glucose determination using serum or plasma), marble top tube (silicone gel; for separating serum from blood cells), and black (oxalate; for clotting studies using plasma).

Handling of Blood Specimens

Proper handling of blood specimens, from collection to testing, is absolutely necessary in order to ensure accurate results. Inaccurate results can lead to unwarranted treatment procedures, cost valuable time, and increase health care costs. Blood specimens should be labeled properly, and any pertinent information that may affect the test results should be noted on the label.

People who handle blood or blood products should (1) always wear gloves and protective eyewear and (2) exercise great care around an exposed needle. Blood tubes must be carefully filled to prevent tube breakage or explosion. As soon as possible after withdrawing the sample, the phlebotomist should replace the needle cover to avoid being stuck and then wash his or her hands. Anyone accidentally cut by a broken tube or stuck by a needle should force the wound to bleed and contact a physician immediately.

International System Units

International system units, commonly referred to as SI units, were established as a common system for medical personnel to use in reporting test results. Despite the attempt to unify test result reporting, many people are reluctant to change and continue to use the conventional system. The laboratory test values provided in this book are reported in both conventional units and recommended International System Units (SI). The SI units appear in parenthesis.

Note

We wish to thank the staff of the Clinical Laboratory at Emerson Hospital, Concord, Massachusetts for reviewing the blood tests in this book for accuracy.

TEST 1
Complete Blood Count (CBC)
(Whole Blood)

The CBC is one of the most frequently requested blood studies. A compendium of blood tests, the CBC provides a complete picture of blood components. Tests that make up the CBC results include:

- Hemoglobin concentration (Hgb)
- RBC count
- Hematocrit (Hct)
- Erythrocyte indices
- Blood smear for examining RBCs and platelets
- Platelet count
- WBC count
- WBC differential

Depending on the results of the CBC, further studies may be required.

Notes

Not all laboratories provide a blood smear with the CBC report. The CBC is usually done if other blood test results indicate it is needed.

Not all laboratories routinely report the WBC differential with the CBC.

TEST 2
Peripheral Blood Smear
(Whole Blood)

The peripheral blood smear provides much useful information: it gives an accurate picture of the different blood cells and any structural abnormalities they have. The smear is examined under microscope to study the morphology of blood cells. (For more information on cellular morphologies, refer to a more detailed hematology text.)

Uses

- To distinguish the morphological features of blood cells

TEST 3
Red Blood Cell Count
(Whole Blood)

The RBC count measures the number of RBCs in a μL or mm^3 of blood. The number is generated by electronic counters that provide fast and accurate results. Prior to the use of electronic counters the count was done manually under a microscope.

Values

The number of RBCs in a μL or mm^3 of blood varies according to the age and sex of the patient as well as the altitude at which the individual lives. The following are normal values for individuals living at sea level:

Adult males: $4.9\text{-}6.2 \times 10^6/\mu L$ $(4.9\text{-}6.2 \times 10^{12}/L)$

Adult females: $4.2\text{-}5.5 \times 10^6/\mu L$ $(4.2\text{-}5.5 \times 10^{12}/L)$

Pregnant females: Somewhat lower

Children: $4.9\text{-}6.8 \times 10^6/\mu L$ $(4.9\text{-}6.8 \times 10^{12}/L)$

Infants: $4.2\text{-}5.5 \times 10^6/\mu L$ $(4.2\text{-}5.5 \times 10^{12}/L)$

Infants about the age of two months: The number drops to $3.5\text{-}3.8 \times 10^6/\mu L$ $(3.5\text{-}3.8 \times 10^{12}/L)$.

Persons living at high altitudes: A higher RBC count. Less O_2 is present in the atmosphere, and more RBCs are needed to transport O_2.

Uses

- To measure the number of RBCs in a μL of blood. The RBC count provides no other information about the RBC.
- To diagnose blood disorders in conjunction with other blood tests
- To furnish numbers for calculating erythrocyte indices, the mean corpuscular volume (MCV), and the mean corpuscular hemoglobin (MCH)

Causes of an Increased RBC Count

Erythrocytosis, or secondary polycythemia. Erythrocytosis is most often found in people with chronic obstructive pulmonary disease (COPD) and children with cyanotic heart disease. Dehydration, or hemoconcentration (Watery diarrhea and shock are common causes.). High altitude. Cardiovascular disease. Polycythemia vera is a blood disease of stem cells (see Ch. 4, Red Blood Cells).

Notes

An increased RBC count can make the blood thick and increase the likelihood of thrombi (clot) formation. Administration of I.V. fluid, such as 0.9% normal saline (NS), may be necessary to decrease blood viscosity and thrombi formation. Cardiovascular status must be assessed first to make sure that the patient can withstand increased fluid volume. The administration of too much fluid puts the individual at risk of congestive heart failure (CHF).

Causes of a Decreased RBC Count

Hemodilution. Hemorrhage more than a day old. Loss of blood. Hemolysis. Deficiencies, such as vitamin, iron (Fe), or growth factor (erythropoietin). Bone marrow suppression from chemotherapy and radiation therapy. Bone marrow tumors. Kidney failure. Some leukemias. Pregnancy. Multiple myeloma. Chronic infections.

Notes

A decreased RBC count is indicative of anemia, which is not a true blood disease but rather an indication of a disease or condition. Depending on the severity of the anemia, the individual may have trouble supplying enough oxygen to the tissues. Signs and symptoms of anemia can include the following: increased heart rate, rapid rate of breathing, and fast pulse, among others.

TEST 4
Hematocrit (Hct, Crit, Packed Cell Volume, PCV)
(Whole Blood)

The Hct is defined as the volume of Packed RBCs in 100 mL or 1 dL of whole blood. Results are reported as a percent. The Hct evaluates the percentage of RBCs in the blood. The test often utilizes a microcapillary tube, for which only a small amount of blood is needed. The microcapillary tube sample is placed in a centrifuge and spun to separate cells and plasma. The level of RBCs indicated by the capillary tube reveals the Hct.

Values

Hematocrit values vary according to many factors—age, sex, and altitude, the size of the RBCs, and the sodium (Na^+) and glucose ($C_6H_{12}O_6$) content of the plasma. High concentrations of Na^+ and/or glucose cause

RBCs to take in fluid and swell, making the RBCs larger and thereby increasing the Hct. The following are normal values:

Adult males: 42-52% (0.42-0.54)

Adult females: 38-46% (0.38-0.46)

Pregnant females: A lower Hct, especially during the last trimester

Children: 30-40% (0.30-0.40)

Infants: 55-68% (0.55-0.68)

Uses

- To furnish numbers for calculating erythrocyte indices
- To aid in establishing fluid balance
- To diagnose blood disorders
- To measure the percentage of RBCs within the circulation
- To determine the amount of blood loss following surgery, trauma, and other conditions

Causes of an Increased Hct

Polycythemia. Erythrocytosis. Hemoconcentration (loss of plasma from the blood). Burns. Late-stage emphysema. Acidosis caused by diabetes. Some obstetrical complications.

Notes

Dehydration, or hypovolemia, gives a higher rather than a true Hct. The Hct is a percentage of red cells to plasma volume and, therefore, any deficit in the plasma volume causes a false increase in the Hct. Causes of decreased plasma volume can include watery diarrhea and decreased fluid intake. An increase in the Hct may require fluid administration to decrease viscosity and to lessen the chances of increased thrombi formation. Cardiac function must always be assessed before the administration of fluid.

Causes of a Decreased Hct

Blood loss. Anemia. Increased levels of RBC destruction (hemolysis). Hemodilution. Absence of necessary chemicals for growth and maturation (iron [Fe], vitamins, erythropoietin). Bone marrow suppression due to chemotherapy, radiation therapy, bone marrow tumors. Some leukemias. Hodgkin's disease. Some malignancies. Liver disease. Kidney failure. Some autoimmune diseases. Some antibiotics. Overhydration. Fluid retention. Poor kidney function.

Signs and Symptoms of Anemia

Paleness of the skin, mucous membranes, eyes, nail beds. Possible increase in blood pressure and pulse rates. Weakness. Fatigue. Frequently, signs of dyspnea (shortness of breath). Increased heart rate. Increased rate of breathing.

Notes

The Hct is approximately 3 times (3x) the Hgb concentration. It is important to determine whether the decreased Hct is due to acute or chronic anemia. Individuals with chronic anemia are better able to tolerate a low Hct because their bodies have learned to compensate for a decrease in RBCs. A decreased Hct may require a blood transfusion to elevate the number of RBCs.

A unit of blood raises the Hct of an adult by about 0.03 (3%). Transfusions can present problems, such as disease transmission, transfusion reaction, or alloimmunization to donor antigens. These factors must be considered before making the decision to transfuse.

TEST 5
Total Hemoglobin (Hgb)
(Whole Blood)

The Hgb test measures the amount of Hgb in 100 mL (1 dL) of whole blood. To determine the amount of Hgb, the blood is converted into a colored compound, which is measured by light. This process is called spectrophotometry or colorimetry.

Values

Adult males: 13.5-18 g/100 mL or dL (135-180 g/L)

Adult females: 12-16 g/dL (120-160 g/L)

Pregnant females: Lower values. These individuals may need iron supplements.

Middle-aged adults: Values drop slightly about this time of life.

Children: 11-13 g/dL (110-130 g/L)

The Hgb concentration varies with the age and sex of the child.

Infants: 15-24 g/dL (150-240 g/L)

Individuals living at high altitudes have increased Hgb.

Normally the Hgb concentration is about 1/3 of the Hct.

Uses

- To furnish numbers for calculating erythrocyte indices
- To follow the course of diseases
- To monitor therapy
- To detect abnormal types of Hgb. After detection, further studies are needed.
- To help identify certain anemias

Causes of an Increased Hgb

An increase in the amount of Hgb in the blood signifies an increase either in the number of RBCs or in the size of the RBC. Normally RBCs contain the maximum amount of Hgb, therefore any increase is abnormal. Dehydration. Polycythemia. High altitudes. Chronic obstructive pulmonary disease (COPD). Congestive heart failure (CHF). Some drugs.

Symptoms

Signs of Dehydration. Thirst. Loss of skin turgor. Dry mucous membranes. Tachycardia. Tachypnea (rapid breathing). Lowered blood pressure.

Causes of a Decreased Hgb

Any decrease in the number of RBCs (anemia) has a direct affect on the Hgb level. Blood loss. Hemolysis. Decreased RBC production. Overhydration. Liver disease. Some malignancies. Some leukemias. Abnormal hemoglobins. Thalassemia. Pregnancy. Some drugs. Fluid retention. Hemodilution. Anemias.

Notes

Certain types of anemia (e.g., iron deficiency, microcytic) are likely to produce cells with less than normal amounts of Hgb. A low Hgb concentration is not considered an indication of anemia until the Hgb concentration is below 13 g/dL in males and 11 g/dL in females.

TEST 6
Hemoglobin Electrophoresis
(Whole Blood)

This is not a routine test. It is used to determine the presence of abnormal types of Hgb, which are not normally in blood. There are many abnormal types of Hgb, but only a small percent cause oxygen transport problems. A sample of blood is placed in an agar gel that is subjected to electrophoresis (an electric current). The different Hgb molecules migrate from the negative pole to the positive pole. As they migrate, they form different bands in the agar gel. An appearance of more than three bands (Hgb A, A_2, and F) indicates abnormal types of Hgb. The result of the Hgb electrophoresis is compared with normal Hgb bands to identify abnormal Hgbs. Once abnormal Hgbs are identified, further studies may be required. Some types of abnormal Hgb are electrophoretically undetectable and can be detected only by staining RBCs with methyl violet or other specific dyes.

Hgb A makes up about 95% of adult Hgb, with Hgb F and Hgb A_2 making up less than 5%.

Values

Hgb A: 95%

Hgb A_2: about 1%

Hgb F: < 2%

Uses

▪ To detect various abnormal types of Hgb, such as thalassemia (Hgb F), sickle-cell anemia (Hgb S), and others

Notes

Abnormal Hgbs are more serious if the affected individual is homozygous (has two defective genes) for the defect. If only one defective gene is present, the individual is heterozygous and has the trait. Most forms of abnormal Hgb are genetic. Some, such as Hgb M (methemoglobin) or methemoglobinemia, may be caused by certain drugs, such as oxidizing agents. Abnormal Hgbs may cause hemolytic anemia.

Thalassemia is indicated if elevated levels of Hgb F are found 6 months following birth.

Hgb S, or sickle-cell Hgb, is the most common Hgb abnormality. It is most commonly found in African Americans. Signs and symptoms of Hgb S are weakness, fatigue, dyspnea, swollen joints, chest pain, and bone pain. These symptoms are usually caused by sickled cells blocking the microvasculature of organs.

TEST 7
Sickle-Cell
(Whole Blood)

This test screens RBCs for the presence of the abnormal hemoglobin molecule known as sickle-cell hemoglobin (Hgb S). The test is simple and easy to perform, and the results are accurate. Results are reported as positive or negative. A cloudy suspension in the tube indicates a positive reaction and the presence of Hgb S. Normal hemoglobin (Hgb A) and other Hgb molecules remain in solution. The suspension is unclouded. Therefore the test is negative.

Individuals homozygous for Hgb S carry two defective genes, whereas heterozygous individuals carry one defective gene and one normal gene. Hgb S individuals have life-long hemolytic anemia. Heterozygous individuals usually show no sign of the disease, except in some situations such as low oxygen tension, hypoxia during anesthesia, and pneumonias, among others. Individuals who are not carriers or homozygous for Hgb S have no evidence of Hgb S in their RBCs.

Uses

- To screen individuals for Hgb S
- To aid in genetic counseling

Notes

Sickling of the RBCs occurs in the vasculature. Causes of sickling include the following: release of oxygen to the tissue by Hgb S (deoxyhemoglobin), low serum osmolarity, increased body temperature, and acidosis, among others. Sickled RBCs block the microvasculature of many organs.

TEST 8
Erythrocyte Indices: MCV, MCH, MCHC

Erythrocyte indices include:

A. The Mean Corpuscular Volume (MCV)

B. The Mean Corpuscular Hemoglobin (MCH)

C. The Mean Corpuscular Hemoglobin Concentration (MCHC)

The erythrocyte indices are calculated using the results furnished by three other tests—the RBC Count, Hct, and Hgb. The results of erythrocyte indices provide valuable information about the size, the color (Hgb concentration), and the weight of Hgb in the average RBC.

Values

MCV in adults: 84-98 μ^3 (cubic microns) (80-96 fL [femtoliter])

Children: Decreased values

Newborns: Increased values

MCH in adults: 26-32 pg (picograms) (26-32 pg or 1.7-2.0 fmol)

Children: Same

Newborns: Increased values

MCHC: 30-36% (0.30-0.36 mmol/L)

Uses

- To diagnose blood disorders
- To monitor the course of therapy
- To differentiate different types of anemia

A. The Mean Corpuscular Volume

The MCV determines the size of the average RBC. The result is expressed in a ratio of the Hct to the size of the RBC (see below). The MCV indicates whether the RBCs is normal (normocytic), or increased (macrocytic), or decreased (microcytic) in size.

$$MCV = Hct \times 10/RBC \ (\times 10^6/\mu L).$$

Results

Normocytic Cells   If the MCV is in the range of values, the cells are normocytic. Some types of anemia, such as sickle-cell, can have normal-sized cells.

Microcytic Cells   If the MCV is less than 84 μ^3, the RBC is smaller than normal size. Microcytic cells appear in certain types of anemia, such as iron deficiency anemia, and in a type of thalassemia called Cooley's anemia. Some malignancies. Lead poisoning. Hemoglobinopathies. Following radiation. Rheumatoid arthritis.

Macrocytic Cells   If the MCV is greater than 98 μ^3, the RBCs are larger than normal in size. Macrocytic cells occur in some types of diseases and anemias. Pernicious anemia. Vitamin deficiency anemia.

Abnormal DNA synthesis. Increased reticulocytes (reticulocytosis). Aplastic anemia. Hypothyroidism. Alcoholism. Some drugs.

B. The Mean Corpuscular Hemoglobin (MHC)

The MCH measures the amount of Hgb in a single RBC.

$$MCH = Hgb(g/dL) \times 10/RBCs \ (\times 10^6/\mu L)$$

C. The Mean Corpuscular Hemoglobin Concentration (MCHC)

The MCHC measures the percentage of the RBC occupied by Hgb.

$$MCHC = Hgb \ (g/dL) \times 100/Hct$$

The MCH and MCHC are evaluated together because they indicate the amount of Hgb in RBCs. RBCs can accommodate only so much Hgb, and it is rare for cells to have more than the normal amount.

Normochromic RBCs   Many anemias do not affect the color of the RBC, and are therefore referred to as normochromic. Normochromic anemia can occur, for example, in an individual who has lost a large amount of blood from surgery or trauma.

Hyperchromic RBCs   RBCs that have a redder than normal color due to increased amounts of Hgb are considered hyperchromic. Hereditary spherocytosis, which is a rare genetic disease, causes RBCs to have more Hgb and a redder than normal color.

Hypochromic RBCs   These RBCs have fewer rather than more of the normal number of Hgb molecules. RBCs with a red color lighter than normal are called hypochromic. Hypochromic RBCs are common in iron deficiency anemia, because iron is needed to make Hgb.

TEST 9
Reticulocyte Count
(Whole Blood)

This test measures the number of reticulocytes in blood. The test values are reported either as a percent or in numbers of reticulocytes/μL. Reticulocytes are immature RBCs occasionally found in the circulation. After reticulocytes are released from bone marrow, they mature within the circulation in about 4 days. An increase in their numbers may signify that the therapy for anemia is working or that a disease process may be involved. Reticulocytes provide valuable information regarding bone marrow function and the effectiveness of therapy for anemia.

Values

Adults: About 0.5-2% or 25,000-75,000 cells/μL reticulocytes in circulation

Children: Same

Infants: Slightly higher levels. Levels decrease within the first month after birth.

Pregnant females: May have higher levels than nonpregnant females

Patients with some types of anemia and undergoing therapy for the anemia can have increased reticulocytes. Individuals with certain types of congenital anemias have a higher reticulocyte count due to the constant destruction and production of new RBCs.

Uses

- To distinguish anemias
- To follow patient response to therapy
- To evaluate blood loss
- To evaluate bone marrow function

Causes of Increased Reticulocytes

Anemias. In anemic individuals, reticulocytes are released into the circulation more quickly than normal, most often in response to the increased need for RBCs. Sickle-cell anemia. Increased bone marrow function in response to therapy. Blood loss. Hemolysis. Treatment of iron deficiency anemia. Vitamin B_{12} deficiency. Folic acid deficiency. Some leukemias. HDN (hemolytic disease of the newborn). Pregnancy. Thalassemia. Some hemoglobinopathies.

Causes of Decreased Reticulocytes

Anemias due to decreased bone marrow production (called hypoplastic bone marrow). Defective erythropoiesis, which may be due to bone marrow or kidney disease. Blood loss. Decreased numbers may be present following blood loss, which indicates the bone marrow is not responding to therapy. Radiation therapy. Adrenal hypofunction. Alcoholism. Cirrhosis. Anterior pituitary hypofunction.

TEST 10
Erythrocyte Sedimentation Rate (Sed Rate, ESR)

The Sed Rate measures how fast RBCs descend in a tube of anticoagulated blood. The test value is reported in mm/hr (millimeters/hour). The Sed Rate is nonspecific because it shows the possibility that an infection or malignancy exists but does not provide information about its location. Many conditions cause an increased ESR. Whatever the cause, the RBCs adhere to one another and descend more quickly.

Values

Adult males: 0-9 mm/hr

Adult female: 0-20 mm/hr

Pregnant females: Higher levels

Age 50 and over: 0-30 mm/hr

Children: 0-20 mm/hr

Newborns: 0-2 mm/hr

Uses

- To aid in the diagnosis of infections and malignant diseases
- To aid in the diagnosis of inflammation
- To aid in the diagnosis of some autoimmune diseases

Causes of an Increased ESR

Increased plasma proteins. Microcytic RBCs. Malignancies. Some anemias. Multiple myeloma. Waldenström's macroglobulinemia. Autoimmune diseases. Tissue destruction. Rheumatoid arthritis. Some drugs. HDN. Heart attack. Syphilis. Last two trimesters of pregnancy. Hepatitis. Liver disease.

Notes

During pregnancy certain plasma proteins are increased, which is seen in an increased ESR. The level drops following birth.

An increased ESR may be the first sign of infection.

Causes of a Decreased Sed Rate

Hypoproteinemias. Some anemias. Polycythemias. Hyperviscous plasma. Low levels of fibrinogen and other clotting factors. CHF. SCA (sickle-cell anemia). Factor V deficiency. Angina. Some drugs. Infectious mononucleosis.

Notes

Usually a decreased Sed Rate is not clinically significant.

TEST 11
White Blood Cell Count (WBC Count)

The WBC count is part of the CBC. It measures the number of WBCs in a mm^3 or μl of whole blood. An increased WBC count is called leukocytosis and a decreased count leukopenia. The WBC count is of little value unless the values are compared with the values of the WBC differential. The WBC differential measures the percentage of each WBC type in the sample (see WBC Differential).

Values

Adults and older children: 4.5-11 x 10^3/μL or 4,500-11,000/μL (4.5-11 x 10^9/L)
Newborns and young children: 6-30 x 10^3/μL (6-30 x 10^9/L)

Uses

- To screen for infection and determine the need for further study
- To monitor chemotherapy and radiation therapy
- To follow bone marrow engraftment after bone marrow transplant

Causes of Increased WBC Count

Leukemias. Tissue necrosis due to heart attacks (MIs), malignancies, and burns. Some drugs. Acute infections (appendicitis, abscesses, etc.). Liver disease. Some malignancies. Emphysema. Some anemias. Stress, both physical and emotional. Parasitic infections or diseases.

Causes of Decreased WBC Count

Many viral infections. Bone marrow suppression or disease. Chemotherapy or radiation therapy. Exposure to organic chemicals. Exposure to heavy metals. Alcoholism. Some autoimmune diseases. Malaria.

TEST 12
White Blood Cell Differential (WBC Diff)
(Whole Blood)

The WBC diff and WBC count are done in conjunction with one another and are part of the CBC. The WBC diff is a very important test because it provides the percentage of WBCs in a sample of 100 WBCs. In the WBC diff, the five types of WBCs are distinguished from one another and counted.

Values

Neutrophils: 47-76%; 1900-8300/μL (1.9-8.3 x 10^9/L)

Bands: 0-5%; 0-500/μL (0-.5 x 10^9/L)

Lymphocytes: 16-43%; 650-4500/μL (.65-4.5 x 10^9/L)

Monocytes: 1-9%; 20-1000/μL (0-1.0 x 10^9/L)

Eosinophils: 0.3-7%; 10-760/μL (0-.76 x 10^9/L)

Basophils: 0.2%-2%; 10-250/μL (0-.25 x 10^9/L)

Uses

- To assess the body's response to infection and disease
- To differentiate the types of leukemia
- To assess the severity of infections and allergic reactions

Causes of Increased Neutrophils

Bacterial infections. Some viral diseases or infections. Some types of leukemia. Some types of drugs. Tissue necrosis due to burns or MIs. Certain malignancies. Stress, both physical and emotional. Acute infections. Anemias. Inflammatory diseases. Crush injuries. HDN.

Notes

During an infection the body's demand for neutrophils causes increased numbers of immature neutrophils, called bands, to be released into the circulation. Bands can be distinguished microscopically from mature neutrophils by the shape of their nucleus (unsegmented as opposed to segmented). A "shift to the left" indicates increased numbers of bands in the circulation.

Causes of Decreased Neutrophils

Bone marrow suppression (chemotherapy, radiation therapy). Bone marrow tumors. Many diseases. Some bacterial and viral infections. Some drugs. Collagen diseases. Hypersplenism. Some anemias. Some leukemias.

Note

Individuals with neutropenia must be watched closely to prevent infections, especially bacterial.

Causes of Increased Eosinophils

Antigen-antibody complexes, which can involve the following: allergic reactions, food or drug reactions, parasitic infections, skin diseases, allergies, some tumors, asthma, emphysema, and kidney diseases. Many drugs affect the number of eosinophils, and before they are administered their effect on eosinophils should be checked in the literature. Stress, either physical or emotional. Adrenal hormones. Bone marrow suppression. Various malignancies. Burns. Shock.

Causes of Increased Basophils

The number of basophils in the blood is low to begin with, but numbers increase in certain conditions, including the following: certain types of leukemia, bone marrow diseases, some infections, allergic reactions, some forms of kidney disease, inflammatory reactions, and some hemolytic anemias.

Causes of Decreased Basophils

Decreased numbers are hard to evaluate because basophils are so scarce. Certain situations that cause a decrease include the following: hypersensitivity reactions, some leukemias, pregnancy, steroids, and some types of infections.

Lymphocytes

In the WBC differential count, lymphocytes are grouped together. The majority of lymphocytes are T cells, which make up about 75% of the lymphocytes. The remaining 25% are B cells. Children are likely to have a greater percentage of lymphocytes than neutrophils.

Causes of Increased Lymphocytes

Viral infections. Immune reactions. Many leukemias. Chronic bacterial infections. Multiple myeloma. Hodgkin's disease. Decreased adrenal corticosteroids. Lymphocytosis, which is an infection seen in children that causes an increase of lymphocytes and passes with time.

Causes of Decreased Lymphocytes

AIDS. Long-standing (chronic) illnesses. Chemotherapy and radiation therapy. Renal failure. Abnormal lymphatic system. Immunosuppressive drugs. Some leukemias. Some autoimmune diseases. Nephrotic syndrome.

Notes

Individuals deficient in lymphocytes are vulnerable to serious infections, usually viral, that can be fatal. When lymphocyte counts are down, an individual's susceptibility to opportunistic infections is increased as well.

Causes of Increased Monocytes

Bacterial, viral, rickettsial, and protozoan infections. Autoimmune diseases. Some malignancies. Some leukemias. Some types of lymphomas. Some solid organ tumors. Some anemias.

Causes of Decreased Monocytes

Some leukemias. Some anemias.

TEST 13
T and B Lymphocyte Assay
(Whole Blood)

This assay uses lymphocytes from whole blood. The process recovers lymphocytes, but it does not differentiate between T and B cells. The E-rosette test distinguishes T cells, and immunofluoresence detects B cells. T and B cells are differentiated by natural protein markers on their cell membranes.

Values

Adults: Normally T cells make up about 70-75% and B cells about 25-30% of lymphocytes.

Total lymphocyte count: 650-4500/µL

T cells: 1400-2700/µL

B cells: 250-650/µL

Children: Higher values than adults'

Because this assay has not been standardized, values differ depending on the testing laboratory, which should be asked about the values it defines as normal.

Notes

An abnormal lymphocyte count does not necessarily conclude that a disease process exists. And a normal lymphocyte count does not assume a competent immune system. For example, in autoimmune diseases the lymphocyte count is normal yet the lymphocytes are not functioning properly.

Uses

- To assist in diagnosing immunodeficiency diseases
- To monitor therapy
- To differentiate lymphocyte disorders

Causes of Increased T Lymphocytes

Infectious mononucleosis. Acute lymphocytic leukemia (ALL). Autoimmune disorders.

Causes of Decreased T Lymphocytes

Congenital T cell deficiency diseases, such as DiGeorge's syndrome, AIDS, Wiskott-Aldrich syndrome. Acute viral infections. Immunosuppressive drugs. Certain B cell proliferative disorders. Chronic lymphocytic leukemia (CLL). Waldenström's macroglobulinemia.

Causes of Increased B Lymphocytes

Chronic lymphocytic leukemia (CLL). Multiple myeloma. Waldenström's macroglobulinemia.

Causes of Decreased B Lymphocytes

Acute lymphocytic leukemia (ALL). Some congenital and acquired immunoglobulin deficiency diseases. Agammaglobulinemia. Hypogammaglobulinemia.

TEST 14
Bleeding Time
(Whole Blood)

The bleeding time test measures the time it takes for a small skin incision to form a platelet plug. It measures the functional status of platelets. Individuals with low platelet counts may continue to bleed following the test and should be monitored. Many disorders affect the quality and quantity of platelets. (See Test 15 Platelet Count.)

Values

The following test methods provide different time ranges:

Template method: 2-8 minutes

Modified template: 2-10 minutes

Ivy method: 1-7 minutes

Duke method: 1-3 minutes

Uses

- To evaluate platelet function
- To evaluate bleeding disorders
- Preoperative screening

Causes of an Increased Bleeding Time

Low platelet numbers. DIC. HDN. Some leukemias. Some lymphomas. Liver disease. Coagulation factor deficiencies. Vascular abnormalities. Hemophilia A and B. Some drugs. Some anemias. Anticoagulants. Aspirin and aspirin-containing compounds. Fibrinolytic agents. Wintergreen candy ingestion.

Cause of a Decreased Bleeding Time

Hodgkin's disease.

Notes

Patients with a platelet count of less than 50,000/μL usually have an abnormal bleeding time.

TEST 15
Platelet Count
(Whole Blood)

The platelet count measures the number of platelets in a μL of blood. Once counted by a laboratory technician, the count is now computed with fast and more accurate electronic equipment.

Values

All ages: 150-450 x 10^3/μL (150-450 x 10^9/L)

Following labor and delivery: An increase

Newborns: Low platelet numbers

Infants: 200,000-400,000/μL

Uses

- To measure the number of platelets (thrombocytes)
- To evaluate platelet function, production, and numbers
- To evaluate the response to chemotherapy and radiation therapy

Causes of Increased Platelets (Thrombocytosis, or Thrombocythemia)

Malignancies. Hemorrhage. Some leukemias. Some anemias. Inflammatory diseases. Surgery. Pregnancy. Splenectomy. Bone marrow abnormalities. Primary thrombocythemia. Polycythemia. Some drugs. Pulmonary embolus. Trauma. Fractures. High altitudes.

Notes

When the platelet count remains high, further studies should be done.

Thrombi are likely to occur when platelet numbers are increased.

Increased bleeding is likely to occur when the platelets are of poor quality or not functioning properly.

Causes of Decreased Platelets (Thrombocytopenia)

Some forms of bone marrow diseases. Some leukemias. Some infections. Some malignancies. Vitamin deficiencies. Some drugs. DIC. Injury to platelets. Enlarged spleen. Some anemias. Liver disease. Kidney disease. Multiple myeloma. Some autoimmune diseases. Chemotherapy and radiation therapy. Splenic abnormalities. Some viral infections such as AIDS. Other blood disorders. Abnormal bone marrow function. Bypass surgery, during which platelets are destroyed by the bypass pump (mechanical destruction). Autologous blood recovery (wash systems).

TEST 16
Clot Retraction
(Whole Blood)

This test measures the ability of platelets to form a clot that becomes firm and shrinks away from the sides of the tube. If platelet numbers are low or the platelets are defective, the clot does not become firm and pull away from the sides of the tube.

Values

All ages: 50%-100% within 2 hours of initiating the test

Uses

- To assess platelet ability to form a normal clot
- To diagnose platelet abnormalities
- To detect the presence of fibrinolysins
- To determine whether bleeding disorders are due to a decreased platelet count

Results

An abnormal clot retraction suggests a platelet abnormality or decreased platelet numbers. Von Willebrand's disease. Polycythemia. Anemia. Decreased amounts of fibrinogen (hypofibrinogenemia). Increased levels of fibrin split products (FSPs). Increased fibrinolysins. Waldenström's macroglobulinemia. Thrombocytopenia.

TEST 17
Activated Partial Thromboplastin Time (aPTT)
(Plasma)

The aPTT measures the time it takes for a clot to form in a sample of blood plasma. The test is used when a study of the intrinsic pathway is desired. The "a" stands for activated and indicates that an activator substance has been added to the plasma sample. The activator substance decreases the time it takes a clot to form. The sample clots faster, and the test value can be obtained more quickly.

Values

All ages: 25-35 seconds

Individuals on anticoagulant therapy: Increased time

Females, pregnant and those taking oral contraceptive pills: Lower times

Newborns: Higher than an adult's

Uses

- To monitor heparin therapy
- To detect bleeding disorders of the intrinsic pathway
- To detect minor clotting defects

Causes of an Increased aPTT

A deficiency of clotting factors XII, XI, VIII, or IX. The most common clotting factor deficiency in the intrinsic pathway is indicated by the absence or by a decreased level of factor VIII. Von Willebrand's disease. Hemophilia B (Christmas disease), which is a deficiency of factor IX. Heparin therapy. Autologous blood transfusions. Liver disease. Vitamin K deficiency. DIC. Some leukemias. Malaria. Inhibitors to coagulation factors VIII and IX. Hypofibrinogenemia. Increased levels of FSPs. Increased fibrinolysins (plasmin).

Notes

Individuals with an increased aPTT have a tendency to bleed. They should be watched following blood sampling and advised to avoid situations in which cuts might occur, such as shaving with a razor.

Causes of a Decreased aPTT

Possible blood clot formation. Widespread cancer. Although a decrease in aPTT is not usually clinically significant, it can indicate an increased chance of blood clot formation.

Notes

Individuals with a decreased aPTT are likely to have increased clot formation. Measures should be taken to reduce the incidence of venous stasis (decreased blood flow in the veins, which can occur, for example, by crossing the legs or sitting for extended periods of time.) Pregnant females may have decreased levels of clotting factors and should be particularly careful.

TEST 18
Prothrombin Time (PT, Pro Time)
(Plasma)

The PT measures the amount of clotting factors in the extrinsic system: factors VII, V, X and II. Drugs in the blood may increase or decrease the PT and, therefore, must be checked for their affect on it.

Values

All ages: 10-12 seconds for the control (+ or - 2 seconds)

Females: In pregnant females and women on oral contraceptives, the PT values may be slightly decreased due to increased clotting factor levels.

Infants and newborns: Lower levels of clotting factors, which means that the PT may be increased

Individuals on oral anticoagulants: The PT is maintained at 1.5-2 times the normal.

Notes

Some laboratories report test results as a percentage of activity. For this test as little as 20-30% of activity is normal. Normal values are based on the laboratory's test method, the reagent system, and the patient population.

Uses

- To detect bleeding disorders of the extrinsic system
- To monitor oral anticoagulant response to therapy

Causes of an Increased PT

Liver disease. A deficiency of factors II, V, VII, or X. Vitamin K deficiency. Circulating oral anticoagulants, such as Coumadin™. Certain drugs or medications other than oral anticoagulants. Alcoholism. Some adrenal hormones. FDP. HDN. CHF. Afibrinogenemia.

Causes of a Decreased PT

Certain drugs and medications. Certain malignancies. MI. Thrombophlebitis. Pulmonary embolus.

Notes

Individuals with a decreased PT may have an increased chance of intravascular clot formation.

TEST 19
Activated Clotting Time (ACT)
(Whole Blood)

The ACT is a simple test administered at the bedside or in the surgical unit to monitor the effects of heparin therapy. During cardiac surgery, it is used by the perfusionist to make sure the patient is adequately heparinized. The test is performed using a special sample tube and an automatic timing device. The tube is filled with 2 mL of blood (via syringe) and placed in the device well. The timer is started, and when a clot forms the timer is stopped. The time it takes for the clot to form indicates roughly how much heparin is in the patient.

Values

Normal: 90-120 seconds, depending on the activator substance (which hastens clotting) in the sample tube. These values are increased when anticoagulation is in use.

Uses

- To monitor heparin therapy
- To monitor heparin administration during cardiopulmonary bypass
- To calculate protamine dosage following cardiac surgery

Results

An increased ACT indicates the individual is heparinized. The amount of heparin in the individual determines the time of the ACT.

TEST 20
One-stage Factor Assays for the Extrinsic and Intrinsic Pathways

A. Extrinsic Pathway
(Plasma)

When the PT and the aPTT are abnormal, the One-stage Factor Assay helps determine a deficiency of clotting factors. When the aPTT is normal and the PT is abnormal, a deficiency of factor VII may be indicated. The One-stage Factor Assay measures the activity of factors II, V, VII, and X. It is a useful test because all the factors in the extrinsic pathway and final common pathway can be checked at the same time. A sample of the individual's plasma is placed in four tubes, each of which is missing a factor. The tube that does not clot indicates the factor deficiency.

Values

The range is between 50-150% of normal activity.

FI: 200-400 mg/dL

FII: 10-15% activity

FV: 50-150% activity

FVII: 65-135% activity

FX: 45-150% activity

Uses

- To isolate a specific factor deficiency in the extrinsic and final common pathways
- To identify acquired or congenital factor deficiencies
- To monitor response to factor deficiency therapy

Causes of Decreased Factor Levels

A deficiency of factors II, V, VII, or X may indicate liver disease, DIC, or FSPs. Increased fibrinolysins. Deficiency of vitamin K. Some leukemias. Some drugs. Hypoprothrombinemia. Parahemophilia. HDN.

Notes

It is unlikely that an individual is deficient in all four factors due to a congenital abnormality. In fact, the absence of factor II is fatal.

B. Intrinsic Pathway
(Plasma)

The One-stage Factor Assay helps determine a deficiency of clotting factors when the PT is normal and the aPTT is abnormal. This test is an assay for factors VIII, IX, XI, and XII.

Values

The range is between 50-150% of the normal activity.

FVIII: 55-145% activity

FIX: 60-140% activity

FXI: 65-135% activity

FXII: minimal amount needed

FXIII: 1% concentration

Uses

- To isolate a specific factor deficiency of the intrinsic pathway
- To identify acquired and congenital factor deficiencies
- To monitor response to factor therapy

Causes of Decreased Clotting Factors

A deficiency of factor VIII, which may indicate either hemophilia A or von Willebrand's disease. A deficiency may also occur when there is an inhibitor (antibody) to factor VIII in the blood. An acquired deficiency of factor VIII may occur with DIC or in the presence of excess fibrinolysis (excess plasminogen or plasmin). There are blood tests (e.g., factor VIII antigen and ristocetin cofactor) available that differentiate between hemophilia A and von Willebrand's disease.

A factor IX deficiency, which may be inherited or acquired. An inherited deficiency leads to Hemophilia B (Christmas disease). An acquired deficiency may be caused by DIC, liver disease, an inhibitor to factor IX, low or absent vitamin K, or oral anticoagulants.

A factor XI deficiency, which may occur during times of stress or following surgery.

A factor XII deficiency, which may be inherited or acquired

Factor XI and factor XII deficiencies may occur spontaneously in newborns.

Other Causes of Factor Deficiencies

Some forms of kidney disease. Hypocalcemia. Malabsorption. Multiple transfusions. Multiple myeloma. DIC. Liver disease. Congenital heart disease. Some drugs. Some autoimmune diseases. Agammaglobulinemia.

Notes

Inhibitors (antibodies) occur in patients following factor replacement therapy.

TEST 21
Thrombin Time (TT)
(Plasma)

The TT measures the time it takes for a sample of plasma with platelets removed to form a clot. Thrombin is produced from prothrombin and rapidly converts fibrinogen to fibrin.

Values

Normal time for all ages: 10-15 seconds

Reptilase Time (RT)

The RT is a variation of the TT and can be used when the individual is heparinized or has increased levels of plasmin and FSPs. The result of the RT is not affected by heparin.

Values

12–20 seconds

Uses

- To identify defective fibrinogen or a deficiency of fibrinogen
- To monitor the response to heparin therapy
- To monitor the response to fibrinolytic therapy
- To detect and diagnose DIC or liver disease
- To monitor streptokinase or urokinase therapy

Causes of Increased Thrombin Time

Heparin therapy. Liver disease. Decreased levels of fibrinogen (hypofibrinogenemia). Ineffective fibrinogen (dysfibrinogenemia). Some leukemias. Vitamin K deficiency. Hypoprothrombinemia. Some drugs. Afibrinogenemia. Circulating anticoagulants. HDN. Some malignancies. Some obstetrical problems. Surgery. Increased FSPs. Hemorrhage. Shock. Polycythemia. DIC.

Notes

To rule out or confirm DIC, the fibrin split products test should be conducted as a follow-up. Other more specific studies may also be required.

TEST 22
Fibrinogen Quantification
(Plasma)

This test measures the amount of fibrinogen in blood. Fibrinogen is a clotting protein produced in the liver and is consumed during clot formation. A deficiency of fibrinogen can lead to mild or severe bleeding disorders. Individuals with decreased levels of fibrinogen should be observed closely.

Values

All ages: Normal levels of fibrinogen: 200–400 mg/dL (2.0–4.0 g/L)
Pregnant females: Elevated levels
Newborns: 150–300 mg/dL

Uses

- To diagnose and screen bleeding disorders caused by defective or deficient levels of fibrinogen

- To aid in diagnosing DIC

Causes of Increased Fibrinogen

Some solid organ tumors, such as kidney, stomach, and breast, among others. Some types of pneumonia. Some types of kidney disease. Infections. Persons on heparin and oral contraceptives. Hepatitis. Inflammatory diseases. Collagen diseases.

Causes of Decreased Fibrinogen

Trauma. Some obstetrical complications. Some types of tumors, such as lung, pancreas, and bone marrow, among others. DIC. Liver disease. Increased amounts of FSPs. Burns. Septicemia. Shock or vascular collapse. Snake venom. Hypofibrinogenemia. Some leukemias.

Notes

Fibrinogen congenital deficiencies may cause hypofibrinogenemia (low amounts), dysfibrinogenemia (nonfunctional), or afibrinogenemia (absence).

TEST 23
Fibrin Split Products (FSPs)
(Serum)

This test measures the amount of FSPs within blood. After a blood clot has formed, the fibrinolytic system (plasmin) breaks down the fibrin clot. When clot breakdown occurs, FSPs are released into the blood. Normally FSPs are removed by the reticuloendothelial system. When this system fails or too many FSPs are circulating within the plasma, increased amounts of FSPs interfere with blood clot formation. The fibrin clot is dissolved by the action of plasmin, the active form of plasminogen.

Values

All ages: By assay, the serum contains less than 10 µg/mL of FSPs. Quantitatively the assay shows less than 3 µg/mL of FSPs within the sample.

Plasma D-dimer: Less than 200 ng/mL (less than 200 mg/L)

Uses

- To evaluate fibrinolytic therapy
- To diagnose DIC

- To assess liver function
- To monitor DIC therapy
- To look for FSPs within the circulation

Causes of Increased FSPs

DIC. Tissue necrosis. Liver disease. Obstetrical emergencies such as abruptio placenta, eclampsia, fetal death. Post-heart attack (MI). Burns. Blood clots. Kidney diseases. Renal transplant rejection. Intraoperative autologous blood recovery and reinfusion. Pulmonary embolus. Increased levels of fibrinolysins. Severe injury. Trauma. Shock. Surgical complications. Acute leukemias.

TEST 24
Plasminogen
(Plasma)

Plasmin, the active form of plasminogen, cannot be measured. However, the plasminogen test can measure the level of plasminogen (the precursor of plasmin) to provide information about the fibrinolytic system.

Values

Values may be reported by the following methods:

Immunologic method: 10-20 ng/dL (100-200 mg/L)

Functional method: 80-120 U/dL (800-1200 U/L)

Council on Thrombolytic Agents: 3.8-8.4 CTA

Uses

- To measure the amount of plasminogen in the blood
- To determine acquired or congenital fibrinolytic disorders
- To monitor fibrinolysis
- To diagnose DIC

Causes of Increased Plasminogen

Acute infections. MI. Stress. Surgery. Trauma. Some malignancies. Oral contraceptives.

Causes of Decreased Plasminogen

DIC. Certain malignancies. Some obstetrical emergencies. Liver diseases. Fibrinolytics. Thrombolytic therapy.

TEST 25
Factors VIII and IX Assay
(Plasma)

Factors VII and IX assays measure the amount of clotting factors VIII and IX. A deficiency of factor VIII or an inhibitor to factor VIII causes classic hemophilia, called hemophilia A. A deficiency of factor IX or an inhibitor to factor IX causes hemophilia B, or Christmas disease. Most cases of hemophilia are of the A type.

Values

All ages: The normal range for factor VIII is 50-200% of normal (.5-2.0 μmol/L).

All ages: The normal range for factor IX is 60-140% of normal (0.6-1.4 μmol/L).

Uses

- To measure the levels of factors VIII and/or IX in the plasma
- To diagnose and differentiate between hemophilia A and von Willebrand's disease
- To diagnose Christmas disease

Causes of Decreased Levels of Factors VIII and IX

All cases of hemophilia A or B are caused by a deficiency of either factor VIII or factor IX or an inhibitor (antibody) to these factors. Hemophilia is a genetic disorder carried by females but usually expressed only in male offspring. There are different levels of the disease—mild, moderate, or severe. Factor replacement is administered to decrease bleeding.

TEST 26
Euglobin Lysis Time
(Plasma)

This test measures the amount of time it takes for a clot to dissolve. The time is recorded from the time the sample forms a clot to the time the clot dissolves.

Results

All ages: The normal time for a clot to break down, or lyse, is a minimum of 2 hours.

Uses

- To measure the amount of time it takes for a clot to dissolve
- To evaluate fibrinolysis
- To detect abnormal fibrinolysis
- To assist in diagnosing DIC

Causes of an Increased Euglobulin Lysis Time

Increased levels of plasminogen usually cause clot breakdown within approximately 1 hour. DIC.

TEST 27
Factor XIII Assay
(Plasma)

A plasma sample is mixed with chloracetic acid or urea. The sample is allowed to clot and is then observed for 24 hours. If the blood clot dissolves, a severe factor XIII deficiency is indicated.

Results

A normal value is indicated if the clot does not dissolve.

Uses

- To diagnose a deficiency of factor XIII

Signs of a Factor XIII Deficiency

Prolonged umbilical cord bleeding following birth. Hematomas. Poor wound healing. Repeated spontaneous abortion. Bleeding into joint spaces.

Causes of a Factor XIII Deficiency

A congenital factor deficiency that is transmitted from parents to offspring. An acquired deficiency may result from liver disease or some types of malignancies.

Notes

Bleeding may be immediate following trauma or may occur many hours later. Before treatment begins, other factor deficiencies should be ruled out. Factor XIII deficiency may be treated with Fresh Frozen Plasma or Cryo.

TEST 28
Factor VIII Antigen
(Plasma)

The plasma sample is impregnated into a gel containing factor VIII antibody. The gel is subjected to an electric field. A normal result appears as bands of spikes, which indicates that an immune response between factor VIII antigen and antibody has occurred. A negative result shows no spikes.

Values

Individuals with hemophilia have normal activity: 40-180% of the control.

Individuals with von Willebrand's disease either lack factor VIII antigen or have a deficient amount.

Uses

- To distinguish between hemophilia and von Willebrand's disease

TEST 29
Antithrombin III (AT-III)
(Whole Blood)

The AT-III test determines causes of hypercoaguability. AT-III inhibits the formation of blood clots in the vasculature. Therefore a balance usually exists between AT-III and thrombin. When AT-III levels are low, an imbalance between AT-III and thrombin occurs that will likely lead to clotting.

Values

All ages: Values vary with each laboratory, but should fall between 80-120% of normal activity. This means that the sample should be between 80-120% of the amount of AT-III found in a normal control sample.

Functional assay: 80-120 U/dL (800-1200 U/L)

Immunologic assay: 20-30 mg/dL (200-300 mg/L)

Uses

- To diagnose a deficiency in levels of AT-III
- To detect hypercoaguable states

Causes of Increased Levels of AT-III

Kidney transplant recipients. Oral anticoagulants. Anabolic steroids.

Causes of Decreased Levels of AT-III

Liver disease. DIC. Thromboembolic disorders. Oral contraceptives. Hypercoagulation. Some malignancies. Some forms of kidney disease. Septicemia (viral or bacterial).

Notes

Low levels of AT-III decrease the effects of heparin, which has no anticoagulative effect of its own. Individuals with low AT-III levels may show signs of heparin resistance (i.e., no increase in ACT or aPTT) following heparin administration.

TEST 30
ABO Grouping
(Whole Blood)

ABO blood grouping classifies blood according to the presence or absence of the A and B antigens on the red blood cell (RBC) membrane and the presence or absence of anti-A or anti-B antibodies in the serum. There are two tests involved in grouping. (1) Forward grouping, or direct, which looks for the A or B antigen and (2) reverse grouping, or indirect, which looks for antibody in the serum. The tests are conducted together to determine the blood group. An ABO group is confirmed when the results of both the forward and reverse tests indicate the same blood group.

Uses

- To identify a blood group
- To determine compatibility between donor and recipient prior to a blood transfusion
- To determine compatibility between donor and recipient prior to a solid organ transplant

Forward Grouping Results

In forward grouping, RBCs are mixed with known reagent serum containing anti-A and anti-B antibodies. Forward grouping tests RBCs for the A or B antigen. If agglutination occurs when RBCs are mixed with anti-B serum, the cells contain the B antigen. If agglutination occurs when RBCs are mixed with anti-A serum, the group is A. If agglutination occurs when RBCs are mixed with both anti-A and anti-B serum, the group is AB. If the cells do not clump with either anti-A or anti-B, the group is O.

Reverse Grouping Results

In reverse grouping, serum is mixed with known reagent A and B RBCs. Reverse grouping tests the serum for anti-A or anti-B antibodies. If agglutination occurs when group A RBCs are mixed with a sample of serum, the serum contains anti-A antibody and the blood is group B. If agglutination occurs when group B cells are mixed with serum, the serum contains anti-B and the blood is group A. If agglutination occurs when both group A and B cells are mixed with serum, the serum contains anti-A and anti-B and is group O (group O has neither antigen, but both antibodies). If no agglutination occurs when both A and B cells are mixed with serum, the blood is group as AB (AB contains neither antibody, but both antigens).

TEST 31
Rh Grouping
(Whole Blood)

Rh grouping determines whether RBCs contain the Rh or D antigen on their membranes. All prospective blood donors must be tested before their blood can be used in a transfusion. A transfusion of the wrong Rh group can cause serious problems for some individuals, for example, females of childbearing potential and individuals receiving multiple transfusions.

Uses

- To identify the presence or absence of the Rh, or D, antigen
- To determine compatibility between donor and recipient
- To determine the need for Rh immune globulin

Results

Blood is classified according to the presence or absence of the Rh, or D, antigen on the membranes of RBCs. If the Rh antigen is present, the blood is classified as Rh+; if the Rh antigen is absent, the blood is Rh-.

Notes

Individuals due to receive a transfusion of Rh+ blood or Rh- females who deliver an Rh+ fetus or abort a fetus with an unknown Rh status should receive Rh immune globulin (RhIG). RhIG prevents the possibility of hemolytic disease of the newborn (HDN) in future pregnancies. HDN is most often caused by Rh antibody produced in the mother when Rh+ fetal blood cells cross the placenta and enter the mother's circulation. In future pregnancies, sensitized maternal Rh antibody crosses the placenta and enters the fetal circulation. If the fetus is Rh+, maternal antibody binds to the Rh antigen on the RBC membrane and destroys the RBCs.

RhIG is given to the following individuals:

- Rh- individuals transfused with Rh+ blood or blood component
- Rh+ female who aborts a fetus of unknown Rh status
- Rh- female who gives birth to an Rh+ child

TEST 32
Cross Matching
(Whole Blood)

The cross matching test determines compatibility between a donor and recipient prior to a blood transfusion. It is the best available means for determining whether the recipient's serum contains antibodies against donor RBCs that could cause a hemolytic transfusion reaction. Blood is always cross matched before a transfusion, except in an extreme emergency, in which case, group O- cells are used until a complete cross match can be done. Cross matching can take 30 minutes to 1 hour.

Uses

- To determine compatibility between donor and recipient prior to a blood transfusion

Results

A positive cross match is indicated by agglutination. Donor and recipient blood groups are not compatible, and this donor blood should not be used for transfusion.

A negative cross match indicates donor and recipient blood groups are compatible. This donor blood can be used for transfusion. A negative result is determined by the absence of agglutination.

TEST 33
Fetal-maternal Red Blood Cell Distribution
(Serum)

It is normal for a small amount of fetal RBCs to enter the mother's circulation following birth, abortion, and C-section, among others. This test determines whether significant amounts of fetal RBCs have crossed the placenta and entered the maternal circulation. The test results indicate the amount of Rh immune globulin (RhIG) to administer to a nonsensitized individual. RhIG is administered to mothers who have been exposed to fetal antigen. It should also be administered within 72 hours following the birth of an Rh+ fetus and following the abortion of a fetus with an unknown Rh status.

Results

Normal: Maternal blood contains no fetal RBCs.

Uses

- To determine the presence of fetal blood in maternal circulation
- To determine the need for and the amount of RhIG by the mother

TEST 34
Antibody Screening (Indirect Coomb's, Indirect Antiglobulin)
(Serum)

The antibody screening test detects antibody (other than anti-A, anti-B) in serum directed against antigen on the RBC membrane. The test is sensitive enough to determine, with about 99% accuracy, the presence of antibody. Once antibody is discovered, other tests determine the specific antibody.

Results

Negative or Positive Normally blood contains no antibody (other than anti-A, anti-B) in the serum. Therefore there should be no agglutination. If agglutination occurs, antibody is present and a positive result is indicated. A positive reaction contraindicates transfusion. If antibodies react with RBC antigens, the blood is incompatible for a transfusion.

Rh The antibody screening test is used to detect the presence of Rh antibody in an Rh- pregnant female who has developed antibody to Rh+ blood from a previous transfusion, pregnancy, or transplant. An elevated titer (amount) of Rh antibody may indicate that the fetus has HDN.

Other　Other causes of a positive test are specific antibodies from a previous transfusion, transplant, or pregnancy; acquired hemolytic anemia; and a wide variety of drug reactions.

Uses

- To assist in the diagnosis of hemolytic anemias
- To evaluate the need for RhIG
- To determine the presence of antibodies in serum prior to a blood transfusion
- To establish the presence of Rh antibody in the mother's blood

---

TEST 35
Direct Antiglobulin (Direct Coomb's)
(Whole Blood or RBCs)

The direct antiglobulin test detects the presence of antibody or complement bound to the RBC membrane, for example, the Rh antigen (D antigen).

This test is sensitive enough to detect a very weak antigen-antibody reaction, even when no agglutination is visibly evident. The test does not identify the specific antibody, only that antibody is present.

Results

The absence of antibody or complement on RBCs indicates a normal or negative test. A normal result indicates there are no unexpected antigens on the RBC membrane that could attach to antibody or complement.

Uses

- To assist in diagnosing hemolytic anemias
- To follow the course of a hemolytic transfusion reaction
- To detect hemolytic disease of the newborn (HDN)
- To determine sensitivity to some drugs

Causes of a Positive Test

Some leukemias. Some autoimmune diseases. Certain drugs. Hemolytic anemia. Transfusion reactions. HDN. Lymphoma.

Notes

A positive result from umbilical cord blood indicates that maternal antibody has crossed the placenta and attached to antigen on the RBC membrane of the fetus. If antibody is present, fetal RBCs will likely be destroyed. Blood used to transfuse the fetus should be O, and the serum should be compatible with the mother's.

TEST 36
Leukoagglutinin (White Blood Cell Antibodies)
(Serum)

This test measures the presence of antibodies against antigens on the surface of white blood cell (WBC) membranes. These antibodies can cause a febrile transfusion reaction if administered to a sensitized individual. Antibodies develop only after exposure to antigens through transfusion, pregnancy, or allogeneic transplant.

Results

Normal results show no agglutination, because normally serum contains no antibodies to WBC antigens.

If the test is positive (antibody is present) in a transfusion recipient, the transfusion reaction is febrile rather being than the more serious hemolytic transfusion reaction. If the donor's blood tests positive, leukoagglutinins are present and the reaction in the transfusion recipient is acute, pulmonary edema (fluid accumulation in the lungs).

Uses

- To monitor transfusion reactions
- To rule out hemolytic transfusion reactions
- To detect leukoagglutinins in blood donors following a transfusion reaction in a recipient

TEST 37
Glucose-6-Phosphate Dehydrogenase (G-6-PD)
(Whole Blood)

This test measures the amount of G-6-PD in RBCs. G-6-PD is an enzyme and a part of the biochemical pathway by which sugar (glucose) is broken down to produce energy. When the enzyme is missing, the RBC membrane is fragile and easily hemolyzed. Individuals who lack this enzyme can experience RBC hemolysis when exposed to changes in acid-base balance, some types of infections, and various chemicals (drugs or other). The gene for the deficiency is carried in the female but usually expressed in male offspring. Individuals of African American or Mediterranean descent are more likely to have the deficiency.

G-6-PD deficiency. Individuals with this deficiency are often unaware that they have it unless they have had a hemolytic episode.

Values

All ages: 5-15 IU/g Hgb

Packed RBCs: 125-280 U/dL

250-510 U/10^6 cells

1210-2110 mIU/mL

Some laboratories report results as either normal or abnormal. An abnormal result indicates a deficiency of G-6-PD.

Use

- To determine whether hemolytic anemia is caused by a G-6-PD deficiency

Causes of Increased Hemolysis

Certain drugs cause hemolysis in individuals with a G-6-PD deficiency. Examples of these drugs include: aspirin (ASA), phenacetin, sulfonamides, nitro-containing compounds, and vitamin K compounds. Certain foods, such as fava beans, may cause hemolysis in individuals with G-6-PD deficiency.

TEST 38
Lactate Dehydrogenase (LDH)
(Serum)

Lactate dehydrogenase (LDH) is an enzyme found in body cells that converts lactic acid to pyruvic acid. LDH is then metabolized to produce energy in the form of ATP. Production of ATP occurs in mitochondria of cells. When tissue is destroyed, LDH is released from cells and enters the blood where its presence signifies tissue damage. However, because LDH is found in so many cells, its use as a diagnostic tool is limited.

Different body cells have different LDH enzymes. These different yet similar enzymes are called isozymes, or isoenzymes. Individual isozymes can be identified through electrophoresis, which means a specific tissue injury can be determined. LDH1 and LDH2 are found primarily in the RBCs, heart, and kidneys. LDH3 is found mostly in the lungs. LDH4 and LDH5 are found in body muscles and liver.

LDH isoenzymes are expressed as a percent of the total LDH:

LDH1: 14-26%

LDH2: 29-39%

LDH3: 20-26%

LDH4: 8-16%

LDH5: 6-16%

LDH1:LDH2 ratio < 1

The Lactate Dehydrogenase and the Creatine Kinase (Test 39) tests have no assigned values because standard values have not been established. The normal values for enzymes vary depending on the equipment and methodology used to perform the test. The range of normal values must be obtained from the testing laboratory.

Uses

- To assist with the diagnoses of some forms of anemia, heart attack (MI), liver disease, pulmonary infarct
- To confirm other diagnostic tests
- To follow the effectiveness of some forms of chemotherapy

Conditions That Cause Increased LDH

The isozymes of LDH are released into the blood in certain conditions listed here:

LDH1: in heart injury, shock, and some anemias

LDH2: in heart injury, shock, and some anemias

LDH3: in shock, pulmonary, and hematologic disorders

LDH4: in shock, hematologic, and liver disorders

LDH5: in some cardiac, shock, and liver disease

Hemolytic and macrocytic anemias. Infectious mononucleosis. Leukemias and other malignancies. Hepatitis. Obstetrical complications. Megaloblastic anemia. Bypass surgery. Skeletal muscle diseases. Some drugs. Stroke (CVA). Sickle-cell anemia. Trauma.

Notes

The LDH level rises between 12 to 48 hours following an MI. It peaks around 300-800 U/L, somewhere between 2 to 5 days, and returns to normal within 7 to 10 days, provided tissue necrosis has stopped. Following an MI, the LDH1 isoenzyme is increased over the LDH2 isoenzyme. This increase in LDH1 over LDH2 is referred to as the "flipped" LDH ratio because normally LDH2 is greater than LDH1.

TEST 39
Creatine Kinase (CK)
(Serum)

Creatine kinase is an enzyme essential for energy production found in muscle and brain cells. An elevated level of CK indicates tissues are being destroyed; the enzyme is released from the tissues and detected in the blood. Like many enzymes, CK has different forms, called isoenzymes. Different tissues have different CK isoenzymes, which can be separated into bands and identified. The band that appears indicates what tissue is being destroyed.

Laboratories vary in the reporting of normal CK results.

The following CK isoenzymes are identified by electrophoresis:

CK-I band (BB), which is produced in brain and smooth muscle

CK-II band (MB), which is produced in the heart

CK-III band (MM), which is produced in skeletal muscle

Uses

- To diagnose an MI
- To diagnose muscle diseases
- To monitor chest pain after cardiac procedures

Results

An elevation of CK isoenzymes may indicate the following: Decreased potassium levels (hypokalemia). Carbon monoxide poisoning. Alcoholism. Cardiomyopathy. Skeletal muscle disorders. Stroke (CVA). Many drugs.

CK-I band May be increased in shock, brain tumors, or serious brain injury, stroke, seizures, pulmonary embolus, and some forms of kidney disease, among others.

CK-II band   CK increases following an MI. The level is elevated 3 to 6 hours following the attack and peaks within 24 hours. It may also increase following cardiac surgery, angina, and with decreased amounts of potassium (K+; hypokalemia).

CK-III band   Not necessarily diagnostic, but increased levels indicate further studies are needed. The level may become elevated in polio, muscular dystrophy, and strenuous exercise, among others. It may rise with hypothyroidism and in states of severe agitation.

TEST 40
Alanine Aminotransferase (ALT)
(Serum)

Alanine aminotransferase is an enzyme found in certain body cells. It is very prominent in liver cells, and its presence in the blood is an indicator of hepatocellular (liver cell) damage. The enzyme ALT was previously known as serum glutamic pyruvic transaminase (SGPT). When liver cells are damaged, ALT is released into the bloodstream. It may appear in the blood before jaundice appears in the skin.

Values

Adults and children: 5-20 U/L
Severe liver damage: Numbers may rise to 2000 U/L or higher.
Pregnant females: During labor and delivery, numbers may be elevated.
Infants: 2-3 times an adult's

Uses

- To diagnose liver damage
- To assess drug toxicity affecting the liver
- To monitor the course of liver disease

Causes of Increased Alanine Aminotransferase

Viral hepatitis. Liver necrosis. Cirrhosis. Liver cancer. Alcohol ingestion. Many drugs: antibiotics, narcotics, oral contraceptives, antihypertensives. Infectious mononucleosis. Reye's syndrome. Shock. Congestive heart failure (CHF). Eclampsia. Hydatiform mole. Strenuous exercise. Aspirin.

TEST 41
Erythropoietin
(Serum)

This test measures the amount of erythropoietin by immunoassay. Erythropoietin is a protein hormone released by the kidneys. It acts on stem cells to produce RBCs. The kidneys release erythropoietin when the amount of oxygen in the tissues is low (hypoxia).

Values

For all ages: Up to 24 mU/mL

Uses

- To determine anemia or polycythemia/erythrocytosis
- To aid in the detection of tumors of the kidney
- To determine drug abuse by competitive athletes

Causes of Increased Erythropoietin

Some anemias produced in response to therapy. Polycythemia/erythrocytosis. Certain kidney tumors.

Causes of Decreased Erythropoietin

Certain anemias. Low or absent hormone levels. Some types of kidney disease.

Notes

Erythropoietin may be used by some athletes to increase or enhance their performance. An increase of RBCs transports more oxygen to the tissues. Adverse reactions can include the following: headache, nausea, vomiting, rash, diarrhea, increased blood pressure, and coagulation abnormalities.

TEST 42
Antidiuretic Hormone (ADH)
(Serum)

ADH is released by the posterior pituitary gland found in the brain. This hormone affects the kidneys by causing reabsorption of water into the blood from the nephron (renal tubule). The test measures the amount of ADH in the serum.

Values

Adult: The values range between 1-5 pg/mL, but this value may be elevated if the osmolality is abnormal. If the osmolality is increased (>290 mOsm/kg), ADH may be elevated (>2-10 pg/mL). If the osmolality is decreased (<285 mOsm/mL), ADH may be decreased (<2 pg/mL).

Uses

- To diagnose diabetes insipidus
- To diagnose the syndrome of inappropriate ADH release
- To diagnose renal diabetes insipidus

Causes of Increased Levels of ADH

Syndrome of inappropriate ADH release. Cancer of the lung. Hypothyroidism. Addison's disease. Cirrhosis. Hemorrhage. Circulatory collapse. Infectious hepatitis.

Causes of Decreased Levels of ADH

Pituitary diabetes insipidus. Hypothalamic tumors. Metastatic cancers. Some viral infections. Head injury or trauma. Lung diseases. Syphilis. Brain surgery.

If ADH levels are normal yet the individual shows signs of diabetes insipidus, the cause is probably due to renal diabetes insipidus rather than cerebral diabetes insipidus.

TEST 43
Alpha$_1$-antitrypsin (AAT)
(Serum)

AAT is a liver enzyme detected by electrophoresis, and any deficiency is noted. AAT makes up the major fraction of the alpha$_1$-globulin proteins found in plasma. The function of AAT is to inhibit dying cells from releasing proteases into the blood. When AAT is deficient proteases are released into the blood and cause damage, such as emphysema.

Values

For all adults: 85-215 mg/dL (0.85-2.15 g/L)

Children: Higher values

Newborns: About the same as an adult's

Uses

- To screen patients for early emphysema
- To identify congenital deficiency of AAT
- To identify tissue necrosis
- To identify infection
- To identify inflammation

Causes of Increased Levels of AAT

Some chronic and acute inflammatory situations. Some types of infections. Tissue necrosis. Later stages of pregnancy. Individuals on oral contraceptives.

Causes of Decreased Levels of AAT

Emphysema or chronic obstructive lung disease at an early age. Liver disease. Malnutrition. Some kidney diseases.

TEST 44
Aldosterone
(Serum)

This test measures the amount of aldosterone in the serum. Aldosterone is a hormone secreted by the adrenal gland (a gland that sits on top of the kidneys). The hormone causes the reabsorption of sodium and chloride in exchange for potassium and hydrogen ion by the nephrons of the kidneys.

Values

Adults: 1–20 ng/dL in a sitting position
          4–30 ng/dL in a standing position
Females: Varying levels of aldosterone

Uses

- To diagnose aldosteronism
- To diagnose hypoaldosteronism (underactive adrenal gland)
- To diagnose other forms of renal disease

Causes of Increased Levels of Aldosterone

Decreased sodium. Dehydration. Cancer of adrenal gland. Hypertension. Cirrhosis. Overactive adrenal glands. Congestive heart failure (CHF).

Some drugs, such as diuretics and others. Primary aldosteronism (Conn's syndrome). Renal hypertension. Later stages of pregnancy.

Causes of Decreased Levels of Aldosterone

Increased sodium. Overhydration. Underactive adrenal glands. Diabetes mellitus. Low sodium diet. Overinfusion of I.V. glucose. Addison's disease. Toxemia during pregnancy. Primary hypoaldosteronism.

TEST 45
Fasting Blood Sugar (FBS)
(Whole Blood)

This test is commonly used to screen for diabetes mellitus. It measures the amount of glucose in the plasma following a 12 to 14 hour fast (no food). The test must be done in a fasting state. Any drugs that affect glucose, such as insulin, must be withheld prior to the test.

Values

Adult serum and plasma: 70-110 mg/dL

Whole blood: 60-100 mg/dL

Pregnant females: May have a slightly higher level

Newborns   Full term: About 30 mg/dL

              Premature: Lower than 30 mg/dL

Children: About the same as an adult's

Uses

- To aid in the diagnosis of diabetes mellitus
- To monitor therapy for diabetes

Causes of Increased Levels of Glucose

Pancreatitis. MI. Cushing's disease. Diabetes mellitus. Acromegaly. Hyperlipoproteinemia. Chronic liver disease. Kidney disease. Brain tumors. Sepsis. Anoxia (lack of O_2). Convulsive disorders. Burns. Congestive heart failure (CHF). Some drugs. Surgery. Following gastrectomy. Diabetic acidosis. Crush injuries.

Causes of Decreased Levels of Glucose

Some types of liver disease. Hyperinsulinism (increased amounts of insulin). Myxedema. Hypopituitarism. Adrenal hyperplasia. Malabsorption syndrome. Some malignancies. Alcoholism. Cirrhosis. HDN. Hypoglycemic reaction.

TEST 46
Two-hour Postprandial Blood Glucose
(Whole Blood)

This test assesses the body's ability to metabolize glucose. It is performed 2 hours following a regular meal. The time the sample is drawn following a meal (2 hours) is crucial to the results.

Values

All ages: A value greater than 140 mg/dL may indicate diabetes mellitus.
Older patients: May have elevated glucose
Children: Slightly lower values than 140 mg/dL

Uses

- To aid in the diagnosis of diabetes mellitus
- To monitor therapy for diabetes

Notes

Increased and decreased levels are the same as for the Fasting Blood Sugar Test.

TEST 47
Cholesterol and Lipoprotein Fractionation
(Serum)

This test measures the levels of cholesterol and lipoproteins in serum. Lipoproteins are lipids (fats) attached to proteins. The main substances measured are chylomicrons, HDL (high density lipoproteins), LDL (low density lipoproteins), IDL (intermediate density lipoproteins), and VLDL (very low density lipoproteins). Elevated levels of cholesterol, specifically high density lipoproteins (HDL) and low density lipoproteins, (LDL) are associated with coronary artery disease.

Values

Normal values for cholesterol vary according to age, sex, ethnicity, and geographic location. Therefore it is necessary to know the values of the testing laboratory.

Cholesterol

Males: Less than 200 mg/dL

Females: Usually lower values than males. Pregnant females have increased levels, 240-300 mg/dL.

Newborns: Around 100 mg/dL. Levels increase around the third month.

Elderly: Tend to have high normal values

Lipoproteins

Adults: 400-800 mg/dL (4-8 g/L)

LDL: 60-160 mg/dL. A risk factor for heart disease exists if values are greater than 160 mg/dL.

HDL: 30-80 mg/dL. An HDL value less than 30 mg/dL indicates a risk factor for heart disease.

Very Low Density Lipoproteins (VLDL): Results are calculated by this formula: VLDL = Plasma triglycerides/2.18

Uses

- To evaluate cholesterol levels
- To aid in detecting individuals at risk for coronary artery disease

Causes of Increased Levels of HDL

Increased levels of HDL usually signify a healthy state, but on occasion may signify hepatitis, alcohol ingestion, or cirrhosis. MI. Multiple myeloma. Eclampsia. Some drugs. Diabetes mellitus.

Causes of Increased Levels of LDL

Diabetes melitus. Hypertension. Lack of exercise. Smoking.

Notes

Increased levels of LDL place an individual at risk of coronary artery disease.

TEST 48
Triglycerides
(Serum)

Triglycerides are the main storage form of lipids, which are stored in adipose, or fatty, tissue. The triglyceride test measures the amount of triglycerides in the blood. Although the test has limited uses, it can indicate hyperlipidemia, which may lead to coronary artery disease or some forms of kidney disease.

Values

Adults: Levels of triglycerides vary according to age and sex. Levels that are acceptable vary.

Males: 40-160 mg/dl (0.40-2.0 mmol/L)

Females: 35-135 mg/dL

Children: Approximately 35-135 mg/dL

Infants: 5-10 mg/dL

Uses

- To screen individuals for increased lipids
- To detect the presence of some forms of kidney disease
- To screen individuals for risk of coronary artery disease

Causes of Increased Levels of Triglycerides

Increased levels of lipoproteins. MI. CVA. Underactive thyroid. Cirrhosis of the liver. Some forms of kidney disease. Diabetes mellitus. Pancreatitis. Down's syndrome. Increased carbohydrate ingestion. Pregnancy. Stress, both physical and emotional. Hypertension. Some drugs oral contraceptives and estrogen. Obstruction of the bile duct.

Notes

The serum of individuals with extremely high levels of triglycerides may have a cloudy appearance.

Causes of Decreased Levels of Triglycerides

Overactive thyroid. Physical exercise. Malnutrition. Some drugs. Increased vitamin C, or ascorbic acid, ingestion. Overactive parathyroid glands. Overactive thyroid. Congenital abnormality of lipoproteins (lipoproteins stay in tissues and are not released into the blood).

TEST 49
Serum Protein Electrophoresis
(Serum)

This test measures amounts of albumin and globulins in the serum by subjecting an agar gel impregnated with a sample of serum to an electric field. The proteins migrate according to the electrical charge and form bands, or patterns.

Values

Adults: Total protein 6-8 g/dL

Serum albumin: 3-5 g/dL; 50-60% of total protein

Serum globulins: 2-4 g/dL; 40-50% of total protein

Apha-1 globulin: 0.1-0.4 g/dL; 4-7% of total protein

Alpha-2 globulin: 0.4-0.1 g/dL; 7-12% of total protein

Beta-1 globulin: 0.5-1.1 g/dL; 1-9% of total protein

Gamma globulin: 0.5-1.7 g/dL; 13-24%

Children: Tend to have slightly higher amounts than adults

Infants and newborns: About the same as an adult's

Pregnant females: An overall decrease in amounts of proteins

Uses

- To diagnose liver disease
- To diagnose kidney disease
- To diagnose malnutrition
- To diagnose protein deficiency
- To diagnose certain malignancies

Causes of Increased Albumin (Hyperalbuminemia)

Dehydration. Multiple myeloma. Stressful exercise.

Causes of Decreased Albumin (Hypoalbuminemia)

Liver disease. AIDS. Kidney disease. Severe burns. Obstetrical complications. Severe malnutrition. Cirrhosis. Congestive heart failure. Occasionally, protein deficiency (more common) in some African American and Latino women.

Notes

If an individual loses albumin, a decrease in osmotic pressure results, possibly leading to edema.

Causes of Increased Globulins (Hypergammaglobulinemia)

Infection. Inflammatory response to injury. Burns. Liver disease.

Autoimmune disease. Some malignancies. Some leukemias. Multiple myeloma. Some anemias. Some kidney diseases. Radiation therapy. Some environmental toxins. Acute MI. Collagen diseases. Pregnancy.

Causes of Decreased Globulins (Hypogammaglobulinemia)

Emphysema. Some kidney diseases. Some leukemias. Congenital or acquired hypogammaglobulinemia. Agammaglobulinemia. (Refer to a more detailed hematology text for a discussion of specific immuno-globulin deficiencies.)

TEST 50
Alpha Fetoprotein
(Serum)

This test is usually performed during weeks 16 to 20 of gestation. Alpha fetoprotein is the major protein produced by fetal tissue and tumors that develop from embryonic structures. The protein can cross the placenta and, therefore, increased levels may be found in maternal circulation. As fetal development approaches term, levels should begin to decrease in maternal circulation. The protein may also be found in certain malignant and nonmalignant conditions.

Values

Fetus: 200-400 mg/dL

Pregnant females: Serum levels increase to 2-16 µg/dL.

Following infancy (after 1 year): Less than 30 ng/dL

Immunoassay test: 6.4 IU/mL or < 15 ng/mL in males and nonpregnant females.

Uses

- To monitor therapy for some neoplasms
- To determine the need for amniocentesis in pregnant females
- To detect the likelihood of twins
- To determine low birth weight infants
- To determine birth defects

Causes of Increased Levels of Alpha-fetoprotein

In utero fetal death. Neural tube abnormalities (spina bifida or anaceph-aly). Down's syndrome. Duodenal atresia. Omphalocele. Turner's syndrome. Tetralogy of Fallot. Rh sensitization. Anacephaly. Intrauterine death.

In nonpregnant individuals the following: Liver malignancy. Germ cell tumors. Cancer of the pancreas. Absence of pregnancy. Alcoholic cirrhosis. Cancer of the stomach. Biliary malignancies. Chronic hepatitis.

TEST 51
Haptoglobin
(Serum)

This test measures the level of haptoglobin within the serum. Haptoglobin is a glycoprotein that binds free hemoglobin (Hgb) and prevents accumulation in the plasma. Plasma-free Hgb (Hgb that is not in the RBC) is of no value in transporting oxygen. When Hgb binds to haptoglobin it can be removed by the reticuloendothelial system (RES). In the event of intravascular hemolysis, haptoglobin levels may be low for a number of days. Intravascular hemolysis is increased by bacteria, antibody, anemias, mechanical trauma (e.g., heart valves), and complement proteins.

Values

All ages: 60-270 mg/dL (0.6-2.7 g/L)
Children: Much lower levels

Uses

- To measure the amount of hemolysis
- To monitor transfusion reactions
- To differentiate between hemoglobin and myoglobin in plasma

Causes of Increased Haptoglobin

Some malignancies. Chronic inflammatory diseases. Steroid therapy. Acute infections. Acute MI. Hodgkin's disease. Some kidney diseases. Some autoimmune diseases. Burns.

Causes of Decreased Haptoglobin

Hemolysis. Liver disease. Transfusion reactions. Infectious mononucleosis. DIC. Malaria. Some anemias. Some platelet disorders.

Notes

Haptoglobin may be absent in some African Americans, a condition called ahaptoglobinemia. If serum levels are very low, the physician watches for signs and symptoms of a transfusion reaction, such as chills, fever, back pain, rapid breathing (tachypnea), rapid heart rate (tachycardia), and decreased blood pressure (hypotension).

TEST 52
Serum Creatinine
(Serum)

This test measures the amount of creatinine in the blood. Creatinine is a breakdown product of creatinine phosphate, a high energy compound found in muscle cells. The level of creatinine in the blood is a good indicator of renal function. Creatinine is filtered in the glomeruli and given off in the urine. Increased levels in the blood indicate that the nephrons are not functioning. It is a more sensitive indicator of kidney function than the blood urea nitrogen (BUN) test.

Values

Adult males: 0.5-1.5 mg/dL (45-130 µmol/L). Higher numbers are due to greater muscle mass.

Adult females: 0.5-1.0 mg/dL (45-90 µmol/L)

Children: 0.5-1.0 mg/dL (45-90 µmol/L)

Infants: Lower than children's

Uses

- To aid in diagnosing kidney disease
- To determine kidney function
- To assess glomerular filtration

Causes of Increased Creatinine

Kidney disease. Some malignancies. Hodgkin's disease. Some leukemias. Some autoimmune diseases. MI. Many drugs. Diabetes that has progressed to nephropathy. CHF. Shock.

Causes of Decreased Creatinine

Pregnancy. Some obstetrical complications.

TEST 53
Plasma Ammonia (NH₃)
(Serum)

This test measures the amount of ammonia in plasma. It should be noted on the blood sample tube whether the individual is taking antibiotics.

Ammonia is formed in the intestine by the action of bacteria on proteins. It enters the portal circulation to the liver where it is converted to urea. The body uses ammonia as a source of nitrogen for making proteins. Ammonia is converted to urea which is excreted by the kidneys. In many forms of liver disease, damage to the liver cells prevents the breakdown of ammonia, which then accumulates in plasma.

Values

Adults: Less than 50 µg/dL (range 10-45 µg/dL) (11-35 µmol/L)

Children: Slightly higher levels

Newborns: Significantly higher levels than an adult's

Uses

- To assist in detecting liver disease
- To monitor therapy for liver disease
- To diagnose hepatic coma

Causes of Increased Ammonia

Liver disease. Hemolytic disease of the newborn (HDN). Emphysema. Acidosis. Gastrointestinal bleeding. Congestive heart failure (CHF). Reye's syndrome. Individuals with a portal-caval shunt, which redirects blood to bypass the liver. Some drugs, especially diuretics. Individuals with liver failure on a high protein diet.

Causes of Decreased Ammonia

Kidney failure. Individuals on antibiotics. Hypertensive individuals. Some drugs.

TEST 54
Blood Urea Nitrogen (BUN)
(Serum)

The BUN measures the percentage of nitrogen contained in urea. Urea is a breakdown product of ammonia, which is a breakdown product of protein metabolism. Urea makes up about 40 to 50% of the blood's nonprotein nitrogen. The BUN reflects the amount of protein taken into the body and the amount excreted by the kidneys. The test is invalidated if the individual has liver disease, is overhydrated, or is dehydrated. The test may also be invalidated by certain drugs, such as some antibiotics and diuretics.

Values

Adults: 8–25 mg/dL

Pregnant females and newborns: May be slightly lower

Elderly: May have slightly higher values

Uses

- To diagnose kidney disease
- To evaluate kidney function
- To aid in evaluating fluid balance

Causes of an Increased BUN

Liver disease. Severe malnutrition. Low protein diet. I.V. administration of dextrose (glucose). Phenothiazines (drugs). Renal disease. Urinary tract obstruction. Increased protein catabolism (breakdown) that occurs with burns, for example.

Causes of a Decreased BUN

Liver damage. Overhydration. Malnutrition.

Notes

A correlation exists between the BUN and the Creatinine, and is referred to as the BUN:Creatinine Ratio. The ratio is 10:1–15:1. A ratio of less than 10:1 signifies malnutrition, liver disease, low protein diet, renal dialysis, or overhydration. A ratio greater than 15:1 signifies kidney disease, inadequate blood flow to the kidneys, shock, dehydration, GI bleeds, steroids, or some antibiotics.

TEST 55
Sodium (Na$^+$)
(Serum)

This test measures the amount of Na$^+$ in the blood.

Values

All age groups: 138-148 mEq/L (138-148 mmol/L)

Uses

- To aid in determining acid-base balance
- To assess kidney and adrenal function
- To assess fluid and electrolyte balance
- To assess neuromuscular function

Causes of Increased Sodium (Hypernatremia)

Low levels of H_2O (water) in the body. Loss of H_2O from the body that occurs, for example, in diarrhea and vomiting. Poor kidney function. Long periods of hyperventilation. Diabetes insipidus due to a central nervous system (CNS) disorder. Aldosteronism, which causes increased Na^+ (sodium) retention. Neonatal exchange transfusion with bank blood (bank blood has increased levels of Na^+). Liver failure. High Na^+ diet. A wide variety of drugs. Fever. Respiratory infections. Osmotic diuretics. Hypothalamic disorders. Overhydration with an I.V. of normal saline. Seizures. Administration of sodium bicarbonate ($NaHCO_3$). Na^+ retention.

Signs of Hypernatremia

Thirst. Increased temperature. Restlessness. Dry mouth and mucous membranes. Small amounts of urine produced (oliguria) or no urine produced (anuria). Poor muscle reflexes. Redness of the skin (flushing). Dry tongue. Rapid heart rate (tachycardia). Edema.

Notes

Hospitalized patients with an I.V. of normal saline running should be closely monitored for overhydration.

Hypervolemia may occur with hypernatremia. Signs of hypervolemia include the following: distended neck veins, dry cough, shortness of breath (dyspnea), chest rales (crackling sound in lungs), increased blood pressure (hypertension), edema, and others.

Causes of Decreased Sodium (Hyponatremia)

Heavy sweating. Gastric suctioning. Vomiting. Burns. Adrenal gland insufficiency. Overhydration. Some diuretics. Low Na^+ diet. Surgery. Pain. Some kidney diseases. Tissue injury. Inflammatory reactions. Excess of water. Increased levels of ADH. Some drugs. Addison's disease, which is caused by the lack of adrenal corticosteroids, causes the kidneys to excrete water and Na^+. Solute loss or water retention. A depletion of circulating blood volume. ADH secretion. Polydipsia (excessive fluid intake). Hypothyroidism.

Notes

Decreased levels of Na^+ cause hypovolemia. Hypovolemia is due to loss of water and electrolytes caused by diarrhea, vomiting, septicemia, burns, edema, kidney disease, and other conditions.

Signs of Hyponatremia

Headache. Tachycardia. Muscle twitches. Low blood pressure. Anxiety. Restlessness. Nausea. Seizures. Coma.

TEST 56
Potassium (K^+)
(Serum)

This test measures the amount of K^+ in the blood.

Values

All ages: 3.5-5.2 mEq/L (3.5-5.2 mmol/L)

Uses

- To assess acid-base balance
- To assess kidney function
- To assess glucose metabolism
- To evaluate hyperkalemia (increased K^+) and hypokalemia (decreased K^+)
- To assess neuromuscular and endocrine disorders
- To assess cardiac arrhythmias

Causes of Increased Potassium (Hyperkalemia)

Most commonly due to inadequate renal output of K^+. Overmedication with medicine containing K^+. Massive cell destruction that occurs, for example, in burns, crush injuries, and following a myocardial infarction. Decreased levels of aldosterone and other steroids. Increased retention of K^+ within the body caused by some diuretics. Diabetic ketoacidosis. Decreased Na^+ excretion due to kidney failure. Addison's disease, which causes decreased amounts of aldosterone. Little or no urine production (oliguria or anuria). A variety of drugs. Kidney failure. K^+ in intravenous fluids. Some types of acidosis in which the kidneys must excrete more H^+, which causes retention of K^+. Lack of insulin in diabetic ketoacidosis. This condition increases hyperkalemia because K^+ needs insulin to enter the cell. Insulin deficiency. Trauma. Cardiac surgery. Digitalis intoxication. Hypoaldosteronism.

Signs of Hyperkalemia

Generalized weakness. Nausea. Abdominal cramps. Diarrhea. Malaise. Oliguria (decrease in urine production). Flaccid muscles. Slow heart rate (bradycardia). EKG signs are peaked T waves, wide QRS complex, widened P-R interval, and S-T depression. Gastrointestinal symptoms can include anorexia, stomach distension, and signs of an ileus (diminished bowel sounds).

Notes

If a hyperkalemic individual needs a transfusion, the blood bag date must be checked, because stored blood that is over 2 weeks old has an increased amount of K^+.

Causes of Decreased Potassium (Hypokalemia)

Aldosteronism, or Cushing's disease. Diuretic therapy. Excessive amounts of licorice ingestion. Vomiting. Diarrhea. Dehydration. Malnutrition. Some types of diets. Burns. Some forms of kidney disease. Excessive amounts of glucose. A wide variety of drugs. Polyuria. Large doses of corticosteroids, which cause Na^+ retention and, therefore, a loss of K^+. Inadequate intake of K^+. Excessive loss of K^+. Certain tumors. Alkalosis. Hypothermia. Delirium tremens (DTs). Hypercalcemia. Acute leukemia. Metabolic acidosis. Increased sweat loss.

Signs of Hypokalemia

Vertigo (dizziness). Hypotension (low blood pressure). Cardiac arrhythmias. Nausea. Vomiting. Diarrhea. Abdominal cramping. Abdominal distension due to decreased peristalsis. Muscle weakness. Leg cramps. Behavioral changes. Irritability. Confusion. Depression.

Notes

The most accurate diagnosis of hypokalemia comes from the EKG report. EKG changes associated with hypokalemia show a flat T wave, S-T depression, and the appearance of the U wave. If the K^+ is very low, ventricular fibrillation, respiratory muscle paralysis, and cardiac arrest can occur.

TEST 57
Calcium (Ca^{++})
(Serum)

This test measures the amount of Ca^{++} in the blood.

Values

Adults: Total Ca^{++}: 8.5-10.5 mg/dL or 4.5-5.5 mEq/L (2.3-2.8 mmol/L)
Ionized Ca^{++}: 4.5-5.0 mg/dL or 2.2-2.5 mEq/L (1.1-1.2 mmol/L)
Newborns, infants, and children: Higher values
Pregnant females: Lower values

Most laboratories report total Ca^{++}.

Uses

- To assess neuromuscular disorders
- To aid in diagnosing acid-base imbalances
- To evaluate blood clotting
- To diagnose cardiac arrhythmias
- To assess skeletal and endocrine disorders

Notes

In acidosis, most Ca^{++} is ionized. In alkalosis, most Ca^{++} is bound to protein and cannot be ionized.

Causes of Increased Calcium (Hypercalcemia)

Dehydration. Increased amounts of parathyroid hormone (PTH), which causes persistently high serum Ca^{++}. High Ca^{++} levels may be a sign of bone disease, because bone that is being destroyed releases Ca^{++}. Long-term immobilization. Thiazide diuretics. Vitamin D intoxication. Increased Ca^{++} can lead to kidney stones (individuals with increased Ca^{++} must be well hydrated to prevent formation of stones). Parathyroid tumors. Paget's disease. Multiple myeloma. Some malignancies. Multiple bone fractures. Kidney disease. Adrenal disease. Increased Ca^{++} ingestion (too much antacid). Bone malignancies. Alcoholism.

Signs of Hypercalcemia

Bone pain. Flaccid muscle. Flank pain due to kidney stones. Nausea. Vomiting. Dehydration. Coma. Death, possibly, usually due to cardiac arrest. Heart block. Anorexia. Slow reflexes. Nerve fibers with a decreased excitability. Constipation. Confusion. Slow heart rate. Pathologic fractures due to Ca^{++} loss from bones. Fatigue. Memory loss. Disorientation. Loss of consciousness.

Notes

Patients with hypercalcemia who take digoxin (cardiac medication that slows the heart rate) must be monitored closely. Increased Ca^{++} enhances the effect of digoxin. Thiazide diuretics are never used to treat hypercalcemia.

Causes of Decreased Calcium (Hypocalcemia)

Hypoparathyroidism (under active parathyroid glands), which is often found in preterm infants. Kidney failure. Elevated phosphate concentrations (Ca^{++} concentrations are lowered). Pancreatitis. Following blood transfusion, because citrate binds Ca^{++}. Severe malnutrition. Rickets, which is found in children with poor diets and who lose Ca^{++} from bone as a result. Osteomalacia, or soft bones, which develops in the elderly and corresponds to a loss of Ca^{++} from bone. Osteoporosis, which occurs in postmenopausal women and is related to lack of Ca^{++} in the diet. Total removal of the parathyroid. Vitamin D deficiency. Malabsorption of Ca^{++}. Cushing's syndrome. Peritonitis (infection of the peritoneum). Diarrhea. Septicemia. Some drugs. Burns.

Notes

Medical personnel should be aware of the affect of pH on Ca^{++} solubility. In alkalotic states, Ca^{++} is less soluble. Therefore the ionized Ca^{++} level may be low but not be evident in the test results of the total Ca^{++}. The opposite occurs in acidosis. More Ca^{++} is in the ionized state but symptoms of low Ca^{++} may not appear in the patient. Acidosis can mask a hypocalcemic state.

A Ca^{++} deficit increases capillary permeability and fluid leakage. The health care worker should make sure the low Ca^{++} level is not due to a low level of albumin, to which most Ca^{+++} is bound.

Signs of Hypocalcemia

Numbness at the periphery and around the mouth. Rigid muscles (tetany). Muscle twitches. Facial spasm. Muscle cramping. Foot spasms. Cardiac arrhythmias. Possible seizures. Muscle spasms of the hand. Twitching, which is usually a positive sign of hypocalcemia. Pathologic fractures. Depression.

Notes

Calcium gluconate can be administered when a rapid effect is needed to replace Ca^{++}. With replacement therapy, blood samples should be drawn before and after therapy to make sure the Ca^{++} level is not too high.

TEST 58
Chloride (Cl⁻)
(Serum)

This test measures the amount of Cl⁻ in the blood.

Values

Adults: 98-111 mEq/L (98-111 mmol/L)
Infants and children: Slightly higher

Uses

- To monitor acid-base disturbances
- To evaluate fluid balance
- To assess anion-cation balance

Causes of Increased Chloride (Hyperchloremia)

Increased Cl⁻ indicates either an increase in Na^+ or a decrease in HCO_3^-. Aldosterone causes the retention of Na^+ and Cl⁻. A deficit of water or ingestion of large amounts of salt. Some types of kidney failure. The kidneys cannot excrete Cl⁻, which leads to renal hyperchloremic acidosis. Decreased amounts of HCO_3^-. Overhydration with I.V. of normal saline. Dehydration. Kidney failure. Head trauma. Hypernatremia. Hyperparathyroidism. Some malignancies. Multiple myeloma. Burns. Infections. Some drugs. Hyperventilation.

Signs of Hyperchloremia

Weakness. Rapid deep breathing. Stupor. Coma and death are possible.

Causes of Decreased Chloride (Hypochloremia)

Prolonged vomiting, which leads to hypochloremic alkalosis. Gastric suctioning. Kidney failure. Addison's disease. Dilution of plasma. Congestive heart failure. Intestinal fistulas. Dehydration. Hyponatremia. Decreased Na^+ diet. Hypokalemia. Diabetic acidosis. Some drugs. Infections. Burns. Profuse sweating. Metabolic alkalosis due to vomiting, diarrhea, gastric suctioning, or diuretics. As Cl^- is lost, HCO_3^- is retained to balance the anions, a situation that gives rise to metabolic alkalosis. Alkalosis, which can cause a decrease in Cl^-. Patients with chronic lung disease often have decreased levels of Cl^- due to higher HCO_3^- levels that offset increased $PaCO_2$ (acidosis).

Signs of Hypochloremia

Tetany (tense muscles). Decreased rate of breathing. Hyperexcitability. Low blood pressure.

TEST 59
Magnesium (Mg^{++})
(Serum)

This test measures the amount of Mg^{++} in the blood.

Values

Adults: 1.7–2.1 mg/dL (by atomic absorption) or 1.5–2.5 mEq/L
Children: Slightly higher
Pregnant females: Slightly lower values

Uses

- To assess electrolyte status
- To evaluate kidney and/or neuromuscular function

Causes of Increased Magnesium (Hypermagnesemia)

Kidney failure (inability to excrete Mg^{++}). Addison's disease. Dehydration. Diabetes mellitus. Leukemias. Some drugs. Magnesium therapy given to obstetrical patients for preeclampsia or toxemia.

Signs of Hypermagnesemia

Sweating (diaphoresis). Tiredness. Muscle weakness. Low blood pressure. Weak pulse. Shallow respiration. Poor tendon reflexes. Feeling of warmth. Flushing (redness). Diminished reflexes. Sedation. Depression of neuromuscular function. Muscle paralysis. Weak deep tendon reflexes. EKG changes.

Causes of Decreased Magnesium (Hypomagnesemia)

Chronic alcoholism. Diarrhea. Malabsorption syndrome. Some diuretics. Following bowel resection. Long-term gastric or bowel drainage. Burns. Hypoparathyroidism. Increased levels of Ca^{++}. Pancreatitis. Aldosteronism. Protein malnutrition. Cirrhosis. Hypokalemia. Diabetes mellitus. Hypercalcemia.

Signs of Hypomagnesemia

Cramps, especially in the foot and legs. Muscle weakness. Cardiac arrhythmias. Muscle twitching. Seizures. Tremors and tetany. Overactive tendon reflexes.

TEST 60
Phosphate (HPO_4^{--})
(Serum)

This test measures the amount of HPO_4^{--} in the blood.

Values

Adults: 2.5-4.5 mg/dL (by atomic absorption) or 1.8-2.6 mEq/L (0.78-1.5 mmol/L)

Children: Higher levels

Elderly: Lower levels

Pregnant females: Lower levels

Uses

- To assess kidney function
- To evaluate acid-base imbalances
- To assess Ca^{++} imbalances
- To monitor endocrine and skeletal disorders

Causes of Increased Phosphate (Hyperphosphatemia)

Hypoparathyroidism. Bone diseases. Kidney failure. Healing fractures. Intestinal obstruction. Diabetic acidosis. Hypocalcemia. Excess vitamin D. Bone tumors. Some drugs.

Notes

An increased level of HPO_4^{--} rarely causes problems. If an increased level is prolonged, however, bone metabolism is affected, causing deposits of calcium phosphate.

Signs of Hyperphosphatemia

They are the same as those for hypocalcemia.

Causes of Decreased Phosphate (Hypophosphatemia)

Malabsorption syndrome. Malnutrition. Hyperparathyroidism. Renal tubular acidosis. Treatment for diabetic acidosis. Starvation. Hypercalcemia. Hypomagnesemia. Alcoholism. Vitamin D deficiency. Overhydration with I.V. glucose. Some drugs. Some diuretics. Hyperalimentation therapy.

Signs of Hypophosphatemia

Confusion. Irritability. Muscle cramping. Bone pain.

Notes

Children with a decreased level can have abnormal growth.

TEST 61
Anion Gap
(Serum)

This test quantitates the difference between anions and cations in the blood. Sodium is the most abundant cation, and chloride and bicarbonate are the most abundant anions.

Values

All ages: The normal gap is 10-12 mEq/L.

Uses

- To assess kidney function
- To determine the type of acidosis present

Results

The anion gap can be normal, increased, or decreased.

Normal   A normal anion gap does not necessarily indicate the absence of acidosis. It does indicate that no imbalance exists between anions and cations, for example, in hyperchloremic acidosis. Other causes of an anion gap imbalance are hyperkalemic acidosis, which is caused by substances that make the blood more acidic; kidney disease caused by sickle-cell disease; and hydronephrosis.

Increased anion gap acidosis, >12 mEq/L This gap occurs when unmeasured anions are increased, as in metabolic acidosis caused by increased lactic acid. Causes include the following: kidney failure, alcohol ingestion, diabetic acidosis, lactic acidosis, and ingested toxins (aspirin and antifreeze, among others).

Decreased anion gap, <10 mEq/L This condition is rare and usually not clinically significant, although it can indicate other disorders. It can occur with the following: multiple myeloma, hypermagnesemia, metabolic alkalosis, and Waldenström's macroglobulinemia. A decreased anion gap can also occur when the Na^+ concentration decreases without a corresponding decrease in the Cl^- and HCO_3^- concentrations.

TEST 62
Arterial Blood Gas (ABG)
(Whole Blood)

The ABG test is one of the most informative diagnostic tests used in clinical medicine. Understanding the results of the ABG is essential for the care and management of critically ill patients, such as those with cardiac, pulmonary, and renal disease, among others. The ABG test provides important information about (1) the ability of the lungs to provide O_2 to the blood (oxygenation) and (2) the ability of the lungs and kidneys to rid the blood of the by-products of cellular metabolism. If these waste products, which are mostly acids, accumulate in the blood, they interfere with enzymatic reactions essential for life. Measurements obtained from the ABG assist in evaluating the ability of the lungs and kidneys to carry out their functions. When the lungs are damaged, they have difficulty in (1) oxygenating the blood, which results in hypoxemia, and (2) removing CO_2, which causes respiratory acidosis. When the kidneys are damaged they cannot remove fixed acids (acids that cannot be converted to a gas), and metabolic acidosis occurs.

The ABG test requires a sample of heparinized arterial blood. The blood is analyzed in a blood gas analyzer.

The ABG test provides the following results from a sample of arterial blood:

- pH   the measure of acidity
- PaO_2 the partial pressure of oxygen

- $PaCO_2$ the partial pressure of carbon dioxide
- SaO_2 the oxygen saturation of hemoglobin
- HCO_3^- the bicarbonate ion concentration
- BE   the excess or deficit of bicarbonate ion

Components of the Arterial Blood Gas Test

1. pH

The pH is defined as the negative logarithm of the [H^+] (hydrogen ion concentration). There is an inverse relationship between the pH and the [H^+]. The greater the [H^+] is, the lower the pH and the more acidic the solution. The lower the [H^+] is, the higher the pH and the more alkalotic, or basic, the solution. Both the pH and the [H^+] are measures of acidity. Some ABG reports provide the [H^+] instead of the pH. The [H^+] is then reported in nmol/L.

2. $PaCO_2$

The $PaCO_2$ is the partial pressure of CO_2 in arterial blood. The concentration of CO_2 in arterial blood is determined by the rate of tissue metabolism. The $PaCO_2$ indicates whether or not the lungs are able to remove CO_2 from the blood, that is, are functioning properly. When CO_2 is not exhaled but is retained and builds up in the blood, the $PaCO_2$ increases. Any disease or condition that affects the lungs can interfere with the exchange of CO_2 between blood and alveoli.

Respiratory Acidosis   Hypoventilation (decreased rate of breathing) is one cause of increased CO_2 in the blood. An increase in the $PaCO_2$ above 45 mmHg indicates respiratory acidosis. In respiratory acidosis the increased CO_2 reacts with water (H_2O) to form increased H_2CO_3 (carbonic acid). H_2CO_3 dissociates and forms H^+ and HCO_3^-. The increased H^+ in solution increases the pH.

Respiratory Alkalosis   With hyperventilation (increased rate of breathing) a decrease of CO_2 occurs in the blood. This decrease causes the $PaCO_2$ to fall below 35 mmHg, which indicates respiratory alkalosis. Alkalosis occurs because less CO_2 is in the blood.

3. HCO_3^-

HCO_3^- is an anion found in blood. Red cells and kidney cells are the only cells capable of producing HCO_3^-, which they do through the breakdown of carbonic acid (H_2CO_3). The amount of HCO_3^-

in the blood is controlled by the kidneys. When the blood is low in HCO_3^-, there is too much H^+, and metabolic acidosis results. Too much HCO_3^- or too little H^+ results in metabolic alkalosis.

HCO_3^- is the most important buffer within the blood. As long as there is a ratio of 20:1 between HCO_3^- and H_2CO_3, the pH of the blood will remain at 7.40 (see figure below).

4. Base Excess

The base excess (BE) is a measure of the excess HCO_3^- and is evaluated along with the pH and $PaCO_2$. When the BE is negative, there is too little base, and acidosis is indicated. When the BE is positive, there is too much base, and alkalosis is indicated. The BE may also be called the base deficit. A positive (+) base deficit is an excess of HCO_3^-. A negative (-) base deficit is a deficiency of HCO_3^-.

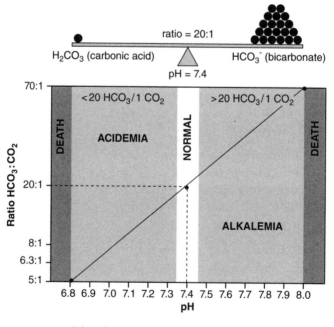

Bicarbonate/Carbon Dioxide Ratio

Adapted from William J. Malley, *Clinical Blood Gases,* 1990, originally appearing in Jacob, S.W., and Fancone, CA: *Structure and Function in Man, 2nd ed.,* W.B. Saunders Company, 1970. Permission granted by Harcourt Brace/W.B. Saunders, Philadelphia.

5. PaO_2

The PaO_2 is the partial pressure, or concentration, of O_2 in arterial blood. The greater the PaO_2, the more O_2 there is bound to Hgb. Thus more O_2 can be delivered to the cells. Pulmonary diseases, such as emphysema, chronic bronchitis, and many others, affect the PaO_2. Other conditions, such as heart attacks, congestive heart failure, chest trauma, damage to chest muscles and the diaphragm, and paralysis, among others, also affect the delivery of O_2 to the tissues.

6. A-a gradient

The A-a gradient is the difference in the partial pressure of O_2 between the alveoli (A) and the pulmonary capillary blood (a). The partial pressure gradient between the alveoli and pulmonary capillary blood is the force that moves O_2 from the alveoli into the pulmonary capillary blood. The A-a gradient is an indicator that blood is being shunted, or redirected, as in atrial septal defects (ASDs) and pulmonary embolus (PE).

7. SaO_2

The SaO_2 is the percentage or quantity of O_2 in arterial blood combined with Hgb. The SaO_2 is the ratio between the amount of O_2 bound to Hgb and the amount of O_2 that could be bound to Hgb.

Acids and Bases

Acids   Acids are substances that add free H^+ to a solution. An example is HCl (hydrochloric acid), which when placed in water ionizes into H^+ ions and Cl^- (chloride ions). The more free H^+ there is, the more acidic the solution.

Body cells constantly produce metabolic by-products from the breakdown of proteins, carbohydrates, and lipids. Most metabolic by-products are acids. Cellular by-products, such as CO_2 and lactic acid (a fixed acid), must be removed from the body. If they are allowed to accumulate in the blood, acidosis occurs. CO_2 is a volatile acid (a gas) removed by the lungs, which excrete more acid than any other organ in the body. Lactic acid and keto acids are fixed acids (they cannot be converted to a gas) and can only be removed by the kidneys.

Bases   Bases are chemicals that add OH^- (hydroxyl ions) to a solution causing it to become more alkaline, or basic. An example of a base, or alkaline solution, is NaOH (sodium hydroxide). When NaOH is placed in water, it ionizes to Na^+ (sodium ions) and OH^- (hydroxyl ions). The more OH^- there are, the more alkaline, or basic, the solution.

Excess bases are removed from the blood by the kidneys. Bases include chemicals such as phosphates and sulfates.

Acid-base Balance

The body must maintain a balance between acids and bases in the blood in order for normal physiologic functions to occcur, such as important enzymatic reactions. Actually, there is not a true balance between acids and bases because the pH of blood is slightly basic. To determine whether there is an imbalance of acids and bases, the clinician must examine the $PaCO_2$, pH, HCO_3^-, and the BE.

The body has three mechanisms for regulating acid-base balance: (1) the action of the lungs, (2) the kidneys, and (3) the blood buffers.

- The lungs help maintain the pH in the normal range by removing CO_2 from the body through exhaling.
- The kidneys help maintain the pH in two ways: (1) they excrete fixed acids in the urine, and (2) they produce HCO_3^-- ions. The kidneys respond to blood HCO_3^- ion concentration either by adding HCO_3^- to the blood when acidosis occurs or by removing HCO_3^- from the blood when alkalosis occurs.
- Blood buffers help maintain pH by absorbing free H+ from solution.

Blood buffers are chemicals that prevent significant changes in acidity or alkalinity of a solution by absorbing H+ and OH- from solution. The major blood buffers are hemoglobin (Hgb) and bicarbonate (HCO_3^-) ion. The main function of blood buffers is to safeguard against an accumulation of acids or bases by quickly removing them from solution.

Compensation in Acid-Base Disturbance

Compensation is the process whereby the organ system not involved in the primary acid-base disturbance (lungs or kidneys) returns the pH toward the normal range. For example, if the lungs are the cause of the acid-base imbalance, the kidneys will either retain or release H+ or HCO_3^- in order to return the pH toward normal.

Compensation may be either partial or complete. When the results of the ABG show no compensation, the acid-base imbalance is acute (new) and compensation has not had time to work.

Respiratory compensation usually happens within minutes after the primary acid-base disturbance occurs. The lungs can rapidly increase or decrease the rate of breathing thereby either blowing off or retaining more CO_2.

Renal compensation occurs usually hours to days after the acid-base disturbance occurs. The kidneys are slower to work in returning the pH toward normal. Although the kidneys are slower to work, they are better able than the lungs to return the pH toward normal.

Values

pH   Arterial: 7.35-7.45   **Venous:** 7.31-7.41
Neonates: Slightly lower

The international standard (SI; International System) for measuring units of pressure is the pascal. Clinical medicine uses the kilopascal (kPa), which is 1000 times more than the pascal.

PaO_2 Arterial: 75-100 mm Hg (10.6 -13.3 kPa) **Venous:** 40 mm Hg
Aged: The PO_2 drops about 5 mm Hg for each 10 years above 30.
Neonates: Lower values, about 60-70 mm Hg

High elevations: Lower values, because the PO_2 is lower. Red cells increase in number in response to the lower O_2 concentration in individuals living at high altitudes (see Ch. 4, Red Blood Cells and Ch. 5, Oxygen and Carbon Dioxide Transport).

$P(A-a)O_2$ gradient   Arterial: 5-10 mm Hg

Gradient: This should be less than 65 mm Hg if the individual is on 100% O_2 therapy.

O_2 Saturation (SaO_2)   Arterial: 95% or greater   **Venous:** 75%

$PaCO_2$ Arterial: 35-45 mm Hg (4.6-6 kPa)   **Venous:** 41-51 mm Hg
Pregnant females: Lower values, especially in the last trimester
Persons at high elevations: The atmospheric pressure is lower, and, therefore, the PCO_2 is lower.

HCO_3^- Arterial: 22-26 mEq/L   **Venous:** 22-26 mEq/L
Pregnant females: Lower values
Neonates: Lower values 20-26 mEq/L

BE   Arterial and Venous: +/- 2 mEq/L of HCO_3^-

The base excess is abnormal if the HCO_3^- is greater than or less than 2 mEq/L. A negative BE is sometimes referred to as a base deficit.

Uses of the Arterial Blood Gas

- To determine the O_2 and CO_2 content of blood
- To monitor acid-base status

- To monitor the effects of respiratory therapy
- To assess ventilatory control (lung function)
- To assess renal function in regulating acid-base balance
- To assess the adequacy of extracorporeal circulation during cardiovascular surgery

Causes of Respiratory Acidosis, or Increased PaCO$_2$

An increase in blood CO$_2$ causes respiratory acidosis. Hypoventilation indicates that not enough CO$_2$ is being removed from the blood. Hypoventilation often occurs with certain drugs that depress the central nervous system (CNS), such as sedatives, anesthetics, and narcotics, or in respiratory diseases, such as emphysema, asthma, and bronchitis. To compensate for the increase, the kidneys retain HCO$_3^-$ and excrete more H$^+$.

An increased PaCO$_2$ can be referred to as hypercapnia or hypercarbia. An increased PaCO$_2$ can be a compensatory mechanism for metabolic alkalosis.

Obstructive lung disorders (emphysema, bronchitis, asthma), pneumonia, and others. Drugs such as sedatives, anesthetics, barbiturates, and others depress the CNS. Muscular disorders, such as myasthenia gravis, polio, some forms of muscular dystrophy, and others. Chest wall injuries. Airway obstruction. Brain injury. Hypoventilation may be due to an improperly adjusted ventilator in individuals who are intubated.

Symptoms

Increased heart rate. Decreased depth and rate of breathing. Cyanosis of the extremities toes, fingers, nail beds, lips, mucous membranes, and others. Mental confusion. Muscle weakness. Fear. Sleepiness. Headache. Possible coma.

Causes of Respiratory Alkalosis, or Decreased PaCO$_2$

Decreased amounts of CO$_2$ in the blood lead to respiratory alkalosis. Hyperventilation (increased rate of breathing) removes too much CO$_2$ from the blood. Anytime the rate of breathing is increased, respiratory alkalosis results. An individual on a respirator for extended periods of time must be monitored to prevent too much CO$_2$ from being removed. A decreased PaCO$_2$ can be a compensatory mechanism in metabolic acidosis.

Some lung disorders. Head trauma or brain injury. Some types of bacterial septicemia. Pulmonary embolus. Improperly adjusted ventilators.

High fever. Aspirin overdose. Strenuous exercise. High altitude. Pain. Pulmonary edema.

Symptoms

Decreased blood pressure. Increased rate of breathing. Tingling (numbness) around mouth and in the extremities. Irregular cardiac rhythms. Mental confusion. Fear. Vertigo (dizziness). Muscle cramping and weakness.

Causes of Metabolic Alkalosis, or Increased HCO_3^-

Any increase in HCO_3^- leads to metabolic alkalosis. Metabolic alkalosis may be caused by a number of conditions, including an imbalance in the electrolytes K^+ and Cl^-. Aside from electrolyte imbalances, the major cause of metabolic alkalosis is the loss of gastric juice from the stomach due to prolonged vomiting or gastric suctioning. The use of sodium bicarbonate (baking soda) as a home remedy for indigestion can cause an increase in the amount of HCO_3^- in the blood. HCO_3^- also increases in the blood as a compensatory mechanism for respiratory acidosis. Compensation is found in individuals with chronic lung disease. These individuals have decreased levels Cl^-, which offsets the increased HCO_3^- in the blood. In metabolic alkalosis the $PaCO_2$ can be increased to compensate for the increased HCO_3^-.

Loss of gastric juice from vomiting (primarily due to loss of K^+, H^+, or Cl^-). Electrolyte imbalance due to diuretics or other causes. Decreased amounts of K^+ (hypokalemia). Corticosteroid therapy. Gastric suctioning. Treatment of acidosis with alkaline substances such as sodium bicarbonate ($NaHCO_3$). Liver disease. Some drugs. Decreased blood volume. Diarrhea.

Symptoms

Seizures, possibly. Muscle weakness and cramping. Irritable behavior. Nausea.

Causes of Metabolic Acidosis, or Decreased HCO_3^-

A decrease in the amount of HCO_3^- is a sign of metabolic acidosis. A decrease can be due to (1) bicarbonate that is being utilized to neutralize acids, or (2) loss of HCO_3^- through the kidneys, or (3) an increase in the amount of Cl- in the blood. Any rapid increase in the amount of acid that enters the body also causes a decrease in HCO_3^-.

Kidney failure. Some poisons. Cardiac arrest (due to a buildup of lactic acid). Shock. Ketoacidosis of diabetes. Alcohol ingestion. Certain parenteral nutrition products. Burns. MI. Starvation.

Symptoms

Loss of appetite. Mental confusion. Low blood pressure. Tiredness. Abnormal heartbeat. Headache. Loss of consciousness. Coma.

■ Interpreting a Blood Gas Report

1. Look at the pH

The pH indicates whether the blood is acidotic or alkalotic.

- Acidosis is indicated when the pH is less than (<) 7.35.
- Alkalosis is indicated when the pH is greater than (>) 7.45.

2. When the pH is < 7.35, acidosis is indicated. To determine whether the acidosis is due to (1) increased CO_2 (respiratory), look at the $PaCO_2$ or (2) to decreased HCO_3^- (renal), look at the HCO_3^-.

- When the $PaCO_2$ is > 45 mm Hg, the acidosis is respiratory in origin.
- When the HCO_3^- is <22 mEq/L, the acidosis is metabolic (renal) in origin.

3. When the pH is > 7.45, determine whether the cause of the alkalosis is respiratory or renal by looking at the $PaCO_2$ and HCO_3^-.

- When the $PaCO_2$ is < 35 mm Hg, the alkalosis is respiratory.
- When the HCO_3^- is > 26 mEq/L, the alkalosis is metabolic or renal.

4. To assess the ability of the lungs to oxygenate the blood, look at the PaO_2.

- A normal PaO_2 is between 75 to 100 mm Hg.
- Hyperoxemia exists when the PaO_2 in the arterial blood is > 100 mm Hg. Hyperoxemia is an increase in the amount of O_2 in the blood and is not usually a problem clinically.
- Hypoxemia exists when the PaO_2 is < 75 mm Hg. Hypoxemia is a decrease in the amount of O_2 in the blood. A low level of O_2 in the blood can be detrimental to the individual.

TEST 63
Bilirubin
(Serum)

This test measures the amount of bilirubin in plasma. Bilirubin is the breakdown product of hemoglobin and the main component of bile. It is formed in the reticuloendothelial system and then bound by albumin.

Albumin transports bilirubin to the liver where it is converted into another substance and excreted along with bile. Bilirubin appears in two forms within the body: (1) direct, or conjugated (soluble), and (2) indirect, or unconjugated (protein-bound). When only one value is reported, it is the total bilirubin.

Values

Total Bilirubin: 0.1-1.2 mg/dL (1.7-20 μmol/L)

Direct: 0.1-0.4 mg/dL (1.7-5.0 μmol/L)

Indirect: 0.1-1.0 mg/dL

Pregnant females: Usually normal ranges of bilirubin during pregnancy

Children: The direct range is higher than an adult's.

Newborns: 1-12 mg/dL

Uses

- To assess liver function
- To monitor jaundice
- To assess the newborn's level of bilirubin
- To assist in detecting hemolytic anemia
- To determine biliary obstruction

Causes of Increased Bilirubin

Direct bilirubin indicates the following: Biliary obstruction. Hepatitis. Bile duct stones. Cirrhosis. Mononucleosis. Liver cancer. Many drugs.

Indirect bilirubin indicates the following: Cellular liver damage. Hemolytic anemia. Congenital enzyme deficiencies. Some drugs, antibiotics, caffeine, and aspirin.

Total bilirubin in the newborn: High levels of bilirubin may indicate the need for exchange transfusion.

TEST 64
Blood Alcohol
(Serum or Plasma)

Ethanol, also called grain alcohol, is the alcohol found in alcoholic beverages. Methanol (not drinkable) is a product of wood. If ingested, it can lead to convulsions, blindness, and even death.

A blood sample for alcohol testing should be packed in ice if it cannot be sent immediately to the testing laboratory. The specimen should be tightly capped to prevent exposure to air.

Results

Normally blood contains no alcohol.

Ethanol

0.00-0.05%; < 50 mg/dL	sober
0.05-0.10%; 50-100 mg/dL	the legal limit is 0.08%
0.10-0.15%; 100-150 mg/dL	intoxication
0.30-0.40%; 300-400 mg/dL	moderate intoxication
0.40-0.50%; 400-500 mg/dL	severe intoxication
0.50%->; > 500 mg/dL	coma and possible death

Methanol (wood alcohol)

25 mg/dL	toxic level
80-120 mg/dL	lethal

Uses

- To detect the presence of alcohol in the blood
- To determine a possible cause of coma

Notes

Most states use 0.08% blood alcohol as the legal standard for driving under the influence (DUI, or OUI). Medical personnel drawing a blood sample to determine the blood alcohol level should be familiar with both state law and the hospital's policy regarding the legal ramifications of testing. If a sample is drawn without consent, or if an error is made, the tested individual may be entitled to file a lawsuit.

TEST 65
Cytomegalovirus (CMV) Antibody Screen
(Serum)

This test is used to determine the presence of antibody to CMV in blood. CMV is a virus of the herpes family that inhabits WBCs, among other cell types. In immunoincompetent individuals the virus can be reactivated and cause serious infections. There are several ways that antibody to CMV can be detected.

Values

Normal antibody titer: Less than 1:5

Negative reaction: The individual with no prior CMV infection has no antibody to CMV.

Positive reaction: The individual is or has been infected with CMV and harbors the virus.

Uses

- To identify prior CMV infection in organ transplant donors and recipients
- To determine prior CMV infection in immunocompromised individuals, especially premature infants receiving transfusions

Notes

Immunosuppressed or immunoincompetent individuals should receive blood or organ transplants from individuals who are seronegative for CMV. CMV-free blood or allogeneic transplants decrease the morbidity and mortality associated with CMV.

TEST 66
Cold Agglutinins
(Serum)

Cold agglutinins are antibodies of the IgM type that aggregate when exposed to low temperatures, for example, in body extremities (fingers and toes). At the inner body temperature, these antibodies do not aggregate and, therefore, pose no problems. But at body temperatures less than 98.6F (37C), they agglutinate RBCs and activate complement proteins. As blood rewarms the antibodies dissolve in plasma. Complement proeins, however, remain on the RBCs and cause hemolysis, which leads to hemolytic anemia.

Values

Normally blood has titers less than 1:32.

The elderly: Increased titers

Uses

- To aid in diagnosing some types of pneumonia
- To prove the existence of cold agglutinins associated with some viral infections and some malignancies

Causes of Increased Cold Agglutinins

A high titer of antibody can occur independently or with some types of pneumonias or lymphomas. The titer is often high with certain infections, such as CMV and infectious mononucleosis, and sometimes in multiple myeloma, pregnancy, malaria, cirrhosis, pulmonary embolus, hemolytic anemias, and peripheral vascular disease. A very high titer of antibody indicates the individual can develop lymphoma. A high titer can present serious clinical problems, such as intravascular agglutination.

TEST 67
Complement Assays
(Serum)

Complement proteins can be measured using several methods. Each method measures the amount of complement in the blood. The assay is not specific and must be considered with other tests.

Values

Total complement: 330-739 CH_{50} units

C1 esterase inhibitor: 8-23 mg/dL

C3: 55-125 mg/dL

C4: 10-54 mg/dL

The elderly: Elevated levels of C1, C3, and C4

Newborns: Lower levels of C1, C3, and C4

Uses

- To aid in diagnosing immune complexes
- To evaluate complement deficiencies
- To monitor therapy
- To detect immunologic diseases

Notes

Complement deficiencies may be genetic or acquired, the latter being more common. The C1 esterase inhibitor is deficient in hereditary angioedema. C3 deficiency is associated with recurrent infections. C4 deficiency is found in patients with systemic lupus erythematosus.

Causes of Increased Complement

Not usually clinically significant. Complement can increase in some inflammatory conditions. Obstructive jaundice. Thyroiditis. Rheumatic fever. Arthritis. Diabetes. MI. Colitis. Some malignancies.

Causes of Decreased Complement

The presence of immune complexes. Insufficient synthesis of complement. Inhibitor formation. Increased breakdown of complement. Cirrhosis. Multiple myeloma. Septicemia. Some anemias. Hypogammaglobulinemia. Solid organ graft rejection. Some kidney diseases.

TEST 68
Folic Acid (Folate)
(Serum)

This test measures the amount of folic acid in the serum. Folic acid is a water soluble vitamin necessary for blood cell development and other body functions. This vitamin must be broken down before it becomes biologically active. Like other water soluble vitamins, it must be taken in with diet. The liver stores only small amounts.

Values

Adults: 3–16 ng/mL
Elderly: Possibly decreased values

Uses

* To diagnose anemia
* To evaluate levels of folic acid

Cause of Increased Levels of Folic Acid

Excessive dietary intake.

Note

An individual with pernicious anemia can show elevated levels.

Causes of Decreased Levels of Folic Acid

Megaloblastic anemia. Other anemias. Malabsorption syndrome. Liver disease. Pregnancy. Some drugs. Some malignancies. Malnutrition. Leukopenia. Thrombocytopenia. Hyperthyroidism. Alcoholism.

TEST 69
Hepatitis B Surface Antigen
(HBsAg, Australian Antigen)
(Serum)

This test detects the presence of HBsAg in the blood of individuals with hepatitis B. The test relies on an immunoassay, which detects the antigen in either an active or carrier state. The HBsAg can be detected from 2 to 24 weeks following exposure to the virus.

Results

Normally individuals are negative for the hepatitis antigen.

Uses

- To screen blood for hepatitis B prior to transfusion
- To aid in the diagnosis of hepatitis
- To screen health care workers susceptible to contracting hepatitis B

Notes

The presence of HBSAg indicates that the individual has hepatitis or is a carrier. Donor blood containing antigen must be discarded to prevent the possibility of transmitting the hepatitis virus to the recipient. Anytime blood tests positive for hepatitis it should be retested, because false-positive results do occur.

Causes of a Positive Test Result

HBSAg can also appear in individuals who have conditions other than hepatitis, such as leukemia, Hodgkin's lymphoma, and hemophilia.

TEST 70
Heterophile Agglutination
(Serum)

This test is primarily used to detect infectious mononucleosis caused by the Epstein-Barr virus (EBV). The test is conducted in two parts because (1) antibody to EBV causes a positive result and (2) Forssman antibody, which is sometimes found in normal serum, also causes a positive result. The first part measures antibody that agglutinates the RBCs of sheep and horses, and the second part distinguishes among different antibodies.

If the second part of the test is positive, a positive diagnosis of infectious mononucleosis can be established.

Values

All ages: The normal titer is less than 1:56

Elderly: May be higher than 1:56

Some laboratories refer to a normal titer as negative or "having no reaction."

Results

In an individual with infectious mononucleosis the antibody titer rises within 2 weeks of infection and peaks within 3 weeks. It can remain elevated for about 6 weeks. The results do not necessarily confirm a positive diagnosis because the titer may be higher than 1:56 in a number of conditions, such as syphilis, lupus erythematosus (LE), cryoglobulinemia, serum sickness, some viral infections, or antibody to treponemata organisms. Other tests can be used to confirm the diagnosis of infectious mononucleosis, such as blood tests that show lymphocytosis (increased lymphocytes).

Use

- To aid in the diagnosis of infectious mononucleosis

TEST 71
Immunoglobins A, G, M
(Serum)

This test measures the amounts of immunoglobulins IgG, IgA, and IgM. Immunoglobulins can be measured by several methods, including immunodiffusion and immunoelectrophoresis.

Values

Adult ranges:

IgG   700-1800 mg/dL (7.0-18.0 g/L)

IgA   70-440 mg/dL (0.7-4.4 g/L)

IgM   60-290 mg/dL (0.6-2.9 g/L)

Uses

- To monitor chemotherapy and radiation therapy

- To determine levels of gammaglobulins
- To diagnose hepatitis and cirrhosis
- To aid in diagnosing plasma protein abnormalities, such as multiple myeloma and Waldenström's macroglobulinemia.

Causes of Increased IgG, IgM, and IgA

IgG: Infections. Liver disease. Poor diet or malnutrition. Rheumatic fever. Sarcoidosis. Hyperimmunization. Some chronic infections. Myeloma. Rheumatoid arthritis. Lupus erythematosus. Pulmonary tuberculosis.

IgM: Some viral infections. Infectious mononucleosis. Some malignancies. Some parasitic diseases. Bacterial infections. Some types of fevers. Waldenström's macroglobulinemia. Hepatitis. Cirrhosis. Some parasitic diseases.

IgA: Liver disease. Chronic infections. Rheumatic fever. Autoimmune disorders. Myeloma. Rheumatoid arthritis. Lupus erythematosus.

Causes of Decreased IgG, IgM, and IgA

IgG: Some leukemias. Some obstetrical complications. Agammaglobulinemia. Some enzyme disorders. Lymphoid aplasia. Macroglobulinemia. Nephrotic syndrome. Some leukemias.

IgM: Same as for IgG.

IgA: Some malignancies. Some leukemias. Aplasia. Ataxia-telangiectasia. Nephrotic syndrome. Agammaglobulinemia.

TEST 72
Prostate-specific Antigen (PSA)
(Serum)

This test measures the level of prostate-specific antigen found in serum. The test helps detect prostatic cancer, and may also be used to track the course of therapy. PSA should be done in conjunction with a digital rectal exam. If increased levels are found, a tissue biopsy should be performed to confirm cancer.

Values

Adult males under 40: The PSA should not exceed 2.5 ng/ml.

Males over 40: The PSA should range from 1-4 ng/mL.

Uses

- To detect prostate cancer
- To monitor a course of therapy

Causes of Increased Levels of PSA

Prostate cancer. Levels may also be increased in benign prostatic hypertrophy.

TEST 73
Serum Osmolality
(Serum)

This test measures the osmolality of serum, which is the concentration of dissolved particles in plasma. Dissolved particles in plasma include the electrolytes, urea, and the sugar glucose. Sodium contributes about 90% to serum osmolality.

This test is useful in determining fluid and electrolyte imbalances. Osmolality may be altered by substances, such as alcohols, in the blood that are not measured by the osmolality test. Therefore this test may be used to screen individuals for alcohol ingestion.

The osmolality of any solution depends on the number of active particles within the solution. The greater the number of active particles there are, the greater the osmolality. Increased osmolality suggests hemoconcentration (dehydration), whereas decreased osmolality indicates hemodilution (overhydration).

Values

Adults: 280-297 mOsm/kg water (H_2O)
Children: Slightly lower values

Uses

- To determine the concentration of solutes in the serum
- To screen for alcohol ingestion
- To determine blood alcohol levels

Causes of Increased Osmolality

Possible fluid volume deficit. Kidneys unable to concentrate urine. Dehydration (hemoconcentration). Diabetes insipidus. Uremia. Hyperglycemia (increased glucose). Hypernatremia (increased Na^+).

Causes of Decreased Osmolality

Overhydration (fluid volume excess). Trauma, stress, drugs, malignancies, and some adrenal disorders can lead to a syndrome in which there is an inappropriate secretion of ADH.

TEST 74
Rapid Plasma Reagin (RPR)
(Serum)

The RPR is a fast and simple test used to screen serum for antibody to the causative agent syphilis. The test is also referred to as the circle card test. It is used to screen for either primary or secondary syphilis.

Results

Normally blood is negative for antibody to the spirochete *Treponema pallidum* that causes syphilis. False-positives may be found in individuals with viral infections, bacterial infections, chronic systemic infections, or infection with nonsyphilitic organisms.

Uses

- To screen serum for antibody to the causative spirochete
- To diagnose primary or secondary syphilis
- To monitor therapy for syphilis

Causes of Increased Levels

Primary or secondary syphilis

Notes

False-positive results can occur with the following: infectious mononucleosis, malaria, leprosy, hepatitis, rheumatoid arthritis, and systemic lupus erythematosus.

TEST 75
Vitamin B$_{12}$
(Serum)

This test measures the level of vitamin B$_{12}$ in serum. The test usually is evaluated in conjunction with folic acid.

Vitamin B$_{12}$ is a water-soluble vitamin that must be replenished through dietary intake. It is essential for blood cell development, skeletal growth, nervous system development, and other body requirements. Vitamin B$_{12}$ is absorbed from the intestine and stored in the liver. A deficiency causes one type of anemia.

Values

Adults: 100-800 pg/mL

Elderly: May have lower values

Uses

- To detect anemias
- To diagnose some central nervous system disorders.

Causes of Increased Vitamin B$_{12}$

Hepatitis. Some leukemias. Oral contraceptives. Polycythemia vera.

Causes of Decreased Vitamin B$_{12}$

Pernicious anemia. Malabsorption. Liver disease. Some drugs. Crohn's disease. Underactive thyroid. Partial removal of stomach. Pancreatic dysfunction.

TEST 76
Human Immunodeficiency Virus (HIV) Antibody Screen
(Serum)

This test, also known as the ELISA (Enzyme Linked Immunosorbent Assay), detects the presence of antibody to HIV.

Results

Normally blood has no antibody to HIV.

A positive test indicates exposure to HIV (Human Immunodeficiency Virus), the virus that causes AIDS. It does not tell anything else regarding the disease process. A positive test should be confirmed by the Western Blot and HIV-1-Ag test before a positive result is reported.

This test is not foolproof. It cannot determine if individuals have recently been exposed to HIV because the antibody titer may not be high enough. The time between a negative test and the development of antibody to HIV is the window, or lag, period.

Uses

- To screen blood prior to a transfusion for HIV
- To aid in diagnosing HIV

TEST 77
Western Blot
(Serum)

The Western Blot confirms the findings of a positive ELISA test for HIV. The test separates viral proteins via an electric current run through an agar gel in which the serum sample has been placed. The formation of bands indicates the individual has been exposed to HIV.

Results

Normally blood contains no antibody to HIV.

Positive reaction: Exposure to HIV is indicated.

Use

- To validate a positive ELISA HIV test

Blot Interpretation

Proteins produced by HIV form a pattern of bands. The protein bands are separated electrophoretically from one another. The major bands include: gp 160, gp 120, and gp 65. (Gp stands for glycoprotein, and the number following gp stands for the molecular weight of the protein in thousands, that is, 65,000.)

Negative blots have no bands present. A positive result shows a specific number of dark-colored bands. Some test results produce bands very light in color or intensity. These bands are indeterminate because they do not indicate a positive test result. An individual with indeterminate bands in the test result should be retested within 6 months.

The Western Blot test is highly sensitive and very specific for antibody to HIV, but the technical difficulty of performing the test, along with its high cost, make it impractical as a screening test.

TEST 78
HIV-1-Antigen (HIV-1-Ag)
(Serum)

In March 1996 the AABB and FDA required that blood and blood components for administration be nonreactive for the HIV-1 antigen. The test shows a positive result before the antibody screening test. The HIV-1-Ag test is the test of choice when screening for HIV.

The HIV-1-Ag test is an enzyme-linked immunosorbent assay that determines the presence of the p24 antigen associated with HIV-1. The patient's serum is mixed with unlabeled serum containing antibodies to HIV-1 antigen. A labeled indicator with the same antibody to p24 binds to any p24 antigen in the serum. A color change indicates a positive result.

Result

All blood and blood components should be negative unless infected by HIV.

Use

To determine whether blood is contaminated with HIV, the virus that causes AIDS

Heparin

Uses in Therapy

Heparin is a polysaccharide that occurs naturally within basophils and mast cells, but its exact physiologic role is unclear. Heparin produced within the body is refered to as endogenous heparin. Exogenous heparin, a drug used therapeutically, is derived from beef lung or pork intestinal mucosa. Exogenous heparin is used as an anticoagulant in certain medical procedures and treatments. However, it is not used in transfusion therapy for either blood collection or storage. The use of heparin prolongs an individual's clotting time and thus prevents unwanted clot formation. Although heparin prevents clot formation, it has no effect on clots already formed. In other words, the drug has no lytic effect. Heparin is the anticoagulant of choice if rapid anticoagulation is needed. The drug is fast-acting and can be reversed or neutralized once its effects are no longer needed.

Heparin is used in such medical procedures as hemodialysis, extracorporeal circulation, autologous blood recovery, and coronary artery angioplasty, among others. This drug prevents blood from clotting in the presence of foreign surfaces, whether they be medical equipment or tissue enzymes. Conditions that require heparin for treatment include pulmonary embolus, deep vein thrombosis, and myocardial infarction.

Individuals receiving heparin therapy must be monitored closely. The drug is administered by parenteral injection, either intravenously (I.V.) or subcutaneously (s.c.; under the skin). Heparin acts more quickly when adminstered by I.V. The dosage is measured in units per mL (U/mL).

Blood Tests That Monitor Heparin Therapy

The aPTT monitors the effectiveness of heparin therapy. The normal aPTT is 25 to 35 seconds.

The Reptilase Time (RT) tests for normal clotting time in the presence of heparin. The RT determines the clotting status of an individual on heparin. When reptilase is added to the sample tube, heparin does not inhibit fibrin formation. The normal RT is between 12 to 20 seconds (see Blood Tests).

531

Heparin and Antithrombin III

In order for heparin to act as an anticoagulant, it first must bind to antithrombin III (AT-III), which is a naturally occurring plasma protein inhibitor of activated clotting proteins. Heparin prevents clot formation by increasing the affinity of AT-III for activated clotting factors.

Heparin does not act as an anticoagulant in individuals deficient in AT-III. A deficiency is suspected when heparin administration does not increase the aPTT. Individuals deficient in AT-III can receive AT-III in fresh frozen plasma (FFP) or recombinant AT-III (Thrombate™).

Heparin Reversal

Once the anticoagulant effect of heparin is no longer needed, heparin is reversed. Reversal prevents the possibility of continued bleeding. The drug protamine, which is administered I.V., reverses the anticoagulative effects of heparin. Heparin, which is an acid, and protamine, which is a base, together form a salt that neutralizes the anticoagulative effect of heparin. Protamine has some anticoagulative effect when injected, but it is never used as an anticoagulant.

Caution must be exercised when using protamine. Because it is made from fish sperm, protamine can cause an anaphylactic reaction in individuals allergic to fish. Protamine can also lower blood pressure when it is administered I.V.

Scientific Symbols and Their Equivalents

>   greater than

<   less than

mm^3 cubic millimeter

L   liter, 1000 mL (approximately 1 quart)
dL   deciliter, 1/10 of a liter
mL   milliliter, 1/1000 of a liter
μL   microliter, 1/1,000,000 of a liter
fL   femtoliter, 1/1,000,000,000,000,000 of a liter

μ micron
mμ millimicron
μ^3 cubic micron

g   gram
kg   kilogram, 1000 grams (approximately 2 pounds)
mg   milligram, 1/1000 of a gram
μg   microgram, 1/1,000,000 of a gram
ng   nanogram, 1/1,000,000,000 of a gram
pg   picogram, 1/1,000,000,000,000 (trillionth) of a gram

mole M, the gram molecular weight of a substance (for example, 1 M of glucose = 180 grams)
mmol millimole, 1/1,000 of a mole
μmol micromole, 1/1,000,000 of a mole
fmol femtomole, 1/1,000,000,000,000,000 of a mole

Osm osmole
mOsm milliosmole, 1/1,000 of an osmole

mEqv milliequivalent, 1/1,000 of an Equivalent

U   unit

BIBLIOGRAPHY

Abbas, Abul K., M.B.B.S.; Lichtman, Andrew H., M.D., Ph.D.; Parker, Gordon S., M.D., Ph.D. *Cellular and Molecular Immunology.* Philadelphia: W.B. Saunders. 1992.

Adams, A.P., M.D.; Hahn, C.E.W., M.D. *Principles and Practice of Blood Gas Analysis.* London: Franklin Scientific Projects. 1979.

American Medical Association, *Drug Evaluations Annual 1994.* Milwaukee: 1994.

Avery, Mary Ellen, M.D.; First, Lewis, R., M.D. *Pediatric Medicine, 2nd ed.* Baltimore: Williams and Wilkins. 1994.

Bannister, Lawrence, H., M.D., *et al. Gray's Anatomy, 38th ed.* London: Churchill Livingstone. 1995.

Beck, William S., M.D., ed. *Hematology, 5th ed.* Cambridge: MIT Press. 1991.

Benjamini, Eli, M.D.; Leskowitz, Sidney, M.D.; *Immunology: A Short Course.* New York: John Wiley & Sons. 1991.

Bergman, Ronald, A., Ph.D, *et al. Histology.* Philadelphia: W.B. Saunders Co. 1996.

Beutler, Ernest, M.D.; senior ed., *et al. Williams Hematology, 5th ed.* New York: McGraw-Hill, Inc. 1995.

Brenner, Barry M., M.D., *The Kidneys, Vols. 1 and 2, 5th ed.* Philadelphia: W.B. Saunders Co. 1996.

Broder, Samuel, M.D., *et al. Textbook of AIDS Medicine.* Baltimore: Williams and Wilkens. 1994.

Bush, Roger K., M.D., ed. *The Medical Clinics of North America.* Philadelphia: W.B. Saunders. 1992.

Cohen, P.T., M.D., *et al. The AIDS Knowledge Base, 2nd ed.* Boston: Little Brown and Co. 1994.

Coltran, Ramzi, M.D., senior ed, *et al. Robbins Pathologic Basis of Disease, 5th ed.* Philadelphia: W.B. Saunders. 1994.

Creasy, Robert, K., M.D. *Maternal Fetal Medicine, 3rd ed.* Philadelphia: W.B. Saunders. 1994.

Cunningham, F. Gary, M.D., senior ed., *William's Obstetrics, 19th ed.* Norwalk, CT: Appleton & Lange. 1993.

De Shazi, Richard D., M.D., senior ed. *Primer on Allergic and Immunologic Disorders.* Prepared by the American Academy of Allergy and Immunology. Journal of the American Medical Association. Nov. 25, 1992. Vol. 268, No. 20.

DeVita, Vincent T., M.D.; Hellman, Samuel, M.D.; Rosenberg, Steven A., M.D., Ph.D., eds. *Cancer Principles and Practice of Oncology, 4th ed.* Philadelphia: J.B. Lippincott Co. 1993.

DeVita, Vincent T., M.D.; Hellman, Samuel, M.D.; Rosenberg, Steven A., M.D., Ph.D., eds. *AIDS Etiology, Diagnosis, Treatment, and Prevention, 3rd ed.* Philadelphia: J.B. Lippincott Co. 1992.

Guyton, Arthur C., M.D., *Textbook of Medical Physiology, 8th ed.* Philadelphia: W.B. Saunders. 1991.

Haskell, Charles M., M.D., ed. *Cancer Treatment, 3rd ed.* Philadelphia: W.B. Saunders. 1990.

Hathaway, William E., M.D.; Goodnight, Scott H. Jr., M.D. *Disorders of Hemostasis and Thrombosis.* New York: McGraw-Hill. 1993.

Henry, John B., M.D. *Clinical Management By Laboratory Methods, 18th ed.* Philadelphia: W.B. Saunders. 1991.

Hoffbrand, A.V., M.D.; Petit, J.E., M.D. *Essential Haematology, 3rd ed.* London: Blackwell Scientific. 1993.

Holland, James F., M.D.; Frei, Emil, III, M.D. *et al. Cancer Medicine, 4th ed.* Philadelphia: Lea and Febiger. 1997.

Jandl, James H., M.D. *Blood Textbook of Hematology, 2nd ed.* Boston: Little Brown and Company. 1996.

Janeway, Charles A.; Travers, Paul. *Immunobiology, 3rd ed.* London: Current Biology Limited/Garland Publishing. 1997.

Jeter, Elaine K., M.D.; Spivey, Mary Ann. *Introduction to Transfusion Medicine: A Case Study Approach.* Bethesda: AABB Press. 1996.

Lawlor, Glen J., M.D.; Fischer, Thomas J., M.D.; Adelman, Daniel C., M.D. *Manual of Allergy and Immunology, 3rd ed.* Boston: Little Brown and Company. 1995.

Lee, Richard G., M.D., *et al; Wintrobe's Clinical Hematology, Vols. 1, 2, 9th ed.* Philadelphia: Lea and Febiger. 1993.

Lewis, Mary senior ed.; *Diagnostic Tests.* Springhouse, PA: Springhouse Corp. 1994.

Loeb, Stanley, senior. ed. *Illustrated Guide to Diagnostic Tests.* Springhouse, PA: Springhouse Corp. 1994.

Malley, William J., M.S., R.R.T., CPFT. *Clinical Blood Gases.* Philadelphia: W.B. Saunders. 1990.

Mandell, Gerald, L., M.D. *et al. Principles and Practice of Infectious Disease, 4th ed.* New York: Churchill Livingstone. 1995.

Mollison, P.L., M.D.; Engelfriet, C.P., M.D.; Contreras, Marcella, M.D. *Blood Transfusion in Clinical Medicine, 9th ed.* London: Blackwell Scientific Publications. 1993.

Moreau, David, senior ed. *Nursing 96 Drug Handbook.* Springhouse PA: Springhouse Corporation. 1996.

Murray, John F., M.D.; Nadel, Jay A., M.D. *Respiratory Medicine, 2nd ed.* Philadelphia: W.B. Saunders. 1994.

Perry, Michael C., M.D. ed. *American Society of Clinical Oncology Educational Book, Spring 1997.* Alexandria, VA: American Society of Clinical Oncology. 1997.

Playfair, J.H.L., M.D. *Immunology at a Glance, 6th ed.* London: Blackwell Scientific. 1996.

Popovsky, Mark A., M.D. ed. *Transfusion Reactions.* Bethesda, MD: AABB Press. 1996.

Ratnoff, Oscar, M.D.; Forbes, Charles, M.D. *Disorders of Hemostasis, 3rd ed.* Philadelphia: W.B. Saunders. 1996.

Reynolds, James E.F., M.D. ed. Martindale. *The Extra Pharmacopia, 30th ed.* London: The Pharmaceutical Press. 1993.

Roitt, Ivan M., M.D. *Essential Immunology, 8th ed.* London: Blackwell Scientific Publications. 1994.

Rossi, Ennio C., M.D.; Simon, Toby L., M.D.; Moss, Gerald S., M.D., eds. *Principles of Transfusion Medicine.* Baltimore: Williams and Wilkens. 1991.

Rudolph, Abraham M., M.D. *Rudolph's Pediatrics, 20th ed.* Stamford, CT: Appleton & Lange. 1996.

Sabiston, David C., M.D., ed. *Sabastion's Textbook of Surgery, 15th ed.* Philadelphia: W. B. Saunders. 1997.

Scanlon, Craig, senior ed. *Egan's Fundamentals of Respiratory Care, 6th ed.* St Louis: Mosby. 1995.

Schiff, Leon, M.D., Schiff, Eugene, R., M.D. *Diseases of the Liver, Vols. 1 and 2, 7th ed.* Philadelphia: J.B. Lippincott Co. 1993.

Shapiro, Barry, A., M.D., *et al. Clinical Application of Blood Gases, 3rd ed.* Chicago: Year Book Medical Publishers, Inc. 1985.

Sherlock, Sheila, M.D.: Dooley, James, M.D. *Diseases of The Liver and Biliary Systems, Vols. 1 and 2, 9th ed.* London: Blackwell Scientific Publications. 1993.

Smith, James J., M.D., Kampine, John P., M.D. *Circulatory Physiology, 2nd ed.* Baltimore: Williams and Wilkins. 1984.

Stites, Daniel P., M.D.; Terr, Abba I., M.D.; Parslow, Tristram G., M.D. *Basic and Clinical Immunology, 8th ed.* Norwalk, CT: Appleton & Lange. 1994.

Valeri, C. Robert, M.D. *Physiology of Blood Transfusion.* Naval Blood Research Laboratory, Boston University School of Medicine. Boston: March 1, 1989.

Vengelen-Tyler, Virginia, ed. *Technical Manual, 12th ed.* Bethesda, MD: AABB Press. 1996.

Voet, Donald; Voet, Judith. *Biochemistry.* New York: John Wiley & Sons. 1990.

Wallach, Jacques, M.D. *Interpretation of Diagnostic Tests, 6th ed.* Boston: Little Brown and Co. 1996.

West, John B., M.D., Ph.D. *Respiratory Physiology, 4th ed.* Baltimore: Williams and Wilkens. 1990.

INDEX

539